Recent Advances in

Surgery 40

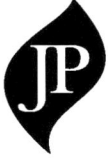

Recent Advances in

Surgery 40

Michael Douek MB ChB, MD, FRCS(Eng),
FRCS (Gen), EBSQ (Breast)
Rosetrees Royal College of Surgeons of England Director of the
Surgical Interventional Trials Unit and Professor of Surgical Sciences
and Breast Cancer, Nuffield Department of Surgical Sciences,
University of Oxford, Oxford, UK

Rachel Hargest BSc MBBS FRCS MD FRCS (Gen)
Clinical Senior Lecturer in Colorectal Surgery
Cardiff China Medical Research Collaborative and
Honorary Consultant Surgeon,
University Hospital of Wales and Velindre Hospital
Cardiff, UK

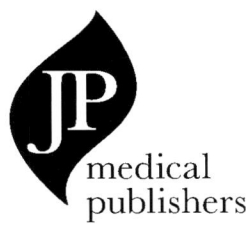

JP
medical
publishers

London • New Delhi

Published by Jaypee Brothers Medical Publishers,
4838/24 Ansari Road, New Delhi, India

Tel: +91 (011) 43574357   Fax: +91 (011)43574390

Email: info@jpmedpub.com, jaypee@jaypeebrothers.com
Web: www.jpmedpub.com, www.jaypeebrothers.com

JPM is the imprint of Jaypee Brothers Medical Publishers.

ISBN: 978-1-78779-162-6

British Library Cataloguing in Publication Data
A catalogue record for this book is available from the British Library

Library of Congress Cataloging in Publication Data
A catalog record for this book is available from the Library of Congress

Development Editor: Nikita Chauhan
Editorial Assistant: Keshav Kumar
Cover Design: Seema Dogra

Typeset, printed and bound in India.

Preface

We are delighted to present this volume of *"Recent Advances in Surgery 40"*. When we began to consider the format of this edition, we could not have known how the world was about to change during 2020. The Coronavirus disease 2019 (COVID-19) pandemic has caused a revolution in the way in which healthcare is delivered worldwide. Surgeons have had to face unprecedented demands this year and it is a tribute to everyone of you that surgeons have shown themselves to be professional, altruistic and compassionate in continuing to deliver surgical care in the most difficult circumstances.

Due to the rapidly changing state of our knowledge of the pathophysiology and consequences of COVID-19, and given the long lead in time of this book, we realised that devoting multiple chapters to management of surgical conditions in COVID-19 positive patients would probably be out of date by the time of publication. Therefore, we have continued to build on the long tradition of the Recent Advances in Surgery series and included chapters on surgery in general, training, and speciality specific updates which we hope will be of interest to a wide range of readers. However, many chapters include recent advances in practice in the light of the pandemic and we trust these will prove useful to busy surgeons in front line practice across the globe, along with those studying for professional examinations at this difficult time.

We are very grateful to our chapter editors for their contributions and patience. It is remarkable that you have been able to find the time to prepare these chapters and we thank you for your efforts.

Finally, we hope that each reader will find something of interest applicable to your daily practice.

Michael Douek
Rachel Hargest
January, 2021

Contents

Contributors

Oshi Abeyakoon MB BS, PhD,FRCR
Consultant Breast Radiologist
University College London Hospital (UCLH)
London, UK

Muneer Ahmed MA, PhD, FRCS (Gen Surg) FEBS
(Breast)
Consultant Oncoplastic Breast Surgeon and
Associate Professor of Surgery, Division of
Surgery and Interventional Science
University College London, Royal Free Hospital
Pond Street, London, UK

Akshay Anand MS
Associate Professor, Department of Surgery
King George's Medical University
Lucknow, Uttar Pradesh, India

Pratusha Babu MBBS MRCPCH AKC DTM&H (RCP)
AFHEA
National Medical Director's Clinical Fellow
NHS England, London, UK

Damon Bizos MBBCH(Wits), FCS(SA), MMed (Surg)
(Wits), FRCS (Eng) (ad eundum)
Adjunct Professor of Surgery and Head of
Surgical Gastroenterology, Department of
Surgery, Faculty of Health Sciences
University of the Witwatersrand
Johannesburg, South Africa

Timothy Briggs CBE MBBS (Hons) MD (Res) MCh
(Orth) FRCS (Ed) FRCS (Eng)
Consultant Orthopaedic Surgeon
Royal National Orthopaedic Hospital NHS Trust
Chair of GIRFT and National Director for Clinical
Improvement, NHS England and Improvement
London, UK

Justina CJ Tai BSc
Medical Student; University College London
Gower Street, London, UK

Ummul Contractor MB BS, MRCS, PgDip
Specialist Registrar in Vascular Surgery
All Wales Higher Surgical Training Scheme
University Hospital of Wales, Cardiff, UK

Andrew Dickenson MBBS BChD PgDipEd FRCS
FDSRCS FRCSEd FDTFEd FAcadMEd
Postgraduate Dental Dean/Oral and Maxillofacial
Surgeon, Health Education England
Westbridge Place, Leicester, UK

Michael Douek MB ChB, MD, FRCS(Eng),
FRCS(Gen), EBSQ (Breast)
Rosetrees Royal College of Surgeons of England
Director of the Surgical Interventional Trials
Unit & Professor of Surgical Sciences and
Breast Cancer, Nuffield Department of Surgical
Sciences, University of Oxford, Oxford, UK

Afsana Elanko BMedSci, BMBS
Director of Education, British Association of
Surgical Oncology, London, UK

Michael Fardy FFDRCS, FDSRCS, FRCS, FFSEM
Consultant Maxillofacial Surgeon
Spire Hospital, Cardiff, UK

Rachel Hargest BSc MBBS FRCS MD FRCS (Gen)
Senior Lecturer and Honorary Consultant
Surgeon, University Hospital of Wales
Henry Wellcome Building, Cardiff University
Heath Park, Cardiff, UK

Jim Khan PhD FRCS
Consultant Surgeon
Associate Professor of Surgery,
Portsmouth Hospital University NHS Trust
Portsmouth, UK

Sunil Kumar MS DNB FRCS (Eng) FRCS (Edin) FIAGES
EFIAGES FFSTEd FACS
Ex-HOD Surgery, Tata Main Hospital
Jamshedpur, India

Ava Kwong MBBS BSc FRCS FRCSEd FCSHK
FHKAM(Surgery)
Daniel CK Yu Professor in Breast Cancer Research
Chief of Division of Breast Surgery, University of
Hong Kong, Hong Kong

Kokila Lakhoo MBCHB, PhD, FRCS (Edin+Eng), FCS (SA), FCS (PAED), MRCPCH(UK)
Professor of Paediatric Surgery Nuffield
Department of Surgical Sciences
University of Oxford, Oxford, UK

Dafydd Locker BMBS MRCS
Specialist Registrar in Surgery
All Wales Higher Surgical Training Scheme
University Hospital of Wales, Cardiff, UK

John Machin MA (Oxf) MB BS MRCS FRCS (Tr&Orth) PGC
Clinical Lead for Litigation, GIRFT
NHS England and Improvement
London, UK

Dennis Mazingi MBBS MMed
Academic Doctor, Centre for Tropical Medicine and Global Health, University of Oxford
Oxford, UK

Akriti Nanda BA (Oxon), BM BCh
Academic Doctor, Oxford University Clinical Graduate School, John Radcliffe Hospital
Oxford, UK

Annakan Navaratnam MBBS BSc (Hons) FRCS (ORL-HNS)
National Medical Director's Clinical Fellow
NHS England, London, UK

Gloria Petralia MD
Consultant Breast Surgeon
Oxford University Hospitals
Oxford, UK

Pankaj Roy MBBS, MS (Gen Surg), MD, FRCS (Glas), FRCS (Gen Surg),
Consultant Breast Surgeon, Oxford University Hospitals, Oxford, UK

Marieke Rutgers MD
Clinical Research Fellow, Portsmouth Hospital University NHS Trust, Portsmouth, UK

Adnan Sharif MD FRCP
Consultant Nephrologist and Transplant Physician
Department of Nephrology and Transplantation
University Hospitals Birmingham NHS Foundation
Trust, Queen Elizabeth Hospital Birmingham
Mindelsohn Way, Edgbaston
Birmingham, UK

Abhinav Arun Sonkar MS FACS FUICC FRCS (England) FRCS (Ireland) FRCS (Glasgow)
Professor and Head of Surgery King George's
Medical University, Lucknow, Uttar Pradesh, India

Michael Stephens MD FRCS
Consultant Transplant and Organ Retrieval
Surgeon, University Hospital of Wales
Cardiff, UK

Arunima Verma MS MRCS FIAGES
Fellowship MAS Upper and Lower GI Surgery
Head of Department of Surgery
Tata Motors Hospital
Jamshedpur, India

Aarathi Vijayashankar MS
Fellow, Centre for Liver and Biliary Sciences
Max Super Speciality Hospital Saket, Delhi
Former Senior Resident, Department of Surgery
King George's Medical University
Lucknow, Uttar Pradesh, India

Richard White FRCR
Consultant Radiologist, Regional Vascular Unit
University Hospital of Wales
Cardiff, UK

Ian Williams MD FRCS
Consultant Vascular Surgeon
Regional Vascular Unit, University Hospital of Wales
Cardiff, UK

Stephanie Wing Yin Yu MBBS, MSc, BA (Hons)
Resident, Department of Surgery
Queen Mary Hospital, Hong Kong

Acknowledgements

The authors wish to thank Dr Jane Lane for proofreading multiple chapters. We also wish to thank the staff at Jaypee Brothers Medical Publishers (P) Ltd. for preparation and publishing of this edition of "Recent Advances in Surgery 40".

Section 1

Surgery in general

Chapter 1

Facemasks in the prevention of infection in surgery

Akriti Nanda, Rachel Hargest, Michael Douek

INTRODUCTION

Surgical facemasks have been part of surgery and operating room (OR) attire for around 100 years. In 2020, due to the coronavirus disease (COVID-19) pandemic, people across the world began wearing facemasks in public spaces, following public health advice and media publicity. This led to growing interest in facemasks, wider choice, evolution and advances in mask design. In this chapter, we review the history, use and evidence for masks within the OR.

HISTORY AND RATIONALE FOR THE USE OF FACEMASKS DURING SURGERY

Masks have been used during operating since the late 19th century (1897) when Johann Mikulicz began wearing a piece of gauze tied with string over his nose and mouth to protect the sterile operating field [1]. The practice was instituted at a time when the local bacteriologist Carl Flügge, with whom Mikulicz had collaborated, had just shown that respiratory droplets carried bacteria [1]. This method of covering the nose and mouth gained popularity across American and European hospitals with a study of > 1,000 photographs of ORs showing most surgeons wore masks by 1935 [2].

At the same time, Capps found masking patients and medical practitioners limited the spread of measles and scarlet fever on hospital wards [3]. The first study of the use of facemasks by healthcare workers (HCWs) in 1918, found lower rates of infection in those who wore a cloth mask [4]. The emigration of masks out of the operating theatre for use in the 1910, Manchurian plague and the 1918, Spanish flu epidemic [1] began the widespread use of facemasks as a means of protecting medical workers and patients from infectious diseases outside of the OR and has since been used to protect HCWs from scarlet fever, measles, influenza, plague and tuberculosis [5]. The rationale for wearing facemasks has moved beyond the original purpose and their use is now two-fold:
- To protect sterile fields from infections
- To limit transmission of infective diseases

How facemasks work

The underlying logic behind facemasks is that they are assumed to act as a physical barrier – retaining and blocking airborne droplets, aerosols, fluid, and particles that may infect others and contaminate surfaces. In surgery, the key surface requiring protection is the surgical wound in order to prevent surgical site infections (SSIs). Studies using tracer particles have shown that bacteria can be shed from hair, exposed skin, and mucous membranes, from both OR personnel and the patient. Hence barriers such as masks, gowns, hood, and drapes are necessary in the OR [6]. Surgical facemasks usually comprise three or four layers, often with two filters which prevent passage of material > 1 μ in diameter, therefore blocking bacteria of that size or larger from contaminating a surgical wound [7].

Critics suggest that facemasks will be penetrated by particles of > 1 μ, an event increased by the exhalation of moist air increasing resistance and infiltration through the mask [8]. Further possible mechanisms to increase infective spread include incorrect use of masks, incorrect removal or touching of mask and subsequent contamination of hands or gloves [9]. At worst, they suggest masks convey liquids containing bacteria via capillary action as well as by collecting and dispersing the wearers' skin scales from the face and thus increase the risk of infection [10].

In terms of protecting the wearer, surgeons know that blood and body fluid exposures occur frequently in the OR. A multicentre study from the United States found that in 8,500 surgical cases, 26% of all blood exposures occurred on the face and neck – thus showing the need for a protective physical barrier for these areas [11]. In terms of limiting transmission of illnesses between patients and theatre personnel, the blockage of bodily fluids, respiratory droplets and aerosols carrying bacterial and viral ribonucleic acid (RNA) is key. A recent study reported that surgical facemasks significantly reduced detection of influenza virus RNA in respiratory droplets and COV RNA in aerosols [12]. Another landmark study found that when patients with known multidrug-resistant tuberculosis breathed on guinea pigs, the rate of infection was significantly reduced in the mask wearing cohort [13]. As with many preclinical studies, it is not possible to assume that the findings can be extrapolated to the clinical setting. The remainder of this chapter will look at the available clinical evidence for the use of facemasks in limiting bacterial and viral transmission in surgery.

SURGICAL SITE INFECTIONS

The benefit of facemasks in preventing SSIs has been studied in two systematic reviews looking at three randomised controlled trials (RCTs) [14,15]. Both reviews highlight that there is a lack of trials and evidence for facemasks in the prevention of SSIs, but the limited studies did not find convincing evidence of the benefit of facemasks in preventing SSIs.

Three studies were included in the reviews. Two were quasi-randomised controlled trials (Q-RCTs) [16,17] conducted prior to 1990, and the third was a RCT [18] in 2010. One Q-RCT [16] was carried out in England during 1984, in which operating teams either wore facemasks or not while operating on 41 women with gynaecological cancer. The trial was stopped early as an increased number of SSIs occurred in the no mask arm. This finding differs from the other trials included in the systematic reviews, which did not demonstrate any statistically significant differences in SSI frequency between the masked and unmasked groups. For example, the Q-RCT from Sweden [17] found that SSIs occurred in 73/537 (4.7%) of operations performed with surgeons wearing facemasks, compared to 53/1,551 (3.5%) of operations without facemasks. This difference was not statistically significant (p > 0.05) and the bacterial species cultured from the SSIs were similar in both groups.

There are however, potential flaws in the methodology of both these Q-RCTs. Chamberlain et al [16] did not specify the criteria used to detect the presence of a wound infection and of course, the discontinuation of the trial after only 7 weeks as result of several infections in the no mask group, creates bias towards the use of facemasks. Tunevall et al [17] only followed patients up until discharge and therefore may be underestimating the number of SSIs.

The most methodologically robust trial with less risk of bias was Webster et al [18], although they only randomised non-scrubbed theatre staff and thus the findings cannot be used to inform personal protective equipment (PPE) guidance for surgeons but rather for our anaesthetic and other non-scrubbed colleagues.

The studies were not deemed appropriate to pool in a meta-analysis as the heterogeneity between studies was great, e.g. due to the time period affecting design of the OR (e.g. air flow rates), type of disposable surgical facemask and staff studied. Overall, it is unclear whether wearing surgical facemasks has any impact on SSIs. The RCTs were in hospitals in England, Sweden and Australia where ORs will have multiple infection control methods. The reason why masks may appear to be insignificant in modern studies may be that other infection control techniques have superseded the benefit of masks making it an insignificant addition for preventing SSIs in the 21st century OR.

To study the theory that masks may be contributing to SSI due to gathering micro-organisms and transferring instead of blocking them, a single clinical study compared facemasks to visors and found no significant clinical difference in incidence of SSIs [19].

Based upon the findings of the reviews, the National Institute for Health and Care Excellence (NICE) advised that 'there is limited evidence concerning the use of non-sterile theatre wear' such as facemasks when reducing rates of SSIs, but there is a 'consensus that wearing non-sterile theatre wear is important in maintaining theatre discipline [20]'. The guidelines are cited as level one evidence since they are based on a systematic review of RCTs. In reality however, due to the GRADE of evidence within the systematic review, the level of evidence is probably four, as it is a recommendation based on expert opinion and formal consensus [21].

Viral transmission

The use of facemasks to limit the transmission of infectious diseases in the OR is less well studied. The basis that facemasks offer a degree of protection to OR staff from patient derived infectious material comes from the fact that facemasks are a physical barrier against blood and bodily fluid splashes during surgery. The observational prospective studies mentioned above show that 25% of bodily fluid exposures during surgery occur on the face and neck [11,22]. Facemasks prevent some of these splashes and any bacteria or viruses carried in them from contaminating the surgeon's face.

Blood and bodily fluids are the carriers of many viruses and surgeons are at high risk of contracting infectious viruses, such as the human immunodeficiency virus (HIV), hepatitis B virus (HBV), and hepatitis C virus (HCV), through exposure to patients' blood [23]. Effective barriers, modified patterns of behaviour and postexposure responses are the best methods for prevention. Masks are part of the barrier protection against the drops of blood, which might be infected with such viruses [17]. However, the use of medications and testing of patients makes elucidating the effect of one type of barrier difficult. Although, there is clear evidence that facemasks act to protect the theatre staff from macroscopic facial contamination, there are studies to suggest that they fail to protect surgeons from potentially hazardous sub micrometre contaminants due to aerosol penetration and leakage of masks [7]. Therefore, the protection that masks confer in the form of macroscopic facial contamination may not necessarily extend to any microscopic infectious agents present within that contamination, therefore not protecting the wearer from becoming infected [24]. Proponents of the surgical facemask may argue that even if they fail to completely negate the risks of infection, they may reduce exposure in a dose-dependant manner. Evidence for this is weak but reports from clinical practice suggest that facemasks fail to confer adequate protection from infection for example due to streptococcal and staphylococcal bacterial species [25] or HBV [24].

Aerosol transmission

It has been proposed that facemasks may protect against another form of viral transmission – that is airborne viral transmission. This is the mode of transmission of many respiratory viral illnesses.

Surgical patients are at higher risk of these infections due to a combination of factors, including surgery-induced immune suppression and immune modulating comorbidities and medication, as well as being surrounded by HCWs who may act as viral shedders and transmitters [26]. Surgical patients who contract respiratory viruses during surgery are at a higher risk of complications and may have a longer postoperative hospital length of stay when compared to matched controls [27]. There are a few studies on the use of masks in protection against respiratory viral transmission for HCWs, but no trials focus specifically on surgeons or staff in the OR and the SSI trials did not evaluate staff infection rates.

PROTECTION OF HEALTHCARE WORKERS

Offedu et al [28] looked at RCTs comparing mask versus no mask in protecting staff against transmission of respiratory viruses (influenza and similar). Two RCTs [5,29] comparing respiratory virus risk in HCWs wearing masks compared to no masks were reported. One RCT compared the use of cloth masks and a control group undergoing 'standard care' [5] but the control group included a significant number of participants who wore cloth masks. The other RCT in this report had a control arm of no masks but this arm was not randomised and instead selected hospitals in this group on the basis that most of their staff did not wear masks (which is not the norm in hospitals in Beijing), which may introduce bias due to the conditions in those hospitals. Results showed that wearing a medical mask or N95-respirator in the hospital conferred significant protection against self-reported clinical respiratory illness (RR 0.59; 95% CI 0.46–0.77) and influenza-like illness (RR 0.34; 95% CI 0.14–0.82) and suggested a protective, but not statistically significant effect against laboratory-confirmed infection (RR 0.70; 95% CI 0.47–1.03). This systematic review contains few studies, with those included being indirect and with a high risk of bias and therefore the conclusions should be interpreted with caution.

A recent systematic review in the Lancet [30] looked at data on the benefit of masks in coronavirus viral transmission. The studies included are of varying quality and due to being observational are at greater risk of bias and heterogeneity. However, the authors justified their use as they focus on coronaviruses [severe acute respiratory syndrome (SARS-CoV-1) = 18 studies, Middle East respiratory syndrome (MERS) = 7 studies and Covid-19/SARS-CoV-2 = 4 studies] and thus the findings are more applicable to the current pandemic. There were 10 adjusted studies (n = 2,647) and 29 unadjusted (n = 10,170) observational studies in this report. The use of both N95-respirators (or similar) and facemasks (e.g., surgical facemask or 12–16-layer cotton facemasks) was associated with a large reduction in risk of infection (unadjusted n = 10,170; RR 0.34; 95%

CI 0.26–0.45 adjusted studies n = 2,647, a OR 0.15; 95% CI 0.07–0.34; AR 3.1% with facemask versus 17.4 with no facemask, RD –14.3%; 95% CI –15.9–10.7; low certainty) with stronger reductions in HCWs (RR 0.30; 95% CI 0.22–0.41) compared with non-healthcare settings (RR 0.56; 95% CI 0.40–0.79).

The findings from these two systematic reviews suggest a protective effect of facemasks for HCWs against respiratory viral illnesses such as influenza and coronaviruses. Given that there are so few studies of facemask use in the prevention of viral transmission in HCWs, with none focussing specifically on OR staff, and most studies using methodology that has a high risk of bias, there is a paucity of robust evidence from RCTs.

THE EVOLUTION OF DIFFERENT MASKS

Medical masks began as cloth and gauze coverings but were replaced by paper masks in the 1930s and disposable synthetic fibre types in the 1960s. The latter are designed to filter incoming and outgoing air, as well as to prevent the spread of droplets as with traditional masks [1]. Another type of mask that has become more prevalent since the beginning of the Covid-19 pandemic, is the N95-respirator, used for protection against smaller particles (**Figure 1.1**).

The filtration efficacy of masks has increased over time. Respirator masks are designed to filter fine particles of 0.01–1 µm in diameter [31]. Consequently, the greater the filtration capacity of a mask, the more it should protect the wearer from infection and limit transmission of micro-organisms.

A recent paper by Bartoszko et al [32] analysed 4 RCTs comparing N95-respirators with medical masks. This meta-analysis found no evidence that medical masks are inferior to N95-respirators in protecting HCWs against laboratory-confirmed influenza infections [OR 0.94 (95% CI 0.73–1.20)] influenza-like illnesses [OR 1.31 (95% CI 0.94–1.85)] and self-reported clinical respiratory illness [OR 1.49 (95% CI 0.98–2.28)]. However, for influenza-like illnesses and clinical respiratory illnesses, the point estimates favoured N95-respirators. The CI are wide and there was considerable heterogeneity in these studies so results should be interpreted with caution. One trial [32] which evaluated coronaviruses separately, found no difference between the two groups (p = 0.49). Due to the heterogeneity of available evidence, the authors suggest

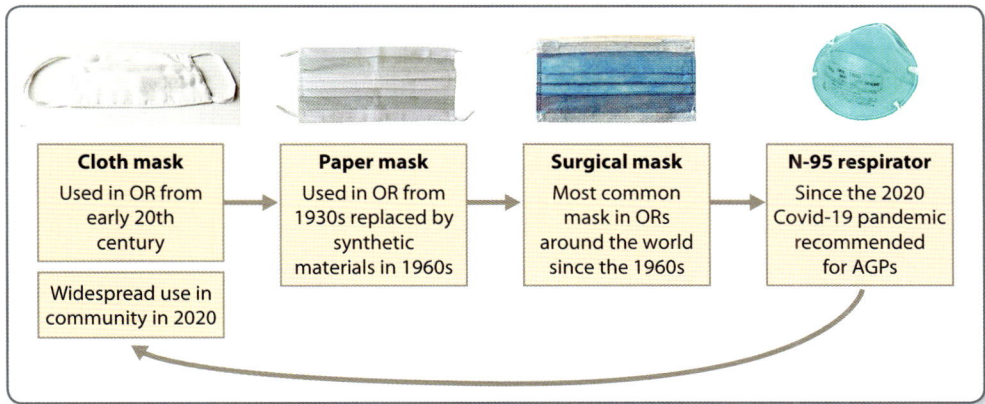

Cloth mask	Paper mask	Surgical mask	N-95 respirator
Used in OR from early 20th century	Used in OR from 1930s replaced by synthetic materials in 1960s	Most common mask in ORs around the world since the 1960s	Since the 2020 Covid-19 pandemic recommended for AGPs
Widespread use in community in 2020			

Figure 1.1 The evolution of facemasks. OR, operating room; AGPs, aerosol generating procedures.

"low certainty evidence that medical masks and N95-respirators offer similar protection against viral respiratory infection including COV in HCWs".

Another recent meta-analysis by Long et al [33] found a protective effect of N95-respirators against laboratory-confirmed bacterial colonisation [RR = 0.58 (95% CI 0.43–0.78)]. This suggests that filtration by the respirators is more effective in limiting transmission of bacteria, which are larger than viruses.

The Lancet systematic review [30] found that protection from COV transmission was more pronounced with N95/any respirators [a OR 0.04 (95% CI 0.004–0.30)] compared to surgical facemasks [a OR 0.33, (95% CI 0.17–0.61)]. The authors state that between-study and within-study comparisons 'we noted a larger effect of N95, or similar, respirators compared with other masks'. The findings of these systematic reviews are conflicting but suggest that N95-respirators may offer some further protection to the wearer against respiratory viruses. This may be due to the stability and transmission of coronaviruses in droplets, or due to better adherence to mask wearing by HCWs during pandemics. Behavioural studies have shown people are more likely to wear masks, if the perceived susceptibility and severity of being afflicted with the disease is high [34]. No studies assessing the benefit of different mask types on SSIs have been reported.

CORONAVIRUS DISEASE-19

The recent pandemic has created a shift from use of traditional surgical masks in ORs to N95-respirators. Large international multicentre observational studies show that surgical patients with COVID-19 have an increased morbidity, mortality and length of hospital stay [35]. At the time of writing, it is therefore imperative to protect both HCWs and patients from transmission. Currently, the World Health Organisation (WHO) and Public Health England (PHE) recommend that a fluid repellent surgical mask should be used when treating any patient. For high-risk patients such as those with confirmed or suspected COVID-19, patients undergoing noninvasive ventilation and those in intensive care units, operating theatres, endoscopy units or those requiring prolonged and close personal care, an N95-respirator should be worn. Likewise a respirator is required during aerosol generating procedures (AGP) such as endoscopy [31]. In general surgery the following have been defined as AGPs:

- *Intubation and extubation* – the anaesthetic staff must be protected. Other personnel must leave the OR or wear N95-respirator
- *Laparotomy* – bowel contents, peritoneal fluid and diathermy smoke have been shown to contain viruses
- *Laparoscopy* – smoke aerosols
- *Endoscopy* – especially upper gastrointestinal

Other than AGPs, the risks of transmission may include the fumes released during open or laparoscopic surgery and contaminated body fluids. The risks of COVID-19 transmission via smoke are not fully known and based on evidence from previous studies with papillomavirus – with documented cases that this viral agent can be contracted from surgical smoke [36]. However, a recent review from the Cardiff team has addressed this issue [37]. The benefit of masks against smoke is not well understood and for this the use of devices with smoke evacuation filters are recommended [38]. Studies have also found that SARS-CoV-1 RNA in plasma and thus protection from blood has been suggested as important though the evidence of this transmission route has yet to be confirmed [39].

Although, the evidence of transmission risks is still developing, the majority of guidance recommends implementing multiple infection control and risk stratification methods (e.g. preoperative swabs, isolation, and modification of surgical techniques to minimise AGPs) to reduce the risk of transmission of SARS-CoV-2 during surgery. It is important to note that facemasks must be combined with correct fitting via fit tests, avoidance of facemask touching, regular hand washing and social distancing to minimise transmission.

RISKS OF WEARING A MASK

Opponents of facemasks have suggested that they provide a false sense of security to the wearer and thus HCWs or patients may engage in more risky behaviour in terms of infection control. There is no evidence for this risk compensation behaviour and infact a recent study found facemasks usage in the general public did not correlate with riskier infection control behaviours [40].

The cost-effectiveness of masks is another point of contention. In 2015, it was estimated that the National Health Service (NHS) spent approximately £9.1 million on masks a year [41] and this will have increased substantially during 2020, with new PPE guidance. Given the uncertainty of their effectiveness in preventing SSIs and viral transmission in the OR it has not been possible to perform any cost-benefit analysis.

Minor harms such as rash, acne and headaches have been associated with prolonged use of masks by healthcare professionals but can be mitigated with rest, skin care, and hydration [42]. Given the minimal harms, policy makers continue to err on the side of caution with facemasks.

CONCLUSION

Although the evidence is conflicting, it is likely that disposable masks and respirators will remain an essential part of OR PPE in the future. Many common medical practices become culturally ingrained despite the absence of robust supporting evidence. With facemasks this is perhaps sensible given the minimal harms and potential benefits. However, this is an area that requires further research in order to provide optimal surgical care to patients and to protect HCWs worldwide in a cost-effective manner.

Key points for clinical practice

- Masks are used in healthcare for two reasons:
  1. To protect sterile fields to prevent infections
  2. To limit transmission of infective diseases
- Evidence for prevention of SSIs by facemasks in RCTs is conflicting and limited
- Impact of masks on SSIs may be insignificant given other modern infection control measures
- Facemasks act as barrier to protect the wearer by retaining and blocking transmission of airborne droplets, aerosols, fluid, and particles
- Facemasks may be beneficial in reducing transmission of respiratory viral illnesses among HCWs
- N95-respirators may confer more protection than traditional facemasks but are currently recommended only in high risk environments and AGPs
- There is no definitive evidence that facemasks limit viral transmission to or from surgeons

REFERENCES

1. Strasser BJ, Schlich T. A history of the medical mask and the rise of throwaway culture. Lancet 2020; 396: 19–20.
2. Adams LW, Aschenbrenner CA, Houle TT, et al. Uncovering the History of Operating Room Attire through Photographs. Anesthesiology 2016; 124:19–24.
3. Capps JA. A new adaptation of the face mask in control of contagious disease. J Am Med Assoc 1918; 70:910–911.
4. Weaver GH. Droplet Infection and its Prevention by the Face Mask. J Infect Dis 1919; 24:218–230.
5. MacIntyre CR, Chughtai AA. Facemasks for the prevention of infection in healthcare and community settings. BMJ 2015; 350:h694.
6. Claudia J, Bearman G. Guide To Infection Control in the Healthcare Setting. Int Soc Infect Control Heal 2018:1–6.
7. Weber A, Willeke K, Marchioni R, et al. Aerosol penetration and leakage charecteristics of masks used in the health care industry. Am J Infect Control 1993; 21:167–173.
8. Romney MG. Surgical face masks in the operating theatre: re-examining the evidence. J Hosp Infect 2001; 47:251–256.
9. Belkin NL. A century after their introduction, are surgical masks necessary? AORN J 1996; 64:602–607.
10. Schweizer RT. Mask wiggling as a potential cause of wound contamination. Lancet 1976; 2:1129–1130.
11. Davies CG, Khan MN, Ghauri AS, et al. Blood and body fluid splashes during surgery–the need for eye protection and masks. Ann R Coll Surg Engl 2007; 89:770–772.
12. Leung NHL, Chu DKW, Shiu EYC, et al. Respiratory virus shedding in exhaled breath and efficacy of face masks. Nat Med 2020; 26:676–680.
13. Dharmadhikari AS, Mphahlele M, Stoltz A, et al. Surgical face masks worn by patients with multidrug-resistant tuberculosis: impact on infectivity of air on a hospital ward. Am J Respir Crit Care Med 2012; 185:1104–1109.
14. Vincent M, Edwards P. Disposable surgical face masks for preventing surgical wound infection in clean surgery. Cochrane Database Syst Rev 2016;4:CD002929.
15. Bahli ZM. Does evidence based medicine support the effectiveness of surgical facemasks in preventing postoperative wound infections in elective surgery? J Ayub Med Coll Abbottabad. 2009; 21:166–170.
16. Chamberlain GV, Houang E. Trial of the use of masks in the gynaecological operating theatre. Ann R Coll Surg Engl 1984; 66:432–433.
17. Tunevall TG. Postoperative wound infections and surgical face masks: a controlled study. World J Surg 1991; 15:383–387.
18. Webster J, Croger S, Lister C, et al. Use of face masks by non-scrubbed operating room staff: a randomized controlled trial. ANZ J Surg 2010; 80:169–173.
19. Norman A. A comparison of face masks and visors for the scrub team. A study in theatres. Br J Theatre Nurs 1995; 5:10–13.
20. National Collaborating Centre for Women's and Children's Health (UK). Surgical site infection: prevention and treatment of surgical site infection. NICE Clinical Guidelines 2008.
21. Burns P, Rohrich R, Chung K. The Levels of Evidence and their role in evidence-based medicine. Plast Reconstr Surg 2011; 128:305–310.
22. White MC, Lynch P. Blood contacts in the operating room after hospital-specific data analysis and action. Am J Infect Control 1997; 25:209–214.
23. Hakeem A, Alsaigh S, Alasmari A, et al. Awareness, Concerns, and Protection Strategies Against Bloodborne Viruses Among Surgeons. Cureus 2019; 11:e4242.
24. Reingold AL, Kane MA, Hightower AW. Failure of gloves and other protective devices to prevent transmission of hepatitis B virus to oral surgeons. JAMA 1988; 259:2558–2560.
25. Ransjö U. Masks: a ward investigation and review of the literature. J Hosp Infect 1986; 7:289–294.
26. Heffernan DS. Influenza and the Surgeon. Surg Infect (Larchmt) 2019; 20:119–128.
27. Spaeder MC, Lockman JL, Greenberg RS, et al. Impact of perioperative RSV or influenza infection on length of stay and risk of unplanned ICU admission in children : a case-control study. BMC Anesthesiol 2011; 11:16.
28. Offeddu V, Yung CF, Low MSF, et al. Effectiveness of Masks and Respirators Against Respiratory Infections in Healthcare Workers: a systematic review and meta-analysis. Clin Infect Dis 2017; 65:1934–1942.

29. MacIntyre CR, Wang Q, Cauchemez S, et al. A cluster randomized clinical trial comparing fit-tested and non-fit-tested N95 respirators to medical masks to prevent respiratory virus infection in health care workers. Influenza Other Respi Viruses 2011; 5:170–179.
30. Chu DK, Akl EA, Duda S, et al. Physical distancing, face masks, and eye protection to prevent person-to-person transmission of SARS-CoV-2 and COVID-19: a systematic review and meta-analysis. Lancet 2020; 395:1973–1987.
31. Jessop ZM, Dobbs TD, Ali SR, et al. Personal protective equipment for surgeons during COVID-19 pandemic: systematic review of availability, usage and rationing. Br J Surg 2020; 10:11750.
32. Bartoszko JJ, Farooqi MAM, Alhazzani W, et al. Medical masks vs N95 respirators for preventing COVID-19 in healthcare workers: A systematic review and meta-analysis of randomized trials. Influenza Other Resp Viruses 2020; 14:365–373.
33. Long Y, Hu T, Liu L, et al. Effectiveness of N95 respirators versus surgical masks against influenza: a systematic review and meta-analysis. J Evid Based Med 2020; 13:93–101.
34. Sim SW, Moey KS, Tan NC. The use of facemasks to prevent respiratory infection: a literature review in the context of the Health Belief Model. Singapore Med J 2014; 55:160–167.
35. COVIDSurg Collaborative. Mortality and pulmonary complications in patients undergoing surgery with perioperative SARS-CoV-2 infection: an international cohort study. Lancet 2020; 396:27–38.
36. Stewart KE, Wright PB, Montgomery BEE, et al. Reducing Risky Sex among Rural African American Cocaine Users: a controlled trial. J Health Care Poor Underserved 2017; 28:528–547.
37 Mowbray N, Ansell J, Horwood J, et al. Safe management of surgical smoke in the age of COVID-19. Br J Surg 2020 ;107:1406–1413.
38. Gloster HM, Roenigk RK. Risk of acquiring human papillomavirus from the plume produced by the carbon dioxide laser in the treatment of warts. J Am Acad Dermatol 1995; 32:436–441.
39. Drosten C, Günther S, Preiser W, et al. Identification of a novel coronavirus in patients with severe acute respiratory syndrome. N Engl J Med 2003; 348:1967–1976.
40. Mantzari E, Rubin GJ, Marteau TM. Is risk compensation threatening public health in the covid-19 pandemic? BMJ 2020; 370:m2913.
41. Da Zhou C, Sivathondan P, Handa A. Unmasking the surgeons: the evidence base behind the use of facemasks in surgery. J R Soc Med.2015; 108:223–228.
42. Elisheva R. Adverse Effects of Prolonged Mask Use among Healthcare Professionals during COVID-19. J Infect Dis Epidemiol 2020; 6:130.

Chapter 2

Quality improvement in surgery

Pratusha Babu, Annakan Navaratnam, John Machin, Timothy Briggs

INTRODUCTION

Before one can understand and develop quality improvement, it is important to consider how to define 'quality' in healthcare. There is no universal definition of quality. However, the United States Institute of Medicine describes it as the 'degree to which health service for individuals and populations increase the likelihood of desired health outcomes and is consistent with professional knowledge'. Healthcare should follow these six dimensions:

1. Safe
2. Timely
3. Effective
4. Efficient
5. Person-centered
6. Equitable

Quality is regarded as a measure of excellence in healthcare [1,2]. Quality improvement is a process of using a defined and structured approach, over a set period of time, to improve patient outcomes and experience [3].

Why do surgeons need to understand quality improvement in healthcare?

Healthcare systems across the world are facing significant financial and operational pressures, with services struggling to maintain standards of care. The aim is to improve quality and deliver better value care (better outcomes at lower cost). Quality improvement is central to this [4].

The professional duties of a doctor in the United Kingdom [5] underline the importance of taking part in quality improvement to promote patient safety. Training programmes and fellowships now recommend (or mandate) involvement with clinical governance, clinical audit, and quality improvement as part of the syllabus and appraisal [6]. Quality improvement empowers anyone to deliver positive changes for patients [3]. Surgeons, within and across specialties, are important in leading and delivering quality improvement.

This chapter will describe in greater detail quality improvement methodology, the importance of data in quality improvement and case study the success of the 'Getting it Right First Time' (GIRFT) programme for both improving patient care and safety resulting in a significant reduction in costs.

QUALITY IMPROVEMENT METHODS

There are numerous approaches to quality improvement in surgery and healthcare in general. No one method is necessarily better than the other and often they can be used simultaneously.

Clinical governance

Clinical governance is a framework through which organisations and their staff are accountable for continuously improving the quality of their services and safeguarding high standards of care, by creating an environment in which clinical excellence will flourish [7]. There are seven pillars of clinical governance:

1. Audit
2. Clinical effectiveness
3. Research
4. Risk management
5. Education and training
6. Patient and public involvement
7. Information

Clinical audit as part of clinical governance questions whether healthcare is provided in line with standards and enables care providers and patients to know where a service is doing well and where there could be improvement [6].

Clinical audit

The role of clinical audit is to check clinical care meets defined quality standards and to implement improvements to address shortfalls identified. This process relies on the existence of established evidence-based clinical standards drawn from best practice and the creation of an audit proforma comprised of measurable outcomes derived from these standards [8]. It also requires a clearly defined population of patients (or sample of this population) whose care will be measured using the proforma.

The clinical audit cycle can be divided into five stages (**Figure 2.1**):

1. Identify the audit topic, based on a clinical problem or issue
2. Set the standard, usually based on a previously determined ideal
3. Collect the data by observing clinical practice
4. Analyse the data and compare it to the standard
5. Implement change to clinical practice to allow an improvement

Interventions are often needed to bring practice in line with these standards in order to improve the quality of care and outcomes [9]. The audit can then be repeated after the intervention has been applied to assess if it has had an impact in improving compliance with a specific clinical standard.

Many hospitals have a clinical audit department and it is advised that all audits are registered with these departments in order for progress to be monitored and also to ensure there is no inadvertent unnecessary replication of work. There are several examples of clinical audit in surgical practice including UK national audits such as the National Emergency Laparotomy Audit [10] and the British Association of Endocrine and Thyroid Surgeons National Audit [11].

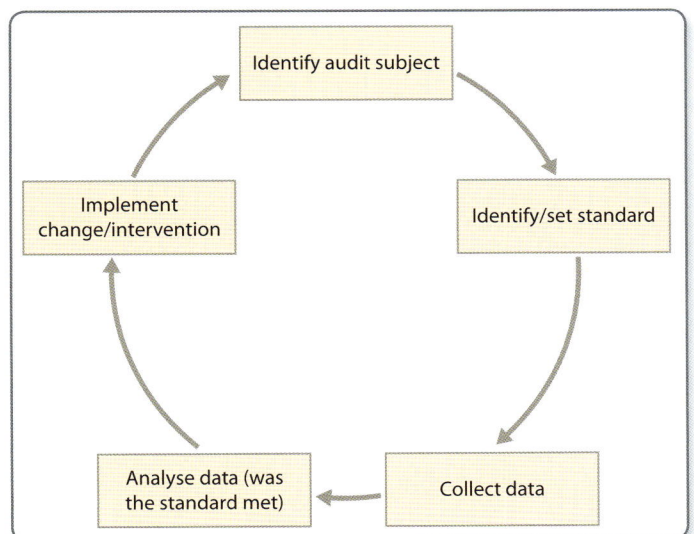

Figure 2.1 Stages of the audit cycle [12].

PLAN-DO-STUDY-ACT

The Plan-Do-Study-Act (PDSA) cycles are a widely accepted and frequently used approach in healthcare improvement [13]. This method of quality improvement involves an iterative process in which potential quality improvements are introduced, tested, and refined on a small scale, prior to wholesale implementation [14]. This approach is particularly effective when a process needs changing or needs to be introduced. PDSA cycles test changes in order to assess their impact. Therefore, this ensures new ideas do actually improve quality before implementation on a wider scale [15].

Making changes to processes can give unexpected outcomes. In order to mitigate against this, it is safer and more efficient to test quality improvements on a small scale before wholesale implementation. Also, this allows a sample of stakeholders involved to assess the proposed changes in action. Interactions with other systems can be tested by the introduction of these small scale changes without causing large scale disruption to service quality. An example of such a change is trialing a new patient preoperative assessment proforma with a limited group of patients before using the proforma for all patients.

The process involves a logical sequence of four repetitive steps (**Figure 2.2**):
1. *Plan phase:* Ideas for improvement are detailed, tasks assigned, expectations confirmed and measures of improvement are selected.
2. *Do phase:* The plan is implemented with any deviation from the plan being recorded. These deviations are often called defects.
3. *Study phase:* The results from the test cycle are examined, and questions are asked regarding what went right, what went wrong, and what will be changed in the next test cycle.

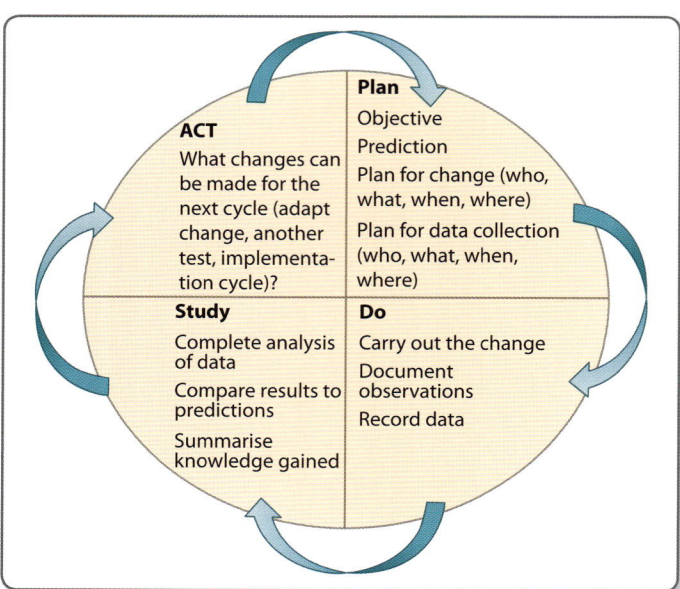

Figure 2.2 The Plan-Do-Study-Act (PDSA) cycle.

4. *Act phase:* Lessons learned from the study phase are incorporated into the test of change, and a decision is made about continuation of the test cycles.

In the subsequent cycle, the aforementioned steps are repeated. PDSA cycles can be used iteratively to test and refine small changes until the process is deemed suitable for large-scale adoption (**Figure 2.3**).

The PDSA cycles have been used to improve compliance with infection control measure in cardiothoracic surgery [16] and reduce complications in endovascular interventions in vascular surgery [17].

MODEL FOR IMPROVEMENT

The model for improvement provides a framework for developing, testing, and implementing changes leading to improvement. It was developed by the Associates in Process Improvement [18] and is advocated by the prestigious Institute for Healthcare Improvement [19]. This model uses PDSA cycles within its framework (**Figure 2.4**). It is a powerful tool for learning from ideas that do and do not work and gives stakeholders the opportunity to see if the proposed change will be successful.

This process of change is safer and less disruptive for patients and staff. When planning any improvement processes, it is essential to know what you want to achieve, how you will measure improvement and to be explicit about the idea to be tested. The key questions that precede the PDSA cycle ensure that a focused aim is set, time frames are clearly articulated and established, and measurable goals are identified at the start of a project.

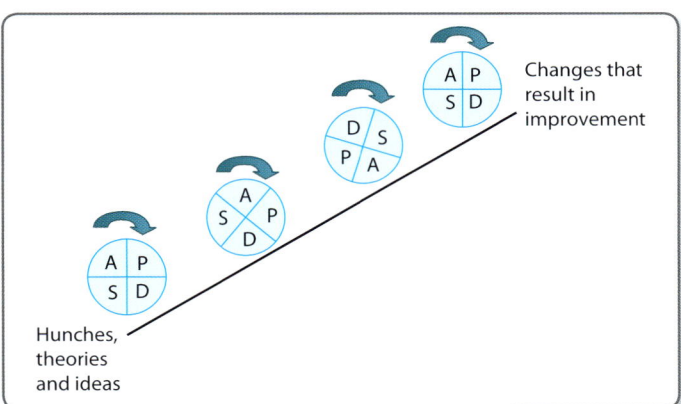

Figure 2.3 Iterative Plan-Do-Study-Act (PDSA) cycles.

Changes that result in improvement

Hunches, theories and ideas

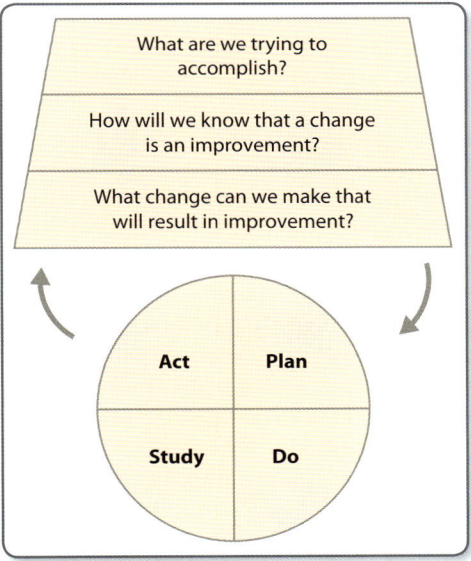

Figure 2.4 Model for improvement.

What are we trying to accomplish?

How will we know that a change is an improvement?

What change can we make that will result in improvement?

Act Plan

Study Do

The framework includes three key questions to answer before testing an improvement concept and a process.

1. **What are we trying to accomplish?** (The aims statement)
   Take the quality issue that has been identified and turn it into an aim, something that is SMART (Specific, Measurable, Achievable, Realistic, Time bound).
2. **How will we know if the change is an improvement?**
   This involves understanding what measures of success will be used. Not only will this include outcomes that are linked to the aims but also the reliability of the measurement processes and the potential unintended consequences that have may be introduced into the system by making these changes.

3. **What changes can we make that will result in improvement?**
    These include the change concepts to be tested.
       The changes are then tested using a PDSA cycle on a small scale. The cyclical nature
    allows the change to be refined and improved through repeated cycles of testing and
    learning. This provides a vehicle for continuous improvement.

An example of this model for improvement in surgical practice is the reducing surgical
complications project from the 1,000 lives campaign in Wales in 2009 [20]. The project used
the model for improvement methodology to implement a National Patient Safety Agency
alert regarding the World Health Organisation (WHO) 'Safer Surgery Checklist [21]'.

PERFORMANCE BENCHMARKING

The performance benchmarking approach drives quality improvement by raising
awareness of local and national performance targets and finding and sharing best practice
across organisations. When local and national performance targets are established and
given organisational importance they can act as drivers for quality improvement. This
quality improvement methodology requires either local or national performance targets as
well as data collection processes for monitoring and a system for sharing this information
with collaborating organisations.

   Performance indicators are used as part of a benchmarking process to raise awareness
of required standards and act as drivers for quality improvement. Hospitals and their
departments strive to meet set standards. Those organisations that perform well can then
demonstrate models of best practice which can be shared, becoming the benchmark
against which future performance is compared.

   Performance may be monitored through provision of data, or evidence of compliance
with standards, to an external agency. Subsequently, league tables or benchmarking charts
can be published, which can also drive quality improvement as organisations aim for lead
positions. Performance indicators should be carefully devised. They are most powerful if
they are active, e.g., focused upon quality improvement initiatives met through evidence
of positive outcomes achieved. The communication of organisational performance against
national benchmarks for context raises awareness of shortfalls within organisations and
stimulates further subsequent quality improvement.

   This is one of the key methods that is utilised by the Getting it Right First Time (GIRFT)
programme in England [22]. Mandatory administrative datasets [Hospital Episode Statistics
(HES)] are used to create specialty specific performance metrics that can be used to
benchmark hospital performance. This data analysis is used in peer-to-peer meetings
between clinicians [23]. Further information regarding the GIRFT programme is provided
in the following text.

   Key performance indicators (KPIs) and benchmarking are also used within healthcare
organisations to compare activity across different departments or units. This can uncover
excellent practice within a hospital and enable sharing of best practice locally to drive
quality improvement.

Statistical process control

Statistical process control (SPC) is a method of quality improvement using statistics
and data to monitor and control a process. It therefore ensures that the process
operates at its full potential so that the required quality is maintained and waste is

minimised. Processes naturally demonstrate controlled variation (common causes) but also uncontrolled variation which is present all the time (special causes). SPC involves understanding the process by constantly mapping it using control charts, then understanding the causes of outliers and variation, and eliminating the sources of special cause variation when they occur. Statistical process control can be applied to any process within which outputs can be measured. It requires considerable data collection, staff training, and statistical analysis.

Statistical process control involves:

- Control charts
- Focus on continuous improvement
- Design of experiments

Statistical process control highlights the degree of variation from required outputs and enables the measurement of the impact of any experimental process change made for improvement. A detailed explanation of the methodology involved in SPC is outside the scope of this chapter but further details can be found on the National Health Service (NHS) Improvement website [24] and in a publication by Timmerman et al [25].

Statistical process control methodology has been utilised in surgical quality improvement programme to reduce surgical-site infections (SSIs) in paediatric surgery [26] and reduce postoperative complications (recurrent laryngeal nerve palsy and hypocalcaemia) in thyroid surgery [27].

SIX SIGMA

This quality improvement methodology was developed within the electronics industry (originating from Motorola Inc in the mid 1980's) and the approach is now widely used in service industries. This is a systematic approach to improving products or processes. It focuses first on understanding how an organisation's customers, or patients, would define "defects" within its products or services. It then works to reduce factors that would be defined as being critical to quality, drawing on statistical methods to develop standards for variation in quality. Quality is measured in terms of defect (error) rates and the aim is reduce this to six standard deviations (sigma or σ) from the process mean. This translates as 99.99966 % error free or 3.4 defects per million opportunities (DPMO).

Quality improvement is achieved by implementing a five-step cyclical process known as define, measure, analyse, improve and control (DMAIC – an advanced form of PDSA):

1. *Define:* State the problem, specify the patient group, identify goals and outline the target process
2. *Measure:* Decide the parameters to be quantified and the best way to measure them. Collect the necessary baseline data and measure again after changes have been made
3. *Analyse:* Identify gaps between actual performance and goals. Then determine the causes of those gaps, determine how process inputs affect outputs, and rank improvement opportunities
4. *Improve:* Devise potential solutions and identify solutions that are easiest to implement. Then test hypothetical solutions and implement required improvements
5. *Control:* Share a detailed solution monitoring plan, observe implemented improvements for success, update on a regular basis and maintain a training routine

Six Sigma is a powerful approach that has been employed in several surgical quality improvement programmes. It has been used to improve operating theatre efficiency by reducing delayed start times and reducing time taken to turn around between cases [28].

Lean

This is a quality management system that draws on the methodology developed by some Japanese car manufacturers, including Toyota, in the way they manage their production processes [29]. The approach focuses on five principles:

1. Patient value
2. Managing the value stream
3. Regulating flow of production (to avoid quiet patches and bottlenecks)
4. Reducing waste
5. Using "pull" mechanisms to support flow. This means responding to the actual demand, rather than allowing the organisational needs to determine output

Lean uses process mapping with associated stakeholders to identify inefficiencies affecting the quality of care and enabling action planning for improvement. In the context of healthcare, process mapping involves reviewing and mapping the whole patient journey or diagnostic pathway with all parties involved. This enables the identification of inefficiencies and opportunities for improvement. It illustrates unnecessary steps, duplication, discrepancies, and variation and stimulates ideas for quality improvement to help create fail-safe systems.

Lean methodology clearly can be utilised in several healthcare processes such as outpatient management and diagnostic pathways. In surgery, operating theatre efficiency has been improved by this approach in reducing the preoperative delays caused when the patient is not ready to be transferred from the ward to theatre [30]. Other examples of the lean methodology in surgical quality improvement projects have included improving perioperative antibiotic therapy [31] and improving surgical clinics experience for patients and staff [32].

SOURCES OF DATA

Key to each methodology of quality improvement is the use of data, either qualitative or quantitative. Data is defined as 'information, especially facts and numbers, collected to be examined and considered and used to help decision-making [33]'. Within healthcare we use a range of data at different levels: patient, service, organisation and population levels [34]. High-quality data allow for identification of trends and patterns, comparisons to be drawn, prediction of future event and outcomes, and evaluation of services [35].

Examples of three sources of surgical service data from the UK and how they have been used to drive quality improvement in surgical services are given below.

National joint registry [36]

A registry is an organised system which uses observational study methods to collect uniform data (clinical and other) to evaluate specified outcomes for a specified population defined by a disease, condition or exposure [37].

Successful registries provide essential clinical and cost-effectiveness data for policy development to help drive improvement in patient care and safety. They can also help develop national and international research collaborations.

The National Joint Registry (NJR), set up in 2002, collects information on hip, knee, ankle, elbow, and shoulder joint replacement surgery and monitors performance of joint replacement implants. It monitors outcomes achieved by brand of prosthesis, hospital and surgeon and if these fall below an expected performance, it allows for prompt investigation and supports follow-up. Additional data related to the patient is provided with the patient's consent.

Over the last 16 years, the NJR has become the largest registry in the world, containing over 3 million records with a quarter of a million records added annually. A Patient Decision Support Tool [38] has been developed using NJR data, for use by patients and clinicians to estimate individual patient outcome, benefits of surgery and risks regarding mortality and revision surgery, based on a number of relevant metrics.

National hip fracture database (NHFD) [39]

This database was commissioned as part of the Falls and Fragility Fracture Audit Programme, a national clinical audit designed to audit care that patients with fragility fractures and inpatient falls receive in hospital [40]. The National Hip Fracture Database (NHFD) collects data on all patients admitted to hospital with hip fractures and improves their care through auditing, which is fed back to hospitals through targeted reports.

Hospitals can access their own organisation's complete data and this enables local health economies to benchmark their performance in hip fracture care against national data. The patient pathway, involves many specialties in addition to surgery, and data fed back includes mortality rates, which anaesthetics are used, hospital length of stay, rates of inpatient pressure ulcers, and reoperations and which operations are being performed for different types of fractures. Quality of patient care is examined using six key performance indicators and the NHFD is designed as a platform to facilitate local quality improvement projects. An example is the recent Hip Fracture Quality Improvement Programme, a multicentre collaborative where five units were recruited and interventions piloted in an 'exemplar unit' were scaled up to these five units. These included better pain management and access to nerve blocks in the Emergency Department and ran over 2 years. Highlighted results include a reduction in 30-day mortality and significantly more people making a good recovery and returning home [41].

Best practice tariffs

Tariffs are prices for units of healthcare (which varies across specialties and services). Providers (hospitals) are reimbursed for services they deliver by the cost of Best Practice, rather than the average cost. There is a large variation in quality of care and therefore, some, but not all, providers provide care in accordance with best practice. The intention of Best Practice Tariffs (BPT) is to introduce a formal financial incentive for complying with known best practice [42], whilst improving the standard of care across all providers to that of the agreed best practice.

The UK National Emergency Laparotomy Audit (NELA) [10] collects data on compliance with evidence-based standards and provides local Trusts (providers) with benchmarked reports on their compliance and performance. One metric that leads to an enhanced tariff (additional payment to providers) if delivered, is that > 80% of high-risk patients undergoing an emergency laparotomy should have a consultant surgeon and consultant anaesthetist present during surgery.

Similar BPT metrics are used in the NJR and NHFD. In the latter, all agreed standards should be met in order to qualify for the extra payment. In the NJR, providers need to use cemented or hybrid prostheses for at least 80% of patients aged over 70 years undergoing hip or knee replacements to obtain the BPT.

GETTING IT RIGHT FIRST TIME [23]

The Getting It Right First Time (GIRFT) programme is designed to improve quality of care in NHS hospitals in England by reducing unwarranted variations in services and practices. By tackling variations in the way services are delivered across the NHS and by sharing best practice between trusts (hospitals), GIRFT identifies changes that will help improve care and patient outcomes, in addition to delivering efficiencies such as the reduction of unnecessary procedures and cost savings.

Getting it right first time methodology

The programme comprises a series of 40 surgical and medical workstreams, each led by a prominent clinician chosen from specialty they are reviewing.

There are four key strands:

1. A broad data gathering and analysis exercise, performed by health data analysts, which generates a detailed picture of current national practice, outcomes, and other related factors
2. A series of discussions between clinical specialists and individual hospital trusts, which are based on the data, providing an unprecedented opportunity to examine individual trust behaviour and performance in the relevant area of practice, in the context of the national picture. This then enables the trust to understand where it is performing well and what it could do better, drawing on the input of senior clinicians
3. A final report that draws on both the data analysis and the discussions with the hospital trusts to identify opportunities for NHS-wide improvement
4. An implementation phase where the GIRFT team supports providers to deliver the improvements recommended after the clinical specialist visits

GETTING IT RIGHT FIRST TIME PROGRAMME REPORTS AND OUTCOMES

It is important to assess the impact of quality improvement programmes. Barret et al. (2017) [43] plan for a mixed methods evaluation of GIRFT in relation to NHS orthopaedic care (the first workstream reviewed in 2012). The example report summaries below not only highlight the methodology in more detail but also the breadth such an initiative can reach to improve patient care and reduce costs.

Getting it right first time general surgery national specialty report (2017) [44]

This report examined key aspects of the way general surgery, defined as the management of patients presenting with elective or emergency abdominal disease, is delivered in the NHS in England. The first aspect of the methodology involves high-quality data driven insight into the specialty drawn on combining different sources. For general surgery, data has been taken from large national audits (National Bowel Cancer Audit, Upper Gastrointestinal Cancer Audit and National Emergency Laparotomy Audit, NELA), Hospital Episode Statistics (HES) and trust reference costs. Patient Reported Outcome Measures (PROMs) are not widely validated in general surgery and less direct indicators such as Friends and Family Scores [45] have been used where good metrics are not yet available. As the programme develops, it is intended to develop more informative and actionable metrics.

This detailed, data-led view of the way General Surgery is currently delivered provides a clear national picture and then allows individual reports for each hospital trust to be generated. Engagement from clinicians and management has been identified as key for embedding a culture of quality improvement and in particular frontline teams are often best placed to develop solutions [46].

Recommendations are examined and then the GIRFT team co-ordinates an implementation programme designed to help trusts address the issues raised and improve quality, which may be at a national or individual hospital level. Although responsibility for implementation rests with each hospital, the GIRFT team ensures there is a range of ongoing support available to help individual providers implement these recommendations locally. Although there are 20 recommendations spread across five themes (data and performance measurement; procurement, choice, commissioning and care pathways; surgical performance; and efficiency and emergency provision) the report highlights three opportunities for improvement. These are opportunities to learn from the trusts where readmission rates following complex surgery are lowest, where the use of day case surgery for less complex procedures is most common and where the proportion of patients with stoma 18 months after surgical resection for colorectal cancer is lowest. If all hospitals reached the national average in these three key areas, it would potentially save the NHS half a million pounds a year but more significantly it would make an enormous positive difference to patients' lives.

Getting it right in orthopaedics: a follow-up on the GIRFT national specialty report on orthopaedics [47]

The GIRFT approach was first used in orthopaedic surgery in 2012, and within 12 months of completing the analysis and visits, led to an estimated £30–50 million savings in orthopaedic care – predominantly through changes that reduced average length of stay and improved procurement. Repeat deep dive visits were undertaken to embed the GIRFT methodology and assess the impact of the initial visits (**Table 2.1**). Key outcome data centred on significant reductions in the rate of revisions for total hip replacements and total knee replacements, average length of stay reduced by a fifth and release of £696 million operational and financial opportunities by trusts to date.

One of the strongest testaments to the success of the GIRFT orthopaedics workstream has been the appetite to reproduce this in the devolved administrations and further afield, as well as in over 40 other specialties. It is worth noting that several aspects of the original report including litigation, SSIs and guideline development have since grown into separate projects in their own right.

Litigation and claims learning [48]

The GIRFT litigation workstream has collaborated to engage trusts and share data regarding their own claims on a specialty-specific basis and through deep dives, better understand the processes that facilitate effective claims prevention, management and learning. As a result, guidance has been produced to enable clinicians and managers to learn from clinical negligence claims to improve current clinical practice. This best practice

Table 2.1 GIRFT orthopaedics in numbers	
336	Deep dive revisits to hospitals
26,880	GIRFT orthopaedics metrics shared with hospitals in deep dive visits
3,064	Actions agreed by hospitals
1,028	Actions completed by hospitals
£696 million	Operational and financial opportunities released by trusts over the course of the programme to date
£165.3 million	Operational and financial opportunities released by trusts in 2018/19
GIRFT, get it right first time	

guidance has been produced in collaboration with national specialist societies to improve documentation for procedures which result in high volumes of litigation to improve care and prevent money being diverted from patient care.

Getting it right first time surgical-site infection survey [49]

Surgical-site infection is an important area of focus, with associated poor patient outcomes, reoperations and they cause significant cost to the NHS and more importantly to patients. Prior to the GIRFT review of General Surgery, there was a lack of awareness of SSI rates by clinicians. The GIRFT SSI programme was set up to review SSI rates and review current practice in prevention of SSIs. This work is ongoing.

CONCLUSION

Quality improvement programmes are an important aspect of (inter)national and local clinical governance to improve the quality of care which patients receive. Different methodologies can be used as tools to drive quality improvement, with emphasis on high-quality data, engagement from clinical and managerial leaders and patient involvement and insight. GIRFT is an initiative that has delivered significant results in improving patient safety and reducing costs through reducing unwanted variation.

Surgeons have a professional obligation to be involved in local and national quality improvement programmes, and as future clinical leaders play an integral part in not only delivering quality services but actively shaping and improving them to provide the best care for their patients.

Key points for clinical practice

- Quality improvement is a process of using a defined and structured approach, over a set period of time, to improve patient outcomes and experience. The following dimensions should be considered when assessing quality of care: Safe, timely, effective, efficient, person-centred, and equitable
- Clinical governance is a framework through which organisations and their staff are accountable for continuously improving the quality of their services and includes seven pillars: Audit, clinical effectiveness, research, risk management, education and training, patient and public involvement and information

- The role of clinical audit is to check clinical care meets defined quality standards and to implement improvements to address shortfalls identified. An example is the National Emergency Laparotomy Audit in the UK
- There are many methods of quality improvement including: PDSA, model for improvement, performance benchmarking, statistical process control, six sigma and lean. It is important to choose the right process for the desired outcome
- Quality Improvement can be incentivised through national registries such as the National Joint Registry and the National Hip Fracture Database, best practice tariffs and improvement programmes
- The GIRFT programme is the largest clinician-led quality improvement and efficiency programme in the history of the NHS and uses performance benchmarking to identify good practice that can be shared and unwarranted variation that can be addressed by focused improvement

REFERENCES

1. Institute of Medicine. Crossing the Quality Chasm. Washington, DC: National Academies Press; 2001.
2. The Health Foundation. (2013). Quality improvement made simple. [online] Available from https://www.health.org.uk/publications/quality-improvement-made-simple. [Last accessed November, 2020].
3. John Hutchinson; Royal College of Surgeons. What is Quality Improvement?. [online] Available from https://www.rcseng.ac.uk/standards-and-research/support-for-surgeons-and-services/quality-improvement-in-surgery/what-is-qi/. [Last accessed November, 2020].
4. The King's Fund. (2017). Making the case for quality improvement. [online] Available from https://www.kingsfund.org.uk/publications/making-case-quality-improvement. [Last accessed November, 2020].
5. General Medical Council. (2018). Domain 2: Safety and quality. [online] Available from https://www.gmc-uk.org/ethical-guidance/ethical-guidance-for-doctors/good-medical-practice/domain-2----safety-and-quality. [Last accessed November, 2020].
6. Intercollegiate Surgical Curriculum Programme. (2017). Assessment of Audit. [online] Available from https://www.iscp.ac.uk/curriculum/surgical/assessment_audit.aspx. [Last accessed November, 2020].
7. General Medical Council. (2018). Domain 2: Safety and quality. [online] Available from https://www.gmc-uk.org/ethical-guidance/ethical-guidance-for-doctors/good-medical-practice/domain-2----safety-and-quality. [Last accessed November, 2020].
8. Benjamin A. Audit: how to do it in practice. BMJ 2008; 336.
9. Burgess R, Moorhead J. New principles of best practice in clinical audit, 2nd edition. London: Taylor & Francis Ltd, 2011.
10. National Emergency Laparotomy Audit. NELA - National Emergency Laparotomy Audit. Available from https://www.nela.org.uk/NELA_home. [Last accessed November, 2020].
11. British Association of Endocrine and Thyroid Surgeons (BAETS). Audit. [online] Available from http://www.baets.org.uk/audit/. [Last accessed November, 2020].
12. Ashley MP, Pemberton MN, Saksena A, et al. Improving patient safety in a UK dental hospital: Long-term use of clinical audit. Br Dent J 2014; 217:369–373.
13. Taylor MJ, McNicholas C, Nicolay C, et al. Systematic review of the application of the plan-do-study-act method to improve quality in healthcare. BMJ Qual Saf 2014; 23:290–298.
14. Speroff T, O'Connor GT. Study designs for PDSA quality improvement research. Qual Manag Health Care 2004; 13:17–32.
15. Berwick DM. Developing and testing changes in delivery of care. Ann Intern Med 1998; 128:651–656.
16. van Tiel FH, Elenbaas TWO, Voskuilen BMAM, et al. Plan-do-study-act cycles as an instrument for improvement of compliance with infection control measures in care of patients after cardiothoracic surgery. J Hosp Infect 2006; 62:64–70.
17. Goodney PP, Chang RW, Cronenwett JL. A percutaneous arterial closure protocol can decrease complications after endovascular interventions in vascular surgery patients. J Vasc Surg 2008; 48:1481–1488.

18. API–Associates in Process Improvement. [online] Available from http://www.apiweb.org/. [Last accessed November, 2020].
19. Institute for Healthcare Improvement. How to Improve. [online] Available from http://www.ihi.org/resources/Pages/HowtoImprove/default.aspx. [Last accessed November, 2020].
20. The 'How to Guide' for Reducing Surgical Complications. [online] Available from http://www.1000livesplus.wales.nhs.uk/sitesplus/documents/1011/Reducing Surgical ComplicationsWHOFinaldraft v2 1.pdf. [Last accessed November, 2020].
21. Haynes AB, Weiser TG, Berry WR, et al. A Surgical Safety Checklist to Reduce Morbidity and Mortality in a Global Population. N Engl J Med 2009; 360:491–499.
22. Timmins N. (2017). Tackling variations in clinical care assessing the Getting It Right First Time (GIRFT) programme. [online] Available from https://www.kingsfund.org.uk/publications/tackling-variations-clinical-care. [Last accessed November, 2020].
23. Getting It Right First Time (GIRFT). Reports. [online] Available from https://www.gettingitrightfirsttime.co.uk/girft-reports/. [Last accessed November, 2020].
24. NHS Improvement. Statistical process control tool. [online] Available from https://improvement.nhs.uk/resources/statistical-process-control-tool/. [Last accessed November, 2020].
25. Timmerman T, Verrall T, Clatney L, et al. Taking a closer look: Using statistical process control to identify patterns of improvement in a quality-improvement collaborative. Qual Saf Heal Care. 2010;19(6):e19.
26. Ryckman FC, Schoettker PJ, Hays KR, et al. Reducing surgical site infections at a pediatric academic medical center. Jt Comm J Qual Patient Saf 2009; 35:192–198.
27. Duclos A, STouzet, Soardo P, et al. Quality monitoring in thyroid surgery using the Shewhart control chart. Br J Surg 2009; 96:171–174.
28. Adams R, Warner P, Hubbard B, et al. Decreasing Turnaround Time between General Surgery Cases: A Six Sigma Initiative. J Nurs Adm 2004; 34:140–148.
29. McCarthy M. Can car manufacturing techniques reform health care? Lancet 2006; 367:290–291.
30. Celik J. Decreasing Preoperative Delays-A Rapid Process Improvement Project. AORN J 2003; 77:737–741.
31. Burkitt KH, Mor MK, Jain R, et al. Toyota production system quality improvement initiative improves perioperative antibiotic therapy. Am J Manag Care 2009; 15:633–642.
32. Waldhausen JHT, Avansino JR, Libby A, et al. Application of lean methods improves surgical clinic experience. J Pediatr Surg 2010; 45:1420–1425.
33. Cambridge University Press. (2008). Cambridge online dictionary. [online]. Available from https://dictionary.cambridge.org/. [Last accessed November, 2020].
34. Shah A. Using data for improvement. BMJ 2019; 364:l189.
35. NHS England. Data quality Improvement. [online] Available from https://www.england.nhs.uk/data-services/validate. [Last accessed November, 2020].
36. National Joint Registry. National Joint Registry. [online] Available from https://www.njrcentre.org.uk. [Last accessed November, 2020].
37. Gliklich RE, Dreyer NA, Leavy MB. Registries for Evaluating Patient Outcomes: a User's Guide [Internet], 3rd edition. Rockville (MD): Agency for Healthcare Research and Quality (US), 2014.
38. National Joint Registry. Patient Decision Support Tool. [online] Available from http://www.njrcentre.org.uk/njrcentre/Patients/Patient-Decision-Support-Tool. [Last accessed November, 2020].
39. The National Hip Fracture Database. The National Hip Fracture Database. [online] Available from https://www.nhfd.co.uk/. [Last accessed November, 2020].
40. Royal College of Physicians (2015). Falls and Fragility Fracture Audit Programme (FFFAP). [online] Available from https://www.rcplondon.ac.uk/projects/falls-and-fragility-fracture-audit-programme-fffap. [Last accessed November, 2020].
41. National Hip Fracture Database. (2019). 2019 Annual Report. [online] Available from https://www.nhfd.co.uk/files/2019ReportFiles/NHFD_2019_Annual_Report_v101.pdf. [Last accessed November, 2020].
42. Gershlick B; The Health Foundation. (2016). Best practice Tariffs. [online] Available from https://www.oecd.org/els/health-systems/Better-Ways-to-Pay-for-Health-Care-Background-Note-England-Best-practice-tariffs.pdf. [Last accessed November, 2020].
43. Barratt H, Turner S, Hutchings A, et al. Mixed methods evaluation of the Getting it Right First Time programme—improvements to NHS orthopaedic care in England: study protocol. BMC Health Serv Res 2017; 17:71.
44. GIRFT. GIRFT General Surgery Report. [online] Available from https://gettingitrightfirsttime.co.uk/wp-content/uploads/2018/08/GIRFT-GeneralSurgery-Aug17-O1.pdf. [Last accessed November, 2020].

45. NHS Choices. (2019). Friends and Family Test (FFT). [online] Available from https://www.nhs.uk/using-the-nhs/about-the-nhs/friends-and-family-test-fft/. [Last accessed November, 2020].

46. The King's Fund. (2017). Embedding a culture of quality improvement. [online] Available from https://www.kingsfund.org.uk/publications/embedding-culture-quality-improvement. [Last accessed November, 2020].

47. GIRFT. (2020). Reflecting on success and reinforcing improvement A follow-up on the GIRFT national speciality report on orthopaedics. [online] Available from https://gettingitrightfirsttime.co.uk/wp-content/uploads/2020/02/GIRFT-orthopaedics-follow-up-report-February-2020.pdf. [Last accessed November, 2020].

48. Machin JT, Navaratnam AV, Ho C, et al. (2020). Learning from Litigation Claims -The Getting It Right First Time (GIRFT) and NHS Resolution best practice guide for clinicians and managers. [online] Available from https://www.gettingitrightfirsttime.co.uk/cross-cutting-stream/litigation/. [Last accessed November, 2020].

49. GIRFT. (2019). Surgical site infection audit. [online] Available from https://www.gettingitrightfirsttime.co.uk/cross-cutting-stream/surgical-site-infection-audit/. [Last accessed November, 2020].

Chapter 3

Paediatric surgery in low- and middle-income countries

Dennis Mazingi, Kokila Lakhoo

RECENT ADVANCES IN THE MANAGEMENT OF APPENDICITIS

INTRODUCTION

Surgically correctable pathology still accounts for a sizeable proportion of the overall global burden of disease. There is still a disparity between the surgical capacity in low- and middle-income countries (LMIC) and those in high-income countries (HIC). Barriers include accessibility, availability, affordability and acceptability of surgical care. The provision of essential paediatric surgical care in LMIC is also different and relatively simple interventions have been shown to prevent death and disability. The best way to illustrate real differences is by reviewing the management of three important surgical conditions in LMICs: appendicitis, gastroschisis, and nephroblastoma.

APPENDICITIS

Appendicitis is the most common reason for emergency abdominal surgery in children worldwide with growing incidence in newly industrialised countries of Asia, the Middle East, Southern America, and Africa [1]. This is in contrast to the incidence in higher-income countries which have a steady or decreasing incidence [1]. It presents most frequently in the second decade of life with a lifetime risk of appendicitis of 6.7–8.6% [2] and boys are more likely to suffer from the disease than girls [2]. In LMICs appendicitis is frequently complicated with a 60% perforation rate and a high rate of re-intervention [3] It is also characterised by treatment delays as a result of late presentation [3]. Appendicitis is the exemplar of the acute abdomen in LMICs and illustrates the importance of sound clinical judgement and rational use of investigations.

Whilst this disease has been exhaustively characterised in the surgical literature, recently debate has intensified about key aspects of diagnosis, and treatment of the condition in children.

> **Key points for clinical practice**
> - The incidence of appendicitis is rising in newly industrialised countries
> - The incidence of appendicitis peaks in the second decade of life

Clinical manifestations and diagnosis

Long-held surgical dogma asserts that diagnosis of appendicitis is strictly clinical, with classical clinical features. However, diagnosis can often be challenging in children because of the difficulty of obtaining a reliable history and eliciting physical signs. In addition, the classical clinical features are neither sensitive nor specific enough in isolation to reliably establish a diagnosis of appendicitis in all children. Nonetheless, the ability to detect a child likely to have appendicitis is an important skill in surgeons particularly in LMICs where ancillary tests are not always available or cost effective. A high index of suspicion should be maintained at all times. Symptoms include abdominal pain that classically starts as a vague, peri-umbilical discomfort that subsequently shifts over the course of hours to days to the right iliac fossa and becomes well localised and sharp reflecting the different innervation of the visceral and somatic peritoneum. Nausea, vomiting, dysuria, diarrhoea and constipation may also develop. Multiple eponymous signs have been described which are primarily attributable to localised or generalised peritoneal irritation (**Table 3.1**). There is a wide clinical spectrum from early appendicitis to advanced appendicitis with either localised or free rupture. Four-quadrant peritonitis is indicative of free rupture of the appendix and is a common presentation [4]. With the typically long delay, the characteristic sequence of symptoms may be difficult to elicit upon anamnesis. Because of limited diagnostic aides available in LMICs, clinical suspicion is paramount. The major diagnostic question to answer—'is emergency surgical exploration required?' Non-specific signs of four-quadrant peritonitis requiring surgery include abdominal rigidity, exquisite tenderness on palpation, a positive Blumberg's sign, and absent bowel sounds.

Laboratory and radiological investigations are also useful adjuncts to diagnosis. A variety of laboratory markers of inflammation such as white cell count (with left shift) and C-reactive protein (CRP) should be routinely requested if available as well as urinalysis [5]. CRP is a particularly useful biomarker in children, CRP > 10 mg/L is a strong predictor of appendicitis in children [6].

Various clinical prediction scores have been developed that aim to improve diagnostic accuracy and reduce negative appendicectomy rates. The Alvarado score was one of the earliest clinical prediction scores described and enjoys widespread usage along with the paediatric appendicitis score of Samuel (PAS) (**Table 3.2**). Whilst both scores are useful, recent consensus guidelines for the diagnosis and treatment of acute appendicitis (the Jerusalem guidelines) recommend against making the diagnosis based on these scores alone [5].

Table 3.1 Selected eponymous signs in appendicitis	
Sign	**Description**
Rovsing's sign	Pain elicited by distending the caecum by applying anti-peristaltic pressure to the left iliac fossa
Psoas test	Abdominal pain elicited by extension of the right thigh with patient in the left lateral decubitus position
Dunphy's sign	Abdominal pain in the RIF elicited by coughing
Obturator test	Hypogastric pain elicited by rotation of the flexed lower limb at the hip
Sitkovsky sign	Increased RIF tenderness elicited by moving from the supine to the left decubitus position
(RIF: right iliac fossa)	

Table 3.2 Comparison of components of clinical prediction scores in children

Clinical feature	Alvarado score	PAS (Samuel score)
Migratory RIF pain	1	1
Anorexia	1	1
Nausea	1	1
Tenderness in the RLQ	2	2
Rebound pain	1	–
Elevated temperature	1	1
Leucocytosis	1	1
Left shift of WBC	1	1
RLQ pain elicited by cough/percussion/hopping	–	2
Total	**10**	**10**

(PAS: paediatric appendicitis score; RIF: right iliac fossa; RLQ: right lower quadrant; WBC: white blood cell)

Table 3.3 Ultrasound features of appendicitis

Aperistaltic, non-compressible, blind-ended tubular structure

Appendiceal diameter > 6 mm

Appendiceal wall thickness > 2 mm

Localised tenderness elicited by graded compression

Presence of a faecalith

Imaging investigations are useful when the clinical likelihood of appendicitis is not high enough to confidently make the diagnosis on clinical grounds or for excluding possible differential diagnoses. The American College of Radiology and the Jerusalem guidelines recommend ultrasonography as the first-line investigation of choice [5]. Real-time compression ultrasonography is performed to identify the appendix and when the appendix has been visualised, has sensitivity and specificity of 98% and 92% respectively. Whilst it is heavily user-dependant it offers the best balance of convenience, price, specificity and sensitivity versus radiation exposure. Sonographic findings in appendicitis are presented in **Table 3.3**. Surgeon-administered point of care ultrasound should be considered an extension of the physical examination and potentially shortens the diagnostic process and decision-making time without reducing accuracy [7]. Plain abdominal X-ray is of limited value and should not be routinely performed. Its utility lies in excluding alternative diagnoses. It may demonstrate a faecalith in up to 7–15% of cases, loss of the psoas shadow, localised ileus with air/fluid levels, and mild scoliosis concave to the right. While computed tomography (CT) scan has excellent sensitivity and specificity it does not appear to have lowered negative appendicectomy rates overall, and therefore does not appear to justify the increased costs, radiation exposure and possible surgical delay.

Treatment

Management of appendicitis should be guided by the clinical state of the child and the expected state of the appendix (i.e., early-unruptured, phlegmon, appendiceal abscess, free rupture) determined by clinical assessment and investigations. Management should focus on initial resuscitation and management of sepsis and thereafter a distinction between early appendicitis and advanced appendicitis is useful to determine further treatment options.

Recent revisions of the surviving sepsis guidelines for children [8] are pertinent in the initial resuscitative phase of treatment and emphasise early (< 3 hours) broad-spectrum anti-microbial therapy, goal-directed fluid resuscitation with balanced crystalloid, emergent source control intervention and vasoactive medications where indicated.

In children with early appendicitis, prompt appendicectomy is the treatment of choice. It has low mortality and is curative. While there is growing evidence that suggests that non-operative management of appendicitis (NOMA) in children is safe, it still has a failure rate of up to 33% at one-year follow-up and depends on careful selection of patients using strict criteria [9,10]. The approach may not be entirely appropriate for LMICs because a higher proportion of children present with complicated disease requiring surgery than in HICs [3]. The approach is also associated with higher rates of emergency department visits and re-admissions [9] which increases overall costs significantly.

Children with advanced appendicitis (which is complicated by perforation or gangrene) require treatment with close attention during the resuscitative phase and expeditious appendicectomy with source control. While laparoscopy is not inferior to laparotomy for complicated appendicitis, laparotomy is a key competency of the LMIC surgeon. It is recognised by the Lancet Commission on Global Surgery as one of the bellwether procedures (acute high-value procedure suggestive of a functional surgical system) [11]. Where laparoscopy is not available or institutional inertia has retarded adoption, laparotomy is a safe and lifesaving procedure. It allows complete exploration of the abdomen to identify concurrent pathology and break up loculated abscesses. Evidence extrapolated from laparoscopy suggests that lavage with copious amounts of saline is not better than suction alone [12]; however adequate source control should be achieved.

IMPROVING THE OUTCOME OF GASTROSCHISIS IN LMICs

GASTROSCHISIS

Gastroschisis is a congenital condition characterised by intestinal protrusion outside the abdomen through an abdominal wall defect. Its name has its roots in the ancient Greek words: *gastro* (of or relating to the stomach) and *schisis* (meaning a separation or cleft) and therefore is a misnomer. For unknown reasons, the birth prevalence of this condition appears to be increasing globally, both in HICs [13] and in LMICs [14], and has been reported as 1:2000–3000. Gastroschisis is particularly illustrative of the stark disparities that exist in surgical care between HIC and LMICs. While survival has steadily increased in HICs (>95%) it still remains remarkably low in many LMICs, as low as 0–33% in some countries [15]. In one hospital this condition was previously considered a non-survivable condition and palliative care was the norm [16]. Antenatal diagnosis rates are low in LMICs (as low as 0–14%) and most affected children are born in distant peripheral health facilities leading to treatment delays [17]. Because of this, pre-referral resuscitation is crucially important, more so than long transfer delays . The answer to improving outcomes in gastroschisis babies likely involves system-wide improvements in transport, training and capacitating district hospital facilities in addition to interventional bundles at the central hospital [18,16].

The diversity of proposed aetiologies reflects the enigmatic nature of the disease. Young maternal age, low socio-economic status, environmental toxins, smoking, drug use and macro- and micronutrient deficiencies have all been implicated however the cause of the disease and its mechanism is still unexplained [19,20]. It may be related to a failure of fusion of the lateral body folds in the 4th week of gestation. Vascular insult may also play a role as evidenced by the frequent association with intestinal atresia.

Clinical features and investigations

The clinical appearance of gastroschisis is striking and distinctive and the diagnosis is often made on sight; however, it should be distinguished from omphalocele, a condition with which it is commonly confused (**Table 3.4**). In gastroschisis, bowel protrudes from

Table 3.4 Differences between gastroschisis and omphalocele		
Feature	**Gastroschisis**	**Omphalocele**
Site of abnormality	Usually right paraumbilical area	Central umbilicus
Sac	Absent A 'pseudosac' may be visible	Present except when ruptured
Contents	Small intestine and colon. Rarely gonads	Liver, intestine, spleen, gonads
Associated systemic anomalies	Rare	Frequent extra-abdominal associations
Outcomes	Dependent on health system and in-hospital management	Dependent on associated anomalies

an abdominal wall defect adjacent to an otherwise normal umbilicus and while individual loops may not be immediately discernible, they are not covered by a true membrane but rather by fibrinous inflammatory peel related to exposure to amniotic fluid. Associated conditions include intestinal atresia and conditions outside of the gastrointestinal system, are rare. Two clinical variants exist: simple or complex (in which necrosis, perforation, volvulus, intestinal atresia or a closing gastroschisis are present). Complex gastroschisis may occur in up to 17% of patients and is associated with increased morbidity and mortality.

Key points for clinical practice

- For gastroschisis, early goal-directed fluid resuscitation and control of hypothermia are crucial for reducing mortality in the pre-hospital phase and thereafter
- In gastroschisis, bowel protection with an improvised plastic covering or silo, prevents fluid losses during patient transfer

---

Management

The initial management of gastroschisis depends on recognition, resuscitation and expeditious and safe referral. This is the major period during which the majority of mortality occurs in LMICs [15] and where opportunities exist for reducing mortality. Further opportunities exist in protocolised care once the child arrives at the central hospital. A pragmatic, home-grown protocol in Uganda has achieved a drop of mortality from 98 to 59% [16].

Route of delivery does not appear to influence outcome and that decision should therefore be made solely based on obstetric indications. In the event that prenatal diagnosis has been made, it may be advantageous to deliver the baby closer to a facility with paediatric surgical expertise particularly in LMICs.

At birth management should focus on prevention of hypothermia and fluid resuscitation. Because of the exposed bowel and the large surface area of the neonate, there is the potential for significant heat and insensible fluid loss. Warmed, balanced intravenous fluids should be administered to maintain hydration and while a fluid deficit should be expected, over-hydration should be avoided. The bowel should be protected from trauma, kinking, fluid and heat loss by being carefully placed within a plastic occlusive dressing or bag. Improvised plastic coverings such as cling film a large urobag or vacolitre bag may be used [16]. Nasogastric tube decompression and urinary catheter insertion should be performed and broad-spectrum antibiotics should be administered. After evaluation for associated anomalies or complications the aim is to achieve full reduction of the bowel into the abdomen while avoiding abdominal compartment syndrome, respiratory compromise and aspiration with as good a cosmetic result as possible [21]. If primary closure cannot be achieved without excessive intra-abdominal pressure, then staged closure should be performed. Primary closure may not be possible in up to 79% of gastroschisis patients [22] because of viscero-peritoneal disproportion or oedema of the bowel. Staged reduction in HICs is performed using preformed spring-loaded silo bags. In LMICs, these are prohibitively expensive and unavailable and improvised silo bags have been made out of sterile urobags, female condoms, sterile saline bags and gloves, for decades [17]. Sutureless closure has been described more recently and purportedly achieves similar outcomes to sutured repair with the added benefit of decreased need for mechanical ventilation and reduced analgesia requirements; however there is a higher incidence of umbilical hernias

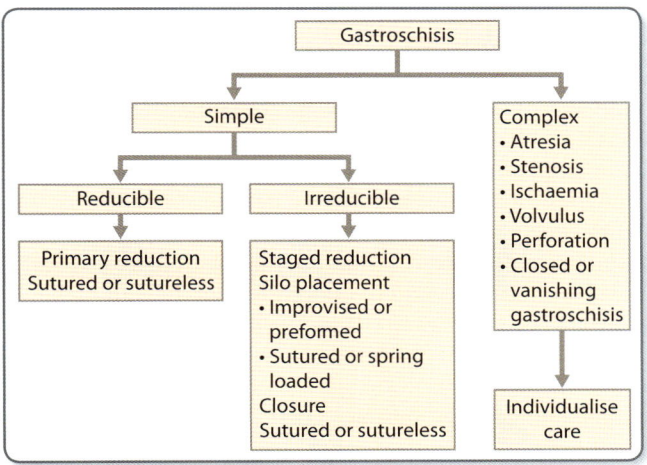

Figure 3.1 Surgical treatment options for gastroschisis, adapted from Petrosyan et al, 2018 [24].

requiring surgery [23]. Once complete reduction has been achieved closure can be done with fascial sutures, using native umbilicus or without sutures using a watertight adherent dressing [24]. Staged reduction and subsequent closure can both be performed safely at the bedside which is an advantage in LMICs where theatre time may be difficult to obtain. Primary reduction appears to allow for earlier enteral feeding and confers a lower risk of infection than staged reduction and predictably, shorter hospital stay [25]. Staged reduction avoids the serious complication of abdominal compartment syndrome. Further challenges in the management of gastroschisis lie in non-availability of total parenteral nutrition (**Figure 3.1**).

Anecdotal experience and empirical evidence from LMICs suggest that quality improvement in gastroschisis treatment requires deliberate, sustained, committed effort from a dedicated team that brings together nurses, paediatricians, surgeons and even caregivers [26,16]. This personal involvement of the entire ward staff compliment and effective teamwork is crucial to success.

Key points for clinical practice

- Adequate resuscitation of neonates with gastroschisis is of utmost importance and more so than prompt referral
- Multiple reduction and closure techniques exist but the aim is to reduce the bowel and close the abdomen in as safe and quick a way as is possible with an acceptable cosmetic result

---

NEPHROBLASTOMA

INTRODUCTION

Childhood cancer is the ninth leading cause of childhood disease burden globally responsible for 11·5 million disability-adjusted life years (DALYs) lost in 2017 [27].

It affects the poorest regions of the world disproportionately with 82% of the global burden of childhood cancer occurring in LMICs [27]. Renal cancers are a major type of childhood cancer and Wilms tumour is the most common intra-abdominal tumour in children, accounting for more than 90% of all paediatric malignant kidney neoplasms. There has been a tremendous improvement in 5-year survival rates for nephroblastoma in HICs since the 20th century, reaching more than 90% in the mid-2010s. This has not happened in LMICs where outcomes have continued to lag behind [28], with 5-year survival rates as low as 0-14%. Postulated reasons for this disparity include: lack of access to treatment, prohibitive costs, late presentation, poor supportive care, abandonment and lack of resources for diagnosis and treatment [29,30]. Recently, the suggestion that biological differences in tumours may contribute at least somewhat to the difference has been broached [31] but not confirmed. Observed infrastructural disparities are pertinent in tailoring management protocols. Differing levels of care for Wilms tumour have been defined to facilitate this. Setting 1 is the major focus of this chapter (**Table 3.5**).

The incidence of Wilms tumour in LMICs is 9.8 age specific rate per million (ASR/million) [29] however, this is likely an underestimate. It is most common in children below the age of 5 years with an almost equal gender distribution [29]. While predominantly a sporadic disease, in a minority of cases it may be associated with multiple malformation syndromes such as the WAGR syndrome, Denys Drash or Beckwith-Wiedemann syndrome.

Table 3.5 Levels of care for treatment of Wilms tumour. Adapted from Gupta et al. [32]

Setting	Medical facilities	Specialists	Drugs	Supportive care	Diagnostic facilities
1. Minimal requirements for curative intent	Paediatric ward Adequate surgical facilities Facilities for perioperative care	Surgeon Paediatric nurse	Vincristine Actinomycin D Doxorubicin	Adequate pain medication Morphine IV Antibiotics Whole blood Social support for impoverished families	Full blood count Ultrasonography Plain chest X-ray
2. Intermediate	Paediatric oncology ward Radiotherapy Pathology Multi-disciplinary care	Pathologist Paediatric surgeon Paediatric oncologist Radiation oncologist Oncology nurse	Doxorubicin Cyclophosphamide Etoposide Ifosfamide Carboplatin	All blood products Central venous access	CT scan
3. State of the art (centre of excellence)	Intensive care unit	Paediatric pathologist Paediatric radiation oncologist Pharmacist (oncology) intensivist		Mechanical ventilation Haemodialysis Pressure support	Special stains Immunohisto-chemistry Cytogenetics

(IV: intravenous)

> **Key points for clinical practice**
>
> - While survival rates in the management of nephroblastoma in HICs are high, they continue to lag behind in LMICs
> - Adequate treatment of nephroblastoma can be achieved even in poorly-resourced LMICs with rational use of available resources

Clinical features and diagnosis

Wilms tumour presents typically as a painless abdominal mass with slow gradual growth over many months that may reach an appreciable size. In LMICs, late presentation is a common problem because of lack of knowledge among parents, financial barriers and seeking care outside of formal medical systems. Scarification marks courtesy of the African traditional healer on the skin should alert the physician that the duration of illness has been long [33,34]. While constitutional symptoms are characteristically uncommon, malnourishment, hypertension, haematuria and fever may also be present. Careful physical examination usually reveals an eccentric, firm, well-circumscribed, non-tender, smooth mass. It is said to be rarely cross the midline and does not move with respiration, facts that may help distinguish it from neuroblastoma, a common differential (**Table 3.6**). Other infrequent clinical features include those attributable to associated congenital syndromes, respiratory embarrassment, mass effect of a large tumour and tumour rupture. A short systolic murmur may indicate vascular involvement with intra-cardiac extension.

Imaging investigations have an important role in establishing the likely diagnosis, excluding differentials, guiding management decisions as well as assessing the state of the contralateral kidney and metastases. While more advanced cross-sectional imaging may be more sensitive, abdominal ultrasound is adequate in resource limited settings and provides a wealth of information. Greyscale ultrasonography can exclude common differentials such as hydronephrosis and multi-cystic kidney disease, establish a renal origin of the mass and characterise the parenchyma as solid, cystic or both. Information about the contralateral kidney is also relevant. In addition, Doppler may give information about vascular involvement including the presence of inferior vena cava (IVC) tumoural thrombi which

Table 3.6 Differences between Wilms tumour and neuroblastoma

Feature	Wilms tumour	Neuroblastoma
Constitutional symptoms	Rare	Common
Crosses the midline	Rare	More likely
Mobility	Mobile	Fixed and immobile
Pain	Rare	More common
Extra-clinical signs	Macroglossia Aniridia Hemihypertrophy	Raccoon eyes–orbital metastases Blueberry muffin skin–cutaneous metastases
Calcification	Uncommon	Common (80–90%)
Vascular involvement	Invades vasculature	Encases vascular structures but does not usually invade them.

CT scan may occasionally miss [35]. Plain chest X-rays are used to detect lung metastases, visible as peripheral rounded opacities [35].

Wilms tumour may be feasibly and effectively managed in LMICs [35]. The minimum requirements for treatment with curative intent have been incorporated into guidelines from the International Society of Paediatric Oncology–Paediatric Oncology in Developing Countries (SIOP PODC) working group for nephroblastoma and are shown in **Table 3.6**. Of note, pathology and radiotherapy services are not considered mandatory. According to the World Health Organisation (WHO) 90% of all imaging requirements in LMICs can be provided for by X-ray and ultrasound services [36] and this is true for Wilms tumour. In recent years, however increasing numbers of LMIC facilities are able to provide more advanced cross-sectional imaging.

Key points for clinical practice

- Nephroblastoma presents as gradual, painless abdominal distention in a generally well child with a smooth large mass that does not typically cross the midline
- For imaging suspected cases of nephroblastoma, ultrasound can provide a wealth of information and is adequate for use where other modalities are unavailable

---

Management

Appropriate therapy of Wilms tumour includes surgery, chemotherapy, radiotherapy and supportive care. Implementation of the context-appropriate guidelines of the SIOP PODC in 5 sub-Saharan African countries demonstrated significant decrease in treatment abandonment and increase in disease-free survival over 2 years [37]. Two approaches exist: The National Wilms Tumour Study/Children's Oncology Group (NWTS/COG) approach which advocates primary surgical resection followed by adjuvant chemotherapy common in the United States and Canada and the SIOP protocol which recommends neoadjuvant chemotherapy followed by surgery. No prospective randomised control trials exist comparing the two and both have excellent outcomes, but there appears to be a slight a preference for the SIOP approach [37,38].

The appropriate surgical procedure for unilateral Wilms tumour with normal contralateral kidney is unilateral radical ureteronephrectomy with lymph node sampling. Surgery should be performed after a multi-disciplinary assessment of patient factors including co-morbidities and malnutrition; tumour factors determining resectability and institutional factors such as blood availability and intensive care beds. Delays in surgery are not uncommon in LMICs and have been implicated in treatment abandonment [35]. Because of this an argument can be made that the NWTS/COG approach may reduce abandonment attributable to surgical delays. However, the SIOP approach downstages tumours before surgery (making resection easier) and reduces the need for radiotherapy which is advantageous in LMICs where late presentation results in large tumours and advanced disease [39]. Post-operative complications include haemorrhage, intraoperative damage to surrounding structures and surgical site infection.

Chemotherapeutic drugs currently used in the management of Wilms tumour include vincristine, actinomycin-D, doxorubicin, ifosfamide, etoposide and cyclophosphamide. The prohibitive cost of some of these drugs has been implicated in poor compliance. Modifications to chemotherapy regimens relevant to LMICs include a reduction in the drug dose or chemotherapeutic agents to two-thirds in severely malnourished children.

Radiotherapy is not available in setting 1 but has a role in three situations. It may reduce the risk of local recurrence in patients with locally advanced disease, it can be used to control lung metastases where there is a poor response to chemotherapy, and as salvage therapy for relapse. These are all plausible scenarios in LMICs and referral to a centrally located, sometimes distant radiotherapy facility may be necessary.

Treatment for Wilms tumour is prolonged, with a risk of non-completion of treatment. Keeping the patient and caregiver in the hospital for the duration of treatment may reduce non-completion rates but time away from family commitments and from gainful employment in LMICs imposes a large social and financial burden on caregivers.

The reasons for the huge disparities in outcomes for Wilms tumour are likely complex and multifactorial. Ultimately improvement in outcomes in Wilms tumour treatment will come from comprehensive, system-wide removal of human resource, infrastructure and resource constraints as well as improvement in the general socio-economic milieu that all contribute to health disparities [39].

Key points for clinical practice

- Two philosophical approaches to the treatment of nephroblastoma exist and while equally effective, there may be practical reasons for preference for one over the other in LMICs
- Treatment of nephroblastoma includes surgery, chemotherapy, radiotherapy and supportive care

---

CONCLUSION

Despite progress made in management of important surgical conditions such as appendicitis, gastroschisis and nephroblastoma, there are still significant differences in their management between LMIC and HIC. These differences are in addition to differences in paediatric surgical capacity and accessibility to surgical care. Future improvements in paediatric surgical care, including future surgical trials, need to consider these differences in order to address them and close this noticeable gap in global paediatric surgical care.

REFERENCES

1. Ferris M, Quan S, Kaplan BS, et al. The Global Incidence of Appendicitis: A Systematic Review of Population-based Studies. Ann Surg 2017; 266:237–241.
2. Körner H, Söndenaa K, Söreide JA, et al. Incidence of Acute Nonperforated and Perforated Appendicitis: age-specific and Sex-specific Analysis. World J Surg 1997; 21:313–317.
3. Kong V, Sartorius B, Clarke D. Acute appendicitis in the developing world is a morbid disease. Annals 2015; 97:390–395.
4. Kong VY, Bulajic B, Allorto NL, et al. Acute appendicitis in a developing country. World J Surg 2012; 36:2068–2073.
5. Di Saverio S, Podda M, De Simone B, et al. Diagnosis and treatment of acute appendicitis: 2020 update of the WSES Jerusalem guidelines. World J Emerg Surg 2020; 15:27.
6. Zouari M, Louati H, Abid I, et al. C-reactive protein value is a strong predictor of acute appendicitis in young children. Am J Emerg Med 2018; 36:1319–1320.
7. Doniger SJ, Kornblith A. Point-of-Care Ultrasound Integrated Into a Staged Diagnostic Algorithm for Pediatric Appendicitis. Pediatr Emerg Care 2018; 34:109–115.

8. Weiss SL, Peters MJ, Alhazzani W, et al. Executive summary: surviving sepsis campaign international guidelines for the management of septic shock and sepsis-associated organ dysfunction in children. Intensive Care Med 2020; 46:1–9.

9. Minneci PC, Hade EM, Lawrence AE, et al. Association of Nonoperative Management Using Antibiotic Therapy vs Laparoscopic Appendectomy With Treatment Success and Disability Days in Children With Uncomplicated Appendicitis. JAMA 2020; 324:581–593.

10. Steiner Z, Buklan G, Stackievicz R, et al. Conservative treatment in uncomplicated acute appendicitis: reassessment of practice safety. Eur J Pediatr 2017; 176:521–527.

11. Meara JG, Leather AJM, Hagander L, et al. Global Surgery 2030: evidence and solutions for achieving health, welfare, and economic development. Lancet 2015; 386:569–624.

12. Gammeri E, Petrinic T, Bond-Smith G, et al. Meta-analysis of peritoneal lavage in appendicectomy. BJS Open 2018; 3:24–30.

13. Alvarez SM, Burd RS. Increasing prevalence of gastroschis repairs in the United States: 1996-2003. J Pediatr Surg 2007; 42:943–946.

14. Arnold M. Is the incidence of gastroschisis rising in South Africa in accordance with international trends? A retrospective analysis at Pretoria Academic and Kalafong Hospitals, 1981–2001. S Afr J Surg 2004; 42:86–88.

15. Wesonga AS, Fitzgerald TN, Kabuye R, et al. Gastroschisis in Uganda: opportunities for improved survival. J Pediatr Surg 2016; 51:1772–1777.

16. Wesonga A, Situma M, Lakhoo K. Reducing Gastroschisis Mortality: a Quality Improvement Initiative at a Ugandan Pediatric Surgery Unit. World J Surg 2020; 44:1395–1399.

17. Oyinloye AO, Abubakar AM, Wabada S, et al. Challenges and Outcome of Management of Gastroschisis at a Tertiary Institution in North-Eastern Nigeria. Front Surg 2020; 7:8.

18. Wright N, Abantanga F, Amoah M, et al. Developing and implementing an interventional bundle to reduce mortality from gastroschisis in low-resource settings. Wellcome Open Res 2019; 4:46.

19. Forrester MB, Merz RD. (2006) Comparison of Trends in Gastroschisis and Prenatal Illicit Drug Use Rates. J Toxicol Env Health, Part A 2006; 69:1253–1259.

20. Bird TM, Robbins JM, Druschel C, et al. Demographic and environmental risk factors for gastroschisis and omphalocele in the National Birth Defects Prevention Study. J Pediatr Surg 2009; 44:1546–1551.

21. Anyanwu LJC, Ajayi NA, Rolle U. Major abdominal wall defects in the low- and middle-income setting: current status and priorities. Pediatr Surg Int 2020; 36:579–590.

22. Risby K, Jakobsen MS, Qvist N. Congenital Abdominal Wall Defects: Staged closure by Dual Mesh. J Neonatal Surg 2016; 5:2.

23. Witt RG, Zobel M, Padilla B, et al. Evaluation of Clinical Outcomes of Sutureless vs Sutured Closure Techniques in Gastroschisis Repair. JAMA Surg 2019; 154:33–39.

24. Petrosyan M, Sandler AD. Closure methods in gastroschisis. Semin Pediatr Surg 2018; 27:304–308.

25. Gurien LA, Dassinger MS, Burford JM, et al. Does timing of gastroschisis repair matter? A comparison using the ACS NSQIP pediatric database. J Pediatr Surg 2017; 52:1751–1754.

26. Apfeld JC, Wren SM, Macheka N, et al. Infant, maternal, and geographic factors influencing gastroschisis related mortality in Zimbabwe. Surgery 2015; 158:1475–1480.

27. Force LM, Abdollahpour I, Advani SM, et al. The global burden of childhood and adolescent cancer in 2017: an analysis of the Global Burden of Disease Study 2017. Lancet Oncol 2019; 20:1211–1225.

28. Paintsil V, David H, Kambugu J, et al. The Collaborative Wilms Tumour Africa Project; Baseline evaluation of Wilms tumour treatment and outcome in eight institutes in sub-Saharan Africa. Eur J Cancer 2015; 51:84–91.

29. Cunningham ME, Klug TD, Nuchtern JG, et al. Global Disparities in Wilms Tumor. J Surg Res 2020; 247:34–51.

30. Ford K, Gunawardana S, Manirambona E, et al. Investigating Wilms' Tumours Worldwide: a report of the OxPLORE Collaboration–A Cross-Sectional Observational Study. World J Surg 2020; 44:295–302.

31. Nyagetuba JKM, Hansen EN. Pediatric solid tumors in Africa: different biology? Curr Opin Pediatr 2017; 29:354–357.

32. Gupta S, Howard SC, Hunger SP, et al. Treating Childhood Cancer in Low- and Middle-Income Countries. In: Gelband H, Jha P, Sankaranarayanan R, Horton S, (Eds). Cancer: Disease Control Priorities, 3rd edition. Washington (DC): The International Bank for Reconstruction and Development/The World Bank; 2015.

33. Osifo OD, Evbuomwan I, Efobi C. Management of Childhood abdominal masses by Nigerian traditional doctors: a worrisome cause of delay in presentation. Pak J Med Sci 2007; 23:809–813.

34. Emordi VC, Aisien E, Osagie OT, et al. Evisceration following Abdominal Scarification in Neonates. J Trop Pediatr 2018; 64:237–240.

35. Israels T, Moreira C, Scanlan T, et al. SIOP PODC: Clinical guidelines for the management of children with Wilms tumour in a low income setting. Pediatr Blood Cancer 2013; 60:5–11.

36. Palmer P, Hanson G, Honeyman-Buck J. (2011). Diagnostic Imaging in the Community A Manual for Clinics and Small Hospitals. Rotary District 6440 and the Pan American Health Organization [online] Available from https://www.paho.org/hq/dmdocuments/2011/HSS-diagnostic-imaging-2011.pdf [Last accessed January, 2021].
37. Israels T, Borgstein E, Pidini D, et al. Management of Children With a Wilms Tumor in Malawi, Sub-Saharan Africa. Journal of Pediatric Hematology/Oncology 2012; 34:606–610.
38. Chagaluka G, Paintsil V, Renner L, et al. Improvement of overall survival in the Collaborative Wilms Tumour Africa Project. Pediatr Blood Cancer 2020; 67:e28383.
39. Carter NH, Avery AH, Libes J, et al. Pediatric Solid Tumors in Resource-Constrained Settings: A Review of Available Evidence on Management, Outcomes, and Barriers to Care. Children (Basel) 2008; 5:143.

Section 2

Surgical training

Chapter 4

Enhancing surgical training through integration of e-learning

Andrew Dickenson

INTRODUCTION

E-learning describes the web-based delivery of educational content, with a robust evidence base that favourably compares learning outcomes to face-to-face methods. This chapter will review the conceptual and theoretical frameworks relevant to digital learning as applied to surgical training. While it is the educational benefits, not the application of technology, that remains the primary objective forelearning, this message can become distracted with the progressive expansion of simulated teaching environments. Ultimately effective education enhances patient safety [1], regardless of delivery mode, but requires engaged educators to adopt and develop interactive and immersive environments which complement clinical training. As the current trend in digital education is moving towards more interactive formats through integration of gamification, as well as augmented and virtual reality (AR/VR), to enhance learner engagement and motivation, this will require a change in how e-learning is delivered. Online teaching platforms have irreversibly transformed the training of the next generation of surgeons [2] through facilitating quality-assured and cost-effective inter-professional learning, independent of location and time constraints. The next challenge in surgical education is to contextualise understanding and encourage integrating e-learning into global clinical training programs [3] while at the same time avoiding widening the health inequalities gap that exists, both within and between countries [4].

BACKGROUND

E-learning has become a universal feature within higher and professional education, with significant investment from Universities, academic medical centres, residency programs, Surgical Boards [5] and Royal Colleges [6]. Millennial trainees have grown up alongside virtual learning environments and expect similar access in their postgraduate studies [7]. This has created a generational gap, with differing learning styles, communication means, and a delineated work-life balance that differentiates them from older colleagues. Trainees anticipate frequent and detailed feedback, with specific career guidance and reassurance around performance. While this can be perceived as a challenge, it offers opportunities for the profession to adapt and innovate.

The requirement for flexible and part-time working, geographical restrictions, and the need for immediately accessible information has made e-learning a valuable resource. Trainees are constantly digitally connected, experienced at searching the internet, and willing to challenge authority. Consequently, they demand accurate information, reliable connectivity in the workplace but less direct trainer interaction [8]. Combined with the rise of smartphone technology and extensive internet coverage, there has been a progressive shift towards social networking in education which has opportunities for surgical e-learning [9].

However, it must be appreciated there is no consistent or agreed definition of e-learning. Different authors and disciplines apply similar concepts, but interchangeably modify the definition [10]. Fundamentally the accepted definition should incorporate the conceptual elements of e-learning:

- Technology
- Delivery systems
- Communication
- Educational paradigms

It is not possible for e-learning to entirely replace direct, workplace-based, and supervised education of surgical trainees; however, a blended approach must be developed to guarantee a comprehensive training. As the concept is still evolving and changing on a regular basis, the most accurate definition for e-learning refers to "learning that utilises electronic means to create a more dynamic and instructive learning environment" **(Table 4.1).**

Traditional acquisition of theoretical knowledge through books, scientific papers, and systematic reviews still applies, but is being supplemented through a diverse array of emerging e-learning tools. The widespread affordability of smartphones, tablets, and multimedia platforms offers innovative and convenient ways for engaging with evidence-based educational materials. E-learning tools range from online textbooks to cognitive stimulators but must always link to robust and approved online curricula. Commonly employed tools are virtual patient cases, digital modelling, tutorial, and webinars, as well as a myriad of open-access recorded surgical procedures. Whatever the method employed, a review of current literature confirms it is an effective adjunct to surgical education [11]. These learning tools can also be integrated with simulation-based training exercises for acquisition and assessment of psychomotor skills (e.g. suture tying) [12]. However, because of restricted contact time in the clinical workplace and the service priorities placed on surgical trainees, the compliance rate continues to be low [13]. It is recommended that appropriate funding for additional resources that can be accessed during working hours will improve learner engagement.

Internet and software-based platforms have been integrated into undergraduate medical, dental, and nursing education. Despite widespread implementation, there is limited evidence to support their effectiveness for surgical training [12]. Various studies have evaluated the effectiveness of e-learning as a teaching tool compared with no intervention and more didactic, clinical-based surgical training [14,15]. Despite significant heterogeneity among platforms, e-learning does appear to be emerging as effective as other training methods.

Table 4.1 E-learning categories

- *Supplemental:* Using e-learning to enhance traditional classroom teaching
- *Replacement:* Hybrid model using e-learning to replace certain parts of a course; can include replacement of some traditional lectures with online content, while retaining essential classroom teaching
- *Fully online:* Entire course is delivered online using a virtual campus

Modern technology is rapidly advancing and allows for an equally increasing array of opportunities in medical education. Most hospitals offer online learning tools and modules for continued professional development [16]. Within UK surgical training, the Royal College of Surgeons of England has dedicated e-learning resources and the Royal College of Surgeons of Ireland (RCSI) mandates surgical trainees to engage with a bespoke learning management system (LMS). The UK medical regulatory body, the GMC, and Department of Health and Social Care resource e-learning as a blended offering for all the National Health Service (NHS) staff statutory and mandatory training [17].

However, there are far wider ranging opportunities for implementing global surgical training through e-learning [18]. The RCSI and the College of Surgeons of East, Central and Southern Africa (COSECSA) have a long established training program which has developed a surgical curriculum, quality assurance processes, membership examinations, a culture for research, financial planning and sustainability, combined with bespoke e-learning resources within a LMS. This resource is available to both surgeons and nonclinicians to address the disparity in the surgical workforce [19].

While e-learning interventions can increase understanding of patient safety methodology, research has not conclusively confirmed a sustained long-term change in clinician attitudes for maintaining patient safety in practice [20]. Potential options for further research could be the inclusion of e-learning alongside face-to-face training or more frequent e-learning refresher modules, possibly linked to mandatory training requirements, to effect a lasting change in attitude. Future programs could focus on validating specific online content, using standardised outcome measures, and assessing long-term knowledge retention after e-learning. While the greatest beneficiaries from this burgeoning library of e-learning content are low- and middle- income countries (LMICs), it is uncertain whether surgical education through e-learning is effective and has yet to demonstrate a direct benefit to patient safety in those countries [21].

PRINCIPLES OF E-LEARNING

E-learning is not a single entity but a combination of teaching methods, which offers scope for novel web-hosted programs, e.g. :

- *Spaced learning:* Repeating the same course material at least once during the course for improved knowledge retention
- *Blended learning:* Online teaching combined with noncomputer-based lectures or tutorials

The variety of e-learning interventions available offers surgical educators the opportunity to select appropriate teaching methods for their specific program without being restrained by the traditional lecture-based model. In the United States for example, the Surgical Council on Resident Education (SCORE) has an established e-learning platform for trainees that fully exploits Web 2.0 features. The SCORE portal is an innovative, nonprofit initiative providing high-quality educational resources within structured self-learning programs, focusing on all areas of general surgery, subdivided by year of training. At present, there are >800 modules across the main competency domains, as well as a "hot topic of the week" section, online textbooks, a multiple-choice question bank for self-assessment, and a large collection of narrated operative videos. While this is not an entirely new approach, SCORE exemplifies opportunities for other surgical educators to emulate.

The identified benefits of online e-learning are often described in terms of the operational and logistical benefits that can be achieved. The Joint Information Council "learning in a digital age" report highlighted emerging practice rather than emerging technology [22], highlighting how online content can be made readily available across a range of platforms, accessible at work or home and not constrained by physical spaces [23]. This flexibility allows trainees to access learning environments at times which are convenient and relevant to their personal training needs, encouraging ownership of their continuing professional development, which remains a statutory expectation of professional regulators in many countries (**Table 4.2**).

Underpinning these developments are economic pressures, financial restrictions, government policies, and changing cultural behaviours influenced by emerging technologies. As a direct consequence, education and training providers have been required to review key aspects of their provision and delivery to ensure it aligns with learner expectations. The quality of the learning experience is now a prime objective, although understanding what defines quality remains the key challenge. Currently e-learning acknowledges that quality outcomes should reflect personalised learning needs, but there is an increasing focus on both learner satisfaction and preparedness for joining the future workforce which must also be considered.

Quality cannot be overlooked as the current generation of surgical trainees have invested heavily in their career and training. Rising university tuition charges, student loan repayments, professional examination application and registration fees have heightened learner expectations from training, with constant focus on quality and consistency of the educational offering. Technology permits personalisation and enhances choice, although it allows access to nonpeer reviewed, and sometimes erroneous, content. If the direction of travel is to reduce face-to-face practical exposure during surgical training, the substituted learning methods must guarantee high quality, reproducible, contemporary, and standardised learning opportunities.

However, the opportunities to simulate real-life situations can be difficult to achieve when there are financial, logistic, or ethical barriers. Economic pressures have required education providers to explore new markets, innovative ways of delivering the curriculum and work across boundaries, both within and outside of healthcare. Innovations, such as moving content online, does not always save money and education providers need to

---

Table 4.2 Benefits of technology in surgical education

- Improved access to up-to-date information
- Faster response to learner enquiries through chat room functions
- Access across a range of platforms, e.g. mobile devices, smartphones
- Easier engagement with end-users, allowing feedback and continuous evaluation
- Regular programme updates that are responsive to learners' needs
- Flexibility in accessing e-learning modules
- Access can be extended to a global audience
- Archive learning and achievements, reflecting continuous professional development
- Bespoke allocation of learning assignments
- Interactive, allowing rapid and timely feedback to learner

ensure they have undertaken a full cost-benefit analysis to secure a return on investment. This requires collaboration between stakeholders, including their target audience, as well as public and commercial partners. The open source community is a clear example of the benefits gained through collaboration, as research and development interests have shown significant benefits [24].

The impact of the European Working Time Directive (2009), escalating clinical workload, restricted study budgets and increased assessments, linked to revalidation, identified that surgical trainees viewed accessible, flexible, and affordable educational content as important [25]. E-learning allows for updated evidence and new protocols to be rapidly accessed, applied, and assessed within a safe and supported setting [26]. This outweighs the inevitable delay incurred with journals and textbooks. In addition, interactive technology with features such as discussion forums, blogs or social media encourages advances to be shared and discussed across the broader medical landscape, permitting networking and global distribution of contemporary information. This knowledge exchange not only ensures a wealth of valuable information and learning is widely disseminated but is also a form of quality assurance.

BENEFITS OF E-LEARNING

As technology improves, the opportunities will also expand, although it remains essential that e-learning encompasses high educational standards to maximise learner outcome. The frequently reported application for e-learning is in the support surgical trainees require during preparation for professional examinations. Discussion rooms, facilitated by expert clinical tutors, permit formative assessment, and feedback on knowledge acquired during completion of structured online packages, which ultimately supports the summative outcome from formal examinations.

The principle benefits can be summarised:

- Inexpensive compared with face-to-face teaching, releasing trainees from time and distance constraints [27]
- Innovative and improving web technology, can incorporate simulation and virtual reality [28]
- Has proven benefits in LMICs [29], where e-learning offers affordable access to high-quality educational content [30]. This can partially offset the shortage of trained healthcare workers through local delivery of essential training [31]
- Sequential improvement in knowledge acquisition has been demonstrated through pre- and post-testing [32]
- Improved learner confidence [33]
- Online teaching platforms that blend online media with traditional classroom methods, such as Zoom or Teams, is encouraged by international technology companies who are now actively developing educational content

While there are inevitable disadvantages, such as dependency on internet speed, high initial design costs, and the need for programming expertise, these are off set in the longer term.

With specific reference to surgical training, most Higher Education Institutes and Royal Colleges offer distance learning surgical qualifications. These range from postgraduate certificate and diploma courses through to Masters level qualifications. Masters courses can be taken in General Surgery (MCh), Medical Education (MMEd), and special surgical fields (MS) [34]. This reduces time away from the workplace and optimises the balance between theoretical and practical training.

MAINTAINING EDUCATIONAL STANDARDS AND PRINCIPLES

With the shift away from didactic teaching in surgical training, considerable research has been undertaken to ensure e-learning conforms to acceptable educational standards. The three essential components for effective e-learning are:

1. Utility
2. Usability
3. Desirability

These areas have been intensively explored through randomised and nonrandomised studies. Product utility ensures e-learning is effective in achieving long-term knowledge retention [35]. As e-learning offers greater opportunity for independent learning, the material must be usable and remain contemporary through frequent updates. However, it remains fundamental that the learning content is closely aligned to clinical practice, as applied e-learning has been demonstrated to promote higher-level thinking and skill scores compared to self-directed learning in isolation [36].

Ensuring the environment meets learners' expectations improves engagement and learning. While trainee satisfaction has been shown to be consistently high [37], it is important that e-learning does not replace educator-directed training. To maintain quality standards, facilitation of online content and assessment is necessary. This is combined with direct workplace supervision by a senior educator as part of an overarching blended-learning strategy [38].

Surgical training remains predicated on the acquisition of knowledge, technical skills, nontechnical skills, and attitudes. As learning is an active process, based on a cycle of experience, reflection, conceptualisation, and experimentation, it is imperative that trainees should be actively challenged to embed knowledge retention [39]. If trainees can be exposed to interactive and multisensory experiences, then their level of recall can be significantly elevated beyond the traditional passive education model [40]. Learners attach most importance to content quality, ease of online accessibility, usability, and availability of gaining attendance credits. However, it is the inconvenience of needing additional software downloads, impact of hospital firewalls, and antivirus programs plus the lack of interaction that deters learners and these issues must be addressed at the design phase (**Table 4.3**).

When applied appropriately, e-learning facilitates the development of knowledge towards the pinnacle of Bloom's taxonomy allowing the learner to both recall information, comprehend, and apply it to a clinical situation. As technology improves, there are greater opportunities to synthesise this information and make decisions and judgments based on the information available. This decision-making process can also be applied within the attitude domain of learning and allows for a safe environment in which learners develop into competent trainees with skills directly relevant to future clinical practice.

All these adaptations will be futile, if the content is not relevant or contemporary. In postgraduate surgical education, it is a requisite that the most up-to-date and critically appraised evidence supports the information included within modules. It is important that content is linked to curriculum outcomes and endorsed by training bodies otherwise this will reduce trainee engagement [41]. It is imperative that the next generation of e-learning

Table 4.3 Standards required for effective e-learning	
Utility	• Will trainees find it useful? • Is it easy to navigate? • Does it offer feedback? • Are learning goals clear? • Does content reflect real-life situations? • Is the content personalised?
Usability	• Will trainees gain more understanding of the subject? • Is it readily accessible? • Is the content readable? • Can the learning be quickly completed? • Are there interactive components and do all the links work?
Desirability	• Does your course topic attract learners? • Does your course appeal to a learners' emotions?

content is coproduced with trainees to ensure the content validity and quality standards match learner expectations [42].

DEVELOPING HIGH-QUALITY E-LEARNING RESOURCES

Creating an effective surgical e-learning environment is time consuming and expensive. Not only does it require a mature understanding of educational principles, but also the ability to critically appraise and assimilate the required information; it also demands creativity and a willingness to explore new ideas and concepts. Time and capacity to invest in content production is a rare commodity for busy surgeons, so the pace of development can be slow [43]. Often it is the end user who invests most to ensure programs are high quality, mandating developers to actively seek and embed user feedback. Surgical trainees often have a clear understanding of technology and its application, having been raised and educated within a connected world. Almost every millennial is connected to the internet, with 19% of them being smartphone-only users, meaning they do not access the internet through a broadband provider. There is an expectation that similar connectivity is readily available within their training program with which, in return, they would be prepared to test the boundaries of possibility [44].

This introduces the concept of learner-cantered experiences within e-learning. In response, this has mandated a fundamental change in mind-set where an educator has become the curator, not the creator, of content. Learners are active in directing content development as they question, analyse, discuss, qualify, and draw their own unique conclusions. This novel approach must be reflected in the content, how it is presented and ultimately assessed. It specifically requires clearly stated objectives, aimed at describing to the learner what they will be able to achieve on completion of the course. Instead of describing the course content in the objectives, the focus must be directed to what learners will be able to do, tasks they should be undertaking and the methods required to achieve the required outcomes.

However, to achieve the expected fidelity and standardisation from an interactive e-learning session will ultimately require collaboration with commercial companies. This has not been a feature of UK surgical education to date, but is a relationship that is fostered and encouraged in Europe [45] and other parts of the world.

APPLICATION OF E-LEARNING IN SURGICAL TRAINING AND EDUCATION

The integration of e-learning in surgery can only be successful if there is a genuine acceptance of immersive technology, moving to a competency-based, patient outcome-orientated training and evolving a multi-professional healthcare environment that aligns to societal expectations [46]. There have been no specific studies exploring the surgical community's acceptance and engagement in developing e-learning content, which has impeded the pace and scale for introducing high-quality adjuncts to conventional training programs.

Increasing financial constraints, quality control and patient safety drivers have relegated the role of the operating theatre as the predominant, standalone, delivery method of surgical training. Regulation and ethical restrictions have also had an impact, for example, in the access to live animal models [47] although substitute blended in-vivo models are starting to appear [48]. In response, surgical educators are having to develop alternative methods for both training and maintaining surgical skills in-line with emerging surgical technologies. Through innovation, there is now the possibility of developing a blended, unified, surgical training program through collaboration with global centres of excellence, transcending the geographic boundaries imposed by physical institutions [49].

Technology enhanced learning (TEL) is based on asynchronous or synchronous delivery formats. The latter, encompassing interactive online lectures via platforms such as Teams, Zoom or WebEx, are becoming increasingly familiar to clinicians. While interpersonal interactivity is essential for knowledge transfer, supported change towards using specific web-based functions such as Web 1.0 (discussion board and email) and Web 2.0 (Wikis and blogs) allows for this to occur synchronously and asynchronously. Until recently, there has been limited enthusiasm for integrating these applications into current surgical training.

Asynchronous e-learning is a learner-cantered approach that permits flexible learning at a time and setting that is convenient, enabling the learner to balance professional development with personal and work commitments. This is self-directed and does not require immediate human contact as the technology facilitates the learning process, although effective mentoring remains an essential component.

Research has identified several key domains that must be incorporated into effective e-learning programs to ensure end-user engagement. These include self-efficacy, user satisfaction, instructional design, knowledge outcomes, clinical skills development, and recognition of barriers to effective implementation. It should be noted that there are inherent issues with e-learning research, not least the use of comparative design studies and this is cited as the reason for reduced learner engagement. Comparing e-learning with traditional teaching methods is flawed as the comparison groups are heterogeneous. It is essential for future research to consider if self-efficacy or knowledge gained through e-learning improves patient outcomes or influences clinical behaviour.

This is the basis of the Kirkpatrick Model for evaluating training and educational outcomes. It considers any style of training, both informal and formal, to determine aptitude based on four criteria [50]. Behaviour change is any practice that is intrinsically linked with the outcomes of the e-learning program undertaken. Most e-learning research has focused on participant experience and knowledge acquisition, outcomes that correspond with the first two levels of Kirkpatrick's model. To date, few studies have examined the effectiveness of internet-based e-learning programs on behaviour, which aligns with Kirkpatrick Level 3. Some studies have used self-reported measures of intention to change behaviour, although self-reporting does not always translate into actual behaviour change. Studies that have not relied on self-reporting have employed various evaluation tools, such as objective structured assessment of technical skills (OSATS), simulation laboratory trainers or in-situ simulation using standardised patients. Due to this inconsistent approach, further research incorporating well-designed randomised controlled trials comparing e-learning against standard teaching is needed. Ideally the research focus should be on identifying whether knowledge gained through e-learning can be translated into clinical practice and influence sustained behaviour changes that improve patient outcomes.

ENHANCING ENGAGEMENT WITH SURGICAL E-LEARNING

There are two further components of effective e-learning; understanding how adults learn and appropriate mentoring [51]. Clinicians, like all adults, have different learning styles which are embedded in andragogic theory and is the standard against which CPD is assessed [52]. Andragogic principles explain why adults have different learning needs in comparison to the pedagogic requirements of children. It is important to appreciate these principles when designing online content, as adult learning is:

- Result-oriented
- Autonomous and self-directed
- Contextualised by life experiences and prior knowledge
- Driven by having a motive to learn
- Practical, with real-life context

Mentoring is therefore important [53], and needs to be in the context of other support offers, with clearly defined outcomes. This is not always integrated with e-learning and it is recommended that every trainee should undergone assessed and agreed needs assessment with their supervisor so that the mentoring process can be defined and bespoke [54]. This initial meeting is more appropriate in person, as online contact does not allow an effective relationship to develop. As a minimum, there needs to be a robust systematic induction, mapping all support mechanisms, a needs assessment, and an agreement on how communication in a blended format will suit both parties [55]. These principles are summarised in **Table 4.4.**

Table 4.4 Principles of virtual mentoring
• Clear mechanisms for actively and regularly engaging the learner
• View learners as individuals
• Regular communication
• Maintain professional communication at all times
• Establish credibility
• Agree learner expectations at the initial meeting
• Proactive, self-directed, learning approach
• Accessible support structure

Defining hybrid or blended education is not easy, as it is influenced by personality and prior experience. The Sloan Consortium describes it as 'integrate online with traditional face-to-face class activities in a planned, pedagogically valuable manner.' While this remains an unclear concept, it seems to suggest that hybrid education is simply the application of online technology to supplement and transform learning.

PLATFORMS

Online platforms were originally introduced by technology companies to provide a simple, easy access, low-cost, interactive solution to deliver mandatory training [56]. The concept of blended learning was a balance between face-to-face teaching with computer-mediated instruction, although initially this required the physical presence of both teacher and students [57].

Blended learning is particularly applicable to surgical education as it allows a combination of skills training integrated with self-directed learning. Blended learning is flexible and includes different components such as instructor-delivered content, elearning, webinars, conference calls, live seminars and can operate across a range of available platforms such as Facebook, chat rooms, podcasts, Twitter, YouTube, Skype and Web boards (such as WhatsApp) [58]. Podcasts are increasingly being used in LMICs where their effectiveness has been evaluated with medical undergraduate training [59]. While yet to be utilised in western education, there are benefits for examination revision, where language issues potentially impact on learning (e.g. when teaching is not in the learners' native language) or supplementing lecture notes [60]. There is also an application for trainees with learning difficulties, such as sensory impairment, where recorded content can be used after the teaching to reinforce learning.

YouTube is a popular supplementary tool for surgical education among medical students and trainees. Unfortunately, issues exist around the quality of content which must be addressed before this platform can be widely recommended for surgical training [61]. Not only is video quality low but there is heterogeneity of content because of the lack of a formal peer review process. To raise the educational quality, requires peer review, preparatory e-learning, and feedback, which could be achieved through an appropriately curated YouTube video library [62].

A virtual learning environment (VLE) is a web-based platform which supports the teaching material for educational institutions. The resources, materials, activities, and interactions are arranged within a course structure and allow trainees to be assessed based on activity. The relationship between VLE engagement and success varies across modules. Frequent engagement with VLE content is linked to course success at undergraduate level and, with some university subjects, this interaction can be used to predict final course grades [63]. VLE usage is more important for instruction-based learning styles but evidence is starting to emerge that a shared platform between surgeons and scientists can enhance collaborative research though a specialist VLE [64].

Massive Open Online Courses (MOOCs) are a recent development within the TEL arena. These offer free-to-access content, normally developed by a University, and hosted on a commercial platform. This enables global access to quality educational content requiring only an internet connected device, which benefits surgical trainees in LMICs. These courses are multi-professional and even accessible to the public as part of the global digital health literacy strategy. However, there is evidence that engagement from surgical trainees is lower than anticipated and an area for further educational research [65,66].

EMERGING E-RESOURCES

Social media is an increasingly important tool for educators although use in surgical education has yet to be quantified [67]. Studies have shown that surgical associations and training organisations, as well as University departments, maintain a visible social media presence but only a minority utilise this for educational purposes [68]. There is emerging evidence that social media augments traditional learning, with postings that have overt educational content attracting greater learner engagement [69]. Further research is needed to assess the efficacy of promoting surgical content via social media platforms but there is an emerging synergy between social media and evidence-based practice that could potentially be exploited within surgical education [70].

Human factors can be delivered and assessed by e-learning [71]. Both the GMC [72] and the WHO [73] recommend integrated delivery of human factors, with assessment of learning outcomes, within the undergraduate curriculum. The use of e-learning for acquiring intravenous cannulation skills in relation to human factors has determined a convincing correlation between preparedness for practice and future clinical performance [74]. In postgraduate surgical education, e-learning can integrate both technical and nontechnical human factors' training [75], where further development for use in multidisciplinary team (MDT) meetings and operating theatres setting would be valuable.

Blended learning has been applied to nontechnical skills acquisition in undergraduate students [76]. Tailor-made, nontechnical skills development though online seminars has been shown to be effective for assessing medical student behaviour, attitudes, and performance during simulated patient treatment [77]. Nontechnical skills seminars should be more broadly embedded within the surgical training curriculum, particularly with the widening access to surgical simulators.

eIntegrity provides global access to the healthcare training materials developed for the UK NHS. This has opened access to high-quality e-learning content to individuals (students, trainees, and qualified practitioners), healthcare providers, colleges, universities, and government bodies across the world. eIntegrity incorporates several surgical specialties, as well as acute and specialist medicine. The programs are collaboration between the UK medical royal colleges, professional organisations, specialist societies, and Health Education England. The content has been authored and peer-reviewed by practicing senior clinicians and regularly updated to reflect the latest clinical developments and guidelines. Importantly, trainees in LMICs s can now directly benefit from the UK's investment in world leading healthcare training, especially with the emergence of m-health through increased internet coverage [78]. At the present time, access has been provided to learners in > 100 countries and reflects the opportunities available to share quality content through access to the internet. As eIntegrity is a community interest company all profits are reinvested back into developing and maintaining content, which continuously benefits healthcare professionals worldwide. This is an essential consideration for high-income countries (HIC) with elective or observership exchange programs for surgical trainees from LMICs. There is an ethical responsibility to prepare visiting surgeons, especially in recognizing unfamiliar conditions endemic in the host country, which can be addressed through appropriately curated e-learning content. It is essential that trainees are supported in understanding covert nontechnical issues that inevitably detract from the overall value of an exchange, particularly the social, cultural, and linguistic challenges. This has been shown to reduce moral distress in visitors, reducing the resulting blame culture, which is ultimately essential for the safe care of patients. From this, a variety of surgical e-learning partnerships are emerging with reverse innovation for training opportunities, allowing HIC trainees to gain benefit from learning across a global platform [79].

FUTURE APPLICATION OF SURGICAL E-LEARNING

Advances in technology will allow e-learning programs to become highly interactive and immersive, whether that involves interactive models, question and answer designs for knowledge acquisition or a more advanced virtual patient model. In the latter design, trainees come face-to-face with an interactive clinical setting and progress through scenarios making appropriate clinical decisions in relation to protocol. Importantly, trainees, and their virtual patient, must justify their decision-making and receive detailed constructive feedback. This safe environment allows for mistakes to be made as a trainee experiments with their understanding of the knowledge and available evidence on a subject, whilst being clinically applicable and realistic. These interactive models can be created within simple structured case scenarios or through high-fidelity simulated models that engage with the learner.

Virtual reality technology is advancing rapidly with realistic virtual reality environments in development. The socialisation of the internet, with the emergence of Web 4.0, as well as the embryonic architectural features of 5.0 make this an exciting prospect for redefining surgical education. Within a generation, it can be anticipated that Web 5.0 will have the capacity to communicate, reason, and allow intelligent interactions between machines and humans. These possibilities will effectively prepare trainees for the clinical environment, rehearse decision-making or practice operative procedures. While the technological advances are exciting, they must not be the sole driving force for the development of interactive tools. Rather, the educational need and evidence of their success should drive development and implementation into surgical training as part of a comprehensive blended learning offering.

The future of surgical e-learning is encouraging and will not develop in isolation from the workplace. Ensuring a surgeon has completed a relevant learning module before attending a face-to-face training event allows for a baseline skill set to be attained, which will facilitate a more meaningful and mentored case-based discussion [80].

The 2020 global Sars-Cov-2 pandemic may prove a pivotal point for the final acceptance and integration of e-learning into surgical training [81]. The immediate and abrupt cessation of training [82], created through the shortage of personal protective equipment, suspension of formal teaching programs, closure of university departments and a significant reduction in elective surgical cases unavoidably impacted on every aspect of surgical education [83]. This saw the rapid emergence of innovative and novel solutions involving the use of e-learning, video consultations, social media discussion forums and telehealth to lessen the impact on medical education. The ultimate benefit of moving to virtual learning has yet to be fully evaluated but there is early evidence of a positive attitude change towards e-learning.

Emerging evidence indicates that the COVID-19 crisis has accelerated innovation within surgical education. With this insight and the experience gained during the crisis, there are new digital learning possibilities that can be exploited by education providers to enhance surgical training. It is predicted that commercial and private educational partnerships will continue to emerge within the crowded e-learning market. While this could pave the way for large-scale, global, and cross-industry co-operation to establish a common educational goal, it raises issues around regulation and quality assurance of the educational content. Equally this could widen inequality as the premise of quality e-learning mandates stable internet access, affordable technology, and necessary skills to use it. This disparity existed pre-COVID and is likely to increase as a direct consequence of the global economic impact in LMICs.

It is too early to judge whether this new hybrid training system will be maintained or whether the short-term adoption of online learning will reflect in reduced performance and revert to established teaching methods. However, the flexibility and responsiveness of e-learning suggests this is now a mainstay in-surgical education, reflected in the steady migration away from an apprentice model. Instead of trying to draw comparisons between e-learning and traditional methods maybe it is time to migrate the effective components of traditional teaching into a virtual environment. It should be acknowledged that learning performance is ultimately influenced by trainee engagement, supervisor contact time, and the subject content. Motivation directly affects transfer performance, even though face-to-face meetings and training contents indirectly influence transfer performance. Effective virtual education must balance teacher-learner interaction, accessible technology, self-motivation, and efficient communication to achieve a lasting culture for online learning.

Key points for clinical practice

- E-learning has considerable potential for use in surgical education, but requires further research.
- Integrating e-learning into surgical training embeds a change towards adult learning theory where educators become the curator, not creator, of content.
- Surgical training must invest in blended learning platforms to give trainees access to innovative web-based virtual patients and interactive knowledge-based teaching material.

REFERENCES

1. Gaupp R, Körner M, Fabry G. Effects of a case-based interactive e-learning course on knowledge and attitudes about patient safety: a quasi-experimental study with third-year medical students. BMC Med Educ 2016; 16:172.
2. Pottle J. Virtual reality and the transformation of medical education. Future Healthc J. 2019;6(3):181–185.
3. Sonesson L, Boffard K, Lundberg L, et al. The challenges of military medical education and training for physicians and nurses in the Nordic countries - an interview study. Scand J Trauma Resusc Emerg Med 2017; 25:38–48.
4. Ruggeri K, Farrington C, Brayne C. A global model for effective use and evaluation of e-learning in health. Telemed J E Health 2013; 19:312–321.
5. Dietl CA, Russell JC. Effects of technological advances in surgical education on quantitative outcomes from residency programs. J Surg Educ 2016; 73:819–830.
6. Kim S. The future of e-learning in medical education: Current trend and future opportunity. J Educ Eval Health Prof. 2006;3:3.
7. Mercer C. How millennials are disrupting medicine. CMAJ 2018; 190:e696–e697.
8. Williams VN, Medina J, Medina A, et al. Bridging the millennial generation expectation gap: Perspectives and strategies for physician and interprofessional faculty. Am J Med Sci 2016; 353:109–115.
9. Quezada J, Achurra P, Asbun D, et al. Smartphone application supplements laparoscopic training through simulation by reducing the need for feedback from expert tutors. Surgery Open Science 2019 1:100–104.
10. Sangrà A, Vlachopoulos D, Cabrera N. Building an Inclusive Definition of e-Learning: An Approach to the Conceptual Framework. Int Rev of Research in Open and Distributed Learning 2012; 13:145–159.

11. Tarpada SP, Morris MT, Burton DA. E-learning in orthopedic surgery training: a systematic review. J Orthop 2016; 13:425–430.
12. Tiew S, Lai MY, Poyser A, et al. A training model for practice of corneal suture tying. Eye (Lond). 2020.
13. De Leeuw RA, Westerman M, Nelson E, et al. Quality specifications in postgraduate medical e-learning: an integrative literature review leading to a postgraduate medical e-learning model. Surg. 2016; 103:1428–1437.
14. Reznek MA, Rawn CL, Krummel TM. Evaluation of the educational effectiveness of a virtual reality intravenous insertion simulator. Academic Emergency Med 2002; 9:1319–1325.
15. Larvin M. E-Learning in surgical education and training. ANZ J Surg 2009; 79:133–137.
16. DoH. (2011). A Framework for Technology Enhanced Learning . [online] Available from https://www.gov.uk/government/publications/a-framework-fortechnology-enhanced-learning. [Last accessed November, 2020].
17. Gajewski J, Bijlmakers L, Brugha R. Global Surgery–Informing national strategies for scaling up surgery in Sub-Saharan Africa. Int J Health Policy Manag 2018; 7:481–484.
18. Henry JA. Global Surgery: Redirecting strategies for a global research agenda. Int J Health Policy Manag 2018; 7:1064–1066.
19. Walsh K. Reflections of health care professionals on e-learning resources for patient safety. Proc Bayl Univ Med Cent 2018; 31:35–36.
20. Frehywot S, Vovides Y, Talib Z, et al. E-learning in medical education in resource constrained low and middle-income countries. Hum Resour Health 2013; 11:4.
21. Ferrell G, Smith R, Knight S. (2012). Learning in a digital age extending higher education opportunities for lifelong learning. [online] Available from https://www.jisc.ac.uk/full-guide/designing-learning-and-assessment-in-a-digital-age [Last accessed November, 2020].
22. Coughlan J, Brinkman W. Design Considerations for delivering e-learning to surgical trainees. International Journal of E-Health and Medical Communications 2011; 2:14–23.
23. Issenberg BS, Ringsted C, Østergaard D, et al. Setting a research agenda for simulation-based healthcare education: a synthesis of the outcome from an Utstein Style Meeting; simulation in healthcare. Simul Healthc 2011; 6:155–167.
24. Butcher K, Bamford R, Burke D. Innovation in e-learning: learning for all. E Cancer Medical Science 2014; 8:467.
25. Pham D, Hardcastle N, Foroudi F, et al. A multidisciplinary evaluation of a web-based elearning training programme for SAFRON II (TROG 13.01): A multicentre randomised study of stereotactic radiotherapy for lung metastases. Clinical Oncology 2016; 28:e101–e108.
26. Payne GW. The role of blended learning in 21st century medical education: current trends and future directions. In: Kitchenham A (Ed). Blended learning across disciplines: models for implementation. Hershey: IGI Global; 2011. pp. 132–146.
27. Mandler AG. Touch Surgery: a twenty-first century platform for surgical training. J Digit Imaging 2018; 31:585–590.
28. Lu J, Cameron B. The effectiveness and challenges of e-learning in surgical training in low- and middle-income countries: a systematic review. Global Health: Annual Review 2020; 1:59–62.
29. Barteit S, Jahn A, Banda SS, et al. E-learning for medical education in sub-Saharan Africa and low-resource settings. J Med Internet Res 2019; 21:e12449.
30. Barteit S, Guzek D, Jahn A, et al. Evaluation of e-learning for medical education in low- and middle-income countries: a systematic review. Comput Educ 2020; 145:103726.
31. DelSignore LA, Wolbrink TA, Zurakowski D, et al. Test-enhanced e-learning strategies in postgraduate medical education: A randomised cohort study. J Med Internet Res 2016; 18:e299.
32. Kaleci D, Akleman E. Assessment of knowledge and confidence for E-learning. World Journal on Educational Technology: Current Issues 2018; 11:104–115.
33. Smith PJW, Wigmore SJ, Paisley A, et al. Distance learning improves attainment of professional milestones in the early years of surgical training. Annals of Surgery 2013; 258:838–843.
34. Walsh K. The utility of e-learning and clinical decision support resources in improving the practice of healthcare professionals in infectious diseases. Med Ed Publish 2018; 7:59. https://doi.org/10.15694/mep.2018.0000059.1
35. Kulier R, Gülmezoglu AM, Zamora J, et al. Effectiveness of a clinically integrated e-learning course in evidence-based medicine for reproductive health training: a randomised trial. JAMA 2012; 308:2218–2225.
36. Brown JM, Kinloch K, Shaw NJ. An investigation into specialty trainee engagement with e-learning. Br J Hosp Med (Lond) 2019; 80:105–108.

37. Sadeghi R, Sedaghat MM, Sha Ahmadi F. Comparison of the effect of lecture and blended teaching methods on students' learning and satisfaction. J Adv Med Educ Prof 2014; 2:146–150.
38. Finnesgard EJ, Aho JM, Pandian TK, et al. Effect of rehearsal modality on knowledge retention in surgical trainees: A pilot study. Journal of Surgical Education 2016; 73:831–835.
39. Madani A, Watanabe Y, Vassiliou MC, et al. Long-term knowledge retention following simulation-based training for electrosurgical safety: 1-year follow-up of a randomised controlled trial. Surg Endosc 2016; 30:1156–1163.
40. Bamford R, Smith FCT, Coulston J. Current concepts in teaching and learning in surgery. Surgery 2018; 36:483–490.
41. Yuen J, Xie F. Medical education during the COVID-19 pandemic: perspectives from UK trainees. Postgraduate Medical Journal 2020; 96:432–433.
42. Patelis N, Matheiken SJ, Beard JD. The challenges of developing distance learning for surgeons. Eur J Vasc Endovasc Surg 2015; 49:237–238.
43. Huynh R. The Role of E-Learning in Medical Education. Academic Medicine 2017; 92:430.
44. Allen T, Donde N, Hofstädter-Thalmann E, et al. Framework for industry engagement and quality principles for industry-provided medical education in Europe. J Eur CME 2017; 6:1348876.
45. Schreuder HW, Oei G, Maas M, et al. Implementation of simulation in surgical practice: minimally invasive surgery has taken the lead: the Dutch experience. Med Teach 2011; 33:105–115.
46. Baran S, Johnson E, Kehler J. An introduction to electronic learning and its use to address challenges in surgical training. Lab Anim 2009; 38:202–210.
47. Maertens H, Vermassen F, Aggarwal R, et al. Endovascular training using a simulation based curriculum is less expensive than training in the hybrid angiosuite. Eur J Vasc Endovasc Surg 2018; 56:583–590.
48. Forgione A, Salman G. The cutting-edge training modalities and educational platforms for accredited surgical training: A systematic review. J Res Med Sci 2017; 22:51.
49. Bamford R, Coulston J. Effective e-learning in surgical education: the core values underpinning effective e-learning environments and how these may be enhanced for future surgical education. E Cancer Medical Science 2016; 10:53.
50. Kirkpatrick DL. Evaluating training programs: The four levels. (1st edition) San Francisco CA Berrett Koehler 1994.
51. Martin D. A guide to critical thinking: implications for dental education. Br Dent J. 2020;229:52–53.
52. Dean B, Jones L, Garfjeld Roberts P, et al. What is known about the attributes of a successful surgical trainer? A systematic review. J Surg Educ 2017; 74:843–850.
53. Tominaga A, Kogo C. Attributes of Good E-learning Mentors According to Learners. Universal Journal of Educational Research 2018; 6:1777–1783.
54. Thompson L, Jeffries M, Topping K. E-mentoring for e-learning development. Innovations in Education and Teaching International 2010; 47:305–315.
55. El Boghdady M, Ewalds-Kvist BM, Alijani A. A review of online platforms in training and surgical education. Eur Surg 2019; 51:41–48.
56. Friesen M. (2012). Report: Defining Blended Learning. [online] Available from https://www.normfriesen.info/papers/Defining_Blended_Learning_NF.pdf [Last accessed November, 2020].
57. Liu Q, Peng W, Zhang F, et al. The effectiveness of blended learning in health professions: systematic review and meta-analysis. J Med Internet Res 2016; 18:e2.
58. De Villiers M, Walsh S. How podcasts influence medical students' learning–a descriptive qualitative study. African Journal of Health Professions Education 2015; 7:130–133.
59. White JS, Sharma N, Boora P. Evaluating the use of podcasting in a general surgery clerkship. Med Teach 2011; 33:941–943.
60. Yiasemidou M, Kordowicz A, de Siqueira J, et al. YouTube as an educational tool: the launch of a simulated surgical procedures channel. J Surg Simulat 2019; 6;23–26.
61. Farag M, Bolton D, Lawrentschuk N. Use of YouTube as a resource for surgical education-clarity or confusion. Eur Urol Focus 2020; 6:445–449.
62. Boulton CA, Kent C, Williams HT. Virtual learning environment engagement and learning outcomes at a 'bricks-and-mortar' university. Computers & Education 2018; 126:129–142.
63. Gilbert L, Wills G, Sim Y, et al. e-Learning within a Collaborative Orthopaedic Research Environment (CORE). Association for Learning Technology 2020; 79–80.
64. Evans CH. Evolving educational techniques in surgical training. Surgical Clinics. 2016;96(1):71–88.
65. Eyigör H, Gürpınar E. A study on the use of massive open online courses in otorhinolaryngology after graduation. Turk Arch Otorhinolaryngol 2019; 57:171–175.

66. Petrucci AM, Chand M, Wexner SD. Social Media: Changing the paradigm for surgical education. Clin Colon Rectal Surg 2017; 30:244–251.
67. Larkins K, Murphy V, Loveday B. Use of social media for surgical education in Australia and New Zealand. ANZ Journal of Surgery 2020; 90:1004–1008.
68. Sterling M, Leung P, Wright D, et al. The use of social media in graduate medical education: a systematic review. Acad Med 2017; 92:1043–1056.
69. Grajales FJ III, Sheps S, Ho K, et al. Social media: a review and tutorial of applications in medicine and health care. J Med Internet Res 2014; 16:e13.
70. Carter H, Hanks S, Gale T. A qualitative study using hybrid simulation to explore the impacts of human factors e-learning on behaviour change. Adv Simul 2020; 5:20.
71. General Medical Council. (2018). Outcomes for graduates. [online] Available from https://www.gmc-uk. org/-/media/documents/dc11326-outcomes-for-graduates-2018_pdf-75040796.pdf [Last accessed November, 2020].
72. World Health Organisation. (2009). WHO Patient Safety Curriculum Guide for medical schools. [online] Available from https://www.who.int/patientsafety/activities/technical/who_ps_curriculum.pdf [Last accessed November, 2020].
73. Carter H, Hanks S, Gale T. A qualitative study using hybrid simulation to explore the impacts of human factors e-learning on behaviour change. Adv Simul 2020;5:20.
74. Villanueva C, Xiong J, Rajput S. Simulation-based surgical education in cardiothoracic training. ANZ Journal of Surgery 2020; 90:978–983.
75. Guapp R, Drazic I, Dinius J, et al. E-learning to develop non-technical skills and attitudes towards patient safety? Findings from 3 years' experience with ELPAS. Resuscitation 2017; 118:e62–e63.
76. Hagemann V, Herbstreit F, Kehren C, et al. Does teaching non-technical skills to medical students improve those skills and simulated patient outcome? Int J Med Educ 2017; 8:101–113.
77. Adepoju IO, Albersen BJ, De Brouwere V, et al. mHealth for Clinical Decision-Making in Sub-Saharan Africa: a Scoping Review. JMIR Mhealth Uhealth 2017;5:e38.
78. Alfa-Wali M, Osaghae S. Practice, training and safety of laparoscopic surgery in low and middle-income countries. World J Gastrointest Surg 2017; 9:13–18.
79. Theodoulou I, Sideris M, Lawal K, et al. Retrospective qualitative study evaluating the application of IG4 curriculum: an adaptable concept for holistic surgical education. BMJ Open. 2020;10(2):e033181.
80. COVID Surg Collaborative. Global guidance for surgical care during the COVID-19 pandemic. Br J Surg 2020; 107:1097–1103.
81. Søreide K, Hallet J, Matthews JB, et al. Immediate and long-term impact of the COVID-19 pandemic on delivery of surgical services. Br J Surg 2020; 10:1002.
82. Dedeilia A, Sotiropoulos MG, Hanrahan JG, et al. Medical and surgical education challenges and innovations in the COVID-19 era: A systematic review. In Vivo 2020; 34:1603–1611.
83. Grant CL, Robinson T, Al Hinai A, et al. Ethical considerations in global surgery: a scoping review. BMJ Global Health 2020; 5:e002319.

Chapter 5

Excellence versus competence in surgical training

Afsana Elanko, Rachel Hargest

INTRODUCTION

It is the duty and privilege of each generation of surgeons to train their successors in the science and craft of surgery. There is the added individual responsibility to learn from one's predecessors and to pass knowledge and skills to one's successors. There is also a corporate responsibility to train a surgical workforce capable of providing surgical care for the population. For many centuries, surgical training consisted of a long apprenticeship with a variety of trainers, each of whom contributed to the development of the trainee's skills. Many older surgeons can attest to the opportunities that this type of system presented and remember with gratitude the inspiration gained from dedicated and skilled surgeons who '*took them under their wing*' at various points in their career.

However, in more recent years, changes to the contractual arrangements for surgeons in many first world and middle-income countries have led to a reduction in working hours for trainees, more regulated training programmes, mandatory assessments and the fragmentation of the traditional surgical 'firm' structure. These factors have reduced the amount of time many trainees now spend learning the craft of surgery. Furthermore, the requirement to complete numerous assessments may lead to a 'box ticking' attitude on the part of both trainer and trainee rather than aspiring to excellence for its own sake.

This chapter will define the terms 'excellence' and 'competence' and review the different philosophies between training for competence versus training for excellence across various surgical subspecialties and geographical regions.
Definitions [1]:
Excellence: 'The quality of being outstanding or extremely good'.
Competence: 'The ability to do something successfully or efficiently'.

KEY ELEMENTS

Excellence

There are three key elements for an individual to develop excellence:
1. Acquisition of a large knowledge base in the area of expertise
2. High level of commitment
3. Practice

In the case of teams which aspire for excellence, there is a fourth element which is essential:
4.   Common goal

Competence

Competence is the safe performance of a task due to the combination of the elements [2]:
- Knowledge
- Training
- Skills
- Experience

Several of the elements are common to both excellence and competence and it is
the degree to which they are pursued and the attitude with which surgical training is
approached which differs.

Knowledge

Both competence and excellence require the acquisition of a body of knowledge relevant
to the discipline. Most countries which have a regulated medical system and postgraduate
specialist training programmes will have a curriculum which defines the mandatory
requirements for theoretical and applied knowledge which a surgeon should acquire
before being certified or licensed as an independent practicing surgeon in that jurisdiction.
Although there are differences in the details of various surgical curricula around the world,
most of them share common elements which are presented in **Table 5.1**.

Many developed countries now have extremely detailed curricula for each specialty
of surgery providing extensive lists of topics, the knowledge of which the trainee surgeon
should acquire and which may be tested by examination or other formal assessment.
However, when training for competence these lists may be viewed as the ceiling of
knowledge which is required in order to obtain career progression. When viewed from
the point of view of training for excellence, such lists will be taken as the floor (minimum)
knowledge required in order to be safe but not sufficient to enable excellence.

Commitment

A career in surgery requires a great deal of commitment and dedication on the part of the
aspiring surgeon. Entry to medical school is competitive and along with high academic
grades, prospective medical students are often expected to have undertaken work
experience in a medical setting, voluntary or community activities and demonstrate good
communication skills and a willingness to collaborate [3,4]. Furthermore, many medical
schools charge significant fees, which along with the cost of accommodation and living

Table 5.1 Knowledge elements in surgical curricula		
Basic science	**Clinical science**	**Surgical technique**
• Anatomy	• Pathology	• Handling properties of tissue
• Embryology	• Microbiology and infection	• Stitch craft
• Physiology	control	• Instruments
• Biochemistry	• Pharmacology	• Technology
• Genetics		
• Statistics		

expenses may deter potential students from less well-off families and influence the career specialty choices of those who do graduate [5-7].

After primary medical qualification, postgraduate training in surgery may take up to 10–12 years depending on the programme undertaken and degree of subspecialisation. The onerous nature of surgical training is one of the reasons which students and junior doctors cite as to why they do not wish to pursue a career in surgery [8]. Therefore, it can be reasonably stated that anyone who embarks on, and completes surgical training must, by definition, have a high level of commitment to their chosen profession.

However, commitment is a continuous variable and although it is not possible to draw a direct correlation between increased commitment and increased excellence, the fields of business and sport have demonstrated that those who succeed at the very highest levels are committed in a way which goes beyond that of many of their peers. A simple internet search will produce thousands of references to motivational speakers, publications and corporate mission statements which define or describe commitment to excellence or the pursuit of excellence. Many of these give tips to the readers on how to succeed in their chosen field. However, there are very few robust scientific studies or publications on the link between commitment and excellence, particularly in the field of medicine or surgery.

One area which does have some experience of this link is sport. Most elite sportsmen and women now work with a sports psychologist to enhance their focus and motivation. However, history demonstrates that the most outstanding athletes of their day were characterised by commitment which surpassed that of their competitors. In 1993, Scanlon and colleagues described the Sport Commitment Model (SCM) [9] which proposed that commitment to sport depended upon factors such as sport enjoyment, involvement alternatives, involvement opportunities, personal investment and social constraints. Each of these constructs was shown to influence the likelihood of commitment to sport and persistence with training. There have been multiple modifications of the SCM over the last 25 years and it is generally accepted that there are two types of sport commitment:

1. *Enthusiastic Commitment (EC):* The desire and resolve to persist in a chosen sport over time
2. *Constrained Commitment (CC):* The perception of an obligation or duty to persist in a chosen sport over time

Table 5.2 illustrates how different constructs can have a positive or negative effect on EC or CC. For some factors the relationship may be complex, for example the influence of social constraints. Although research in this area is lacking, it would not be unreasonable to replace 'sport' with 'surgery' and consider the influence which each of these constructs might have on the commitment of an individual to a career in surgery.

One of the most interesting motivations in sporting achievement is the desire to excel, particularly the construct of mastery achievement. This concept has been described in more detail by O'Regan's team from Leeds in the previous edition of Recent Advances in Surgery [10]. When translated from sport to surgery, one can see how the aspiration to master a skill for its own sake may lead to a greater commitment than when performance of that skill merely needs to be signed off as competent. As the great tennis player, Arthur Ashe said '*You are never really playing an opponent. You are playing yourself. Your own highest standards, and when you reach your limits, that is real joy.*' This desire to continually improve and perform better is what characterises not just elite athletes, but many surgeons who remain committed to developing, refining and improving their surgical skills throughout their long careers.

Table 5.2 Constructs associated with enthusiastic commitment or constrained commitment		
	Enthusiastic commitment	**Constrained commitment**

Positive construct	• Sport enjoyment
	• Valuable opportunities
	• Personal investment
	  – Loss
	  – Quantity
	• Social support
	  – Emotional
	  – Informational
	• Desire to excel
	  – Mastery achievement
	  – Social achievement
	• Social constraints
		• Personal investment
		  – Loss
		  – Quantity
		• Social constraints

Negative construct	Involvement alternatives	Involvement alternatives

Practice

There has long been a debate as to whether excellence in the fields of sport or the arts may occur due to an innate talent or whether, time spent practicing a skill can lead to the same level of performance. The composer Wolfgang Amadeus Mozart is widely thought to be one of the most gifted musicians in the history of the world. His abilities as a pianist whilst still a child, his prodigious and glorious compositions and the wide range of his musical brilliance have led many to term him a 'genius' with the assumption that these skills came naturally to him, with minimal effort on his part. However on delving deeper, it can be seen that he was taught by his father from infancy, and between the ages of 6 and 21 years, it is estimated that he played or composed for up to 16 hours a day. This would give a total number of hours of practice well in excess of the 10,000 hours often quoted as the level required for excellence in any skill (see below). In a letter to his father Leopold he wrote, *"It is a mistake to think that the practice of my art has become easy to me. I assure you, dear friend, nobody has devoted so much time and thought to compositions as I. There is not a famous master whose music I have not industriously studied through many times. You know that I immerse myself in music, so to speak–that I think about it all day long–that I like experimenting–studying–reflecting".*

The reduction in contracted hours for surgical trainees in large parts of Europe and the USA has led to much debate in the medical literature as to whether, it is possible to train surgeons adequately, let alone for excellence, during that time. The more limited range of specialisation of newly appointed consultant and attending surgeons and their greater need for mentoring in the early years bear testament to the difficulty of obtaining mastery of surgical skills when undertaking training programmes for 48–80 hours a week as compared to the 100+ hours per week of former generations of surgeons.

Numerous attempts have been made to try to define how many hours of practice are required in order to master a skill or become excellent in one's chosen field. Chess grandmasters were studied by Simon and Chase [11] who reported that all had spent between 10,000 and 50,000 hours of practice over about 10 years before achieving this status. The psychologist Ericsson made a comprehensive study of how skills in several disciplines were obtained and refined over time, which led to his seminal and extensive publication in 1993 [12]. He contended that many characteristics once believed to reflect innate talent are in fact the result of intensive practice for a minimum of 10 years.

In more recent years, the psychologist Malcolm Gladwell has published extensively including his popular book Outliers: The Story of Success [13]. He reviewed the literature over the last 40 years relating to the factors influencing high achievers, both historical and current, in a range of disciplines including business, sport and the arts. He concluded that they had all dedicated about 10 years of daily practice to their chosen activity, leading him to introduce the term – 'The Ten Thousand Hours Rule'. This emphasises the need for repetitive practice to develop and excel in a skill irrespective of any innate talent.

Although the exact numbers of contracted hours for surgical trainees vary in different countries, and acknowledging that many trainees work in excess of these hours, there is a risk that many European training schemes which apply the 48 hours per week limit of the European Working Time Directive (EWTD) and have 4–6-year training programmes will not provide the minimum 10,000 hours required to master a craft.

Competence-based training in surgery

In many developed countries, there has been a move from time-based to competence-based training. There are very compelling reasons for this transition including:

- Knowledge and skills acquired at different rates by individual trainees
- Varying opportunities offered by different posts
- Ability to define and recognise competence and readiness to progress to the next stage of training
- Possible defence against future legal challenge

Surgical training curricula have become more extensive and detailed in many jurisdictions [14]. The ability to map assessment to each element of the curriculum allows competence to be assessed in a formative manner throughout training.

The Royal College of Surgeons of England has recently introduced a new programme called Improving Surgical Training (IST) which seeks to remedy some of the problems with current training programmes and deliver a future surgical workforce for the United Kingdom [15]. There are many laudable aspirations in this programme but what is noticeable is that trainees appear to be the passive receipts of training which will be delivered to them in order that the 'product of training' can be delivered into the surgical workforce. This contrasts with the vibrant, active and aspirational tone of many American residency programmes which explicitly state that surgical trainees are expected to be intelligent high achievers, action orientated and unique within medicine. The vision of IST states:

'We aim to create a surgical training system that produces competent, confident, self-motivated professionals who are able to provide the highest quality of care to patients in the NHS'.

Whilst it would be impossible to disagree that surgeons should be competent, this contrasts with the American Board of Surgery booklet of information for residents, which in its Mission Statement gives its vision as:

The American Board of Surgery serves the public and the specialty of surgery by providing leadership in surgical education and practice, by promoting excellence through rigorous evaluation and examination, and by promoting the highest standards for professionalism, lifelong learning, and the continuous certification of surgeons in practice.

There is a subtle difference in the tone of these two statements and it is recognised by trainees that the culture within which they work and the expectations that are put before them may lead to either inspiration to excel or disillusionment with the training on offer. The so-called tick box culture has a very demoralising effect on young intelligent, aspirational students and trainees [16]. Furthermore, there is evidence that among many other factors, burnout is more likely when contending with loss of autonomy, lack of progression and a tick box culture of work.

Table 5.3 shows the number of mentions of either excellence or competence in the documents which lay out the curricula, training programmes or examination, and certification requirements for accreditation of surgeons in a variety of surgical specialties across a number of countries throughout the world. This table is not exhaustive and for linguistic reasons only contains documents which are written in English. Despite these allowances, it can be seen that most of these documents make far more mentions of competence (or similar terms, see Table 5.3) than they do of excellence. This is particularly apparent for those programmes emanating from Europe or North America. In contrast, the equivalent documents for surgical training programmes in Asia, the Middle East and Australia make little mention of either of these terms, but do make statements as to their aspirations to provide fully trained surgeons who will provide high-quality surgical care to the population. For example, the opening statement of the College of Surgeons of the Colleges of Medicine of South Africa states that it is "the custodian of the quality of medical care in South Africa".

EXCELLENCE VERSUS COMPETENCE – DOES IT MATTER?

Patient's perspective

It is an incontrovertible fact that 50% of surgeons will be 'below average'. However, no patient would ever consent to surgery with a 'below average' surgeon should they know that to be the case. Therefore, the need for a minimum standard of competence is compelling. Training organisations, professional societies and medical regulators play their part in training, assessing and certifying individuals to practice in specific surgical disciplines. Patients need to be confident that this process is robust and that their surgeon is not just minimally qualified, but is excellent at his/her job. However, it is very difficult to define excellence and therefore surrogate measures of quality which often concentrate on the metrics of process, case mix and measurable outcomes are used [29]. In recent years, patient reported outcome measures (PROMs) have been used to try to assess the quality of surgical care particularly in the fields of orthopaedics and cancer surgery [30]. It is relatively easy to compose a list of PROMs for common conditions and operations where treatment follows standard clinical pathways, surgery involves well-defined operations and outcomes are relatively predictable. However, it is much harder to define PROMs for unusual conditions, emergency presentations or complex situations where co-morbidities and other patient factors may influence outcomes. Very few training schemes assess the ability of surgeons to make decisions under pressure or in complex situations as competence-based curricula usually require trainers to make a pass/fail assessment of the trainee for each skill or topic listed. Cases chosen for these assessments tend to be those where there is just one aspect to be addressed and realistic complex clinical situations are rarely listed in the compulsory competencies which have to be obtained.

Table 5.3 Mentions of competence* or excellence† in documents relating to surgical training and certification listed by geographical area, specialty, and professional body

Region	Document	Professional body	Excellence	Competence	Reference
Europe	Good Surgical Practice 2014	Royal College of Surgeons of England	2‡	11	17
Europe	Improving Surgical Training–2015	Royal College of Surgeons of England	8	41	15
Europe	Work Based Assessment Handbook for Ophthalmology Specialty Training 2014	Royal College of Ophthalmologists	2	23	18
Europe	Improving Surgical Training–Trainee Prospectus 2020	Royal College of Surgeons of England	2	5	19
Europe	Charter on Training in General Surgery 2007	Association of Surgeons of Malta	0	7	20
Africa	Training Curriculum–Fellowship in General Surgery 2017	College of Surgeons of East, Central and Southern Africa	4	9	21
USA/Canada	Score® Inc. Curriculum	• Surgical council on Resident Education • American Board of Surgery	0	1	22
USA/Canada	General Surgery Competencies 2020	Royal College of Physicians and Surgeons of Canada	3	42	23
USA/Canada	Orthopaedic Surgery Competencies 2020	Royal College of Physicians and Surgeons of Canada	3	30	24
Australia/New Zealand	Clinical Curriculum Performance Standards 2014	Royal Australian and New Zealand College of Ophthalmologists	1	1	25
Asia	Training Programme 2018	College of Surgeons of Hong Kong	0	0	26
Asia	Clinical Fellowship Examination in Surgery – Instructions to Candidates	College of Physicians and Surgeons Pakistan	0	0	27
Middle East	Residency	Scientific Council of the Israeli Medical Association	0	0	28

* search terms – competence/competent/competently/competency/competencies
† search terms – excellence/excellent
‡ includes one citation of a publication by National Institute of Health and Clinical Excellence

The Friends and Family test is a simple measure of how likely a patient is to recommend their surgeon/doctor/professional team to a friend or family member. The reasons why patients may make recommendations are ill defined and very variable. The importance which individual patients attach to particular aspects of their care may be based in emotional or idiosyncratic reasons and short-term nonclinical factors may outweigh clinical outcomes which doctors and surgeons may feel are more important long-term. The Friends and Family test has been criticised by a variety of commentators in the literature because of the inability to provide robust evidence regarding the weighting of outcome measures [31-34]. Whatever the merits of different methods of measuring patients' satisfaction with surgical care, we, as surgeons, all know which of our colleagues we would deem 'excellent' and it is our duty to ensure that all patients have access to excellent surgical care.

Surgeon's perspective

It can be argued that providing better outcomes for patients as well as aspiring to surgical excellence is good for the surgeons themselves. As with elite performers in sport, music or other disciplines, there is a degree of affirmation and reward in performing a skill to the very highest level and continually improving and refining one's performance. Burnout is becoming recognised as a significant cause of underperformance and early retirement in many branches of medicine [35]. The causes of burnout are multi-factorial [36]. However, repetitive tasks, loss of autonomy and disengagement are characteristics which may be associated with burnout. Surgical residents are at a higher risk of burnout than attending surgeons in many studies and although this may reflect generational attitudes to work and mental health issues, it is also possible that surgical trainees see their training programmes as a series of hurdles which have to be overcome rather than a pathway to developing their personal knowledge and skills to their highest ability, which can then be put to use in the service of patients.

Many strategies have been proposed to prevent or mitigate burnout in surgeons. The details are beyond the scope of this chapter but include emotional and peer support, maintaining a healthy lifestyle and rebalancing work commitments. No single intervention will address all the problems of burnout, disengagement and early retirement. However, the surgical career is a long-term undertaking and there is some evidence that maintaining an interest in one's work, continuing to learn and improve new skills and enjoying the affirmation of high-level performance can reduce the likelihood of burnout and early departure from the surgical workforce [37].

CONCLUSION

Training in surgery is recognised as a long and arduous undertaking during which the individual acquires a detailed level of knowledge and surgical skill. There is a commitment to the specialty and to providing a high-quality surgical service for patients. The need to assess and certify surgical training programmes has driven the move towards competence-based training. Although this will provide a safety net for patients and ensure that all certified or licensed surgeons are able to provide a minimum standard of care, it runs the risk of causing disillusionment to trainees and trainers and to stifling the commitment and effort required to attain excellence in training and performance. In conclusion, perhaps we should approach surgical training, and indeed the practice of surgery following the philosophy of Oscar Wilde— '*I have the simplest tastes. I am always satisfied with the best*'. [38].

Key points for clinical practice

- Excellence is the quality of being outstanding or extremely good
- Competence is the ability to do something successfully or efficiently
- Both require a high level of knowledge, commitment and practice
- Excellence requires a higher degree of self-motivation
- Competence-based training schemes allow for more definitive recognition of the ability to perform tasks satisfactorily
- Competently trained surgeons can be licensed to provide safe surgical care
- Aspiring to excellence is more likely to inspire and enthuse surgical trainees and retain the engagement and interest of practicing surgeons

---

REFERENCES

1   Simpson JA, Weiner ESC. Oxford English Dictionary. Oxford: Clarendon Press; 1989.
2   Health and Safety Executive. What is competence? [online] Available from http://www.hse.gov.uk/competence/what-is-competence.htm. [Last accessed November, 2020].
3   Soemantri D, Kurthilake I, Yang J-H, et al. Admission policies and methods at crossroads: a review of medical school admission policies and methods in seven Asian countries. Korean J Med Educ 2020; 32:243–256.
4   Medical Schools Council. (2019). Entry requirements to medicine updated for entry in 2020. [online] Available from https://www.medschools.ac.uk/news/entry-requirements-to-medicine-updated-for-entry-in-2020. [Last accessed November, 2020].
5   Pisaniello MS, Asahina AT, Bacchi S, et al. Effect of medical student debt on mental health, academic performance and specialty choice: a systematic review. BMJ Open 2019; 9:e029980.
6   Fritz EM, van der HS, Braman JP. Association between medical student debt and choice of specialty: a 6-year retrospective study. BMD Med Educ 2019; 28:295.
7   Fong JM, Tan YT, Sayampanathan AA, et al. Impact of financial background and student debt on postgraduate residency choices of medical students in Singapore. Singapore Med J. 2018;59:647–651.
8   S Jaunoo, T King, R Baker, et al. A national survey of reasons why students and junior doctors choose not to pursue a career in surgery. Bull RCS 2014; 96:192–194.
9   Scanlon TK, Carpenter PJ, Simons JP, et al. An introduction to the sport commitment model. J Sport Ex Psychol 1993; 15:1–15.
10   Papaspyros S, Lodhia JV, O'Regan. Acquisition of surgical skills—from novice to master; a fresh perspective. Recent Advances in Surgery 39, 1st edition. New Delhi: Jaypee Brothers Medical Publishers (P) Ltd; 2019. pp. 27–36.
11   Simon WG, Chase HA. Skill in Chess. Am Scientist 1973; 61:394–403.
12   Ericsson KA. The role of deliberate practice in the acquisition of expert procedures. Psychol Rev 1993; 100:363–406.
13   Gladwell M. The 10000 hours rule. Outliers: The Story of Success. 2008. Little, Brown and Company; 2008.
14   Drossard S. Structured surgical residency training in Germany: an overview of existing training programs in 10 surgical subspecialties. Innov Surg Sci 2019; 4:15–24.
15   Royal College of Surgeons of England. (2015). Improving Surgical Training—Proposal for a pilot surgical training program. [online] Available from https://www.rcseng.ac.uk/library-and-publications/rcs-publications/docs/improving-surgical-training/. [Last accessed November, 2020].
16   Rehan S, Rehan Z. The pursuit of excellence. Clin Teach 2019; 16:280–282.
17   Royal College of Surgeons of England (2014). Good Surgical Practice. [online] Available from https://www.rcseng.ac.uk/standards-and-research/gsp/. [Last accessed November, 2020].
18   Royal College of Ophthalmologists. (2014). Workplace Based Assessments (WpBA) Handbook for OST. [online] Available from https://www.rcophth.ac.uk/wp-content/uploads/2014/11/WpBA-Handbook-V4-2014.pdf. [Last accessed November, 2020].

19   Royal College of Surgeons of England. (2020). Improving Surgical Training—Trainee Prospectus 2020. [online] Available from https://www.rcseng.ac.uk/-/media/files/rcs/careers-in-surgery/ist/ist-prospectus-2020.pdf. [Last accessed November, 2020].

20   Association of Surgeons of Malta. (2007). Charter on Training in General Surgery. [online] Available from https://www.efort.org/wp-content/uploads/2014/07/Malta-_SAC_Orthopaedic_Surgery_training_requirements-en.pdf. [Last accessed November, 2020].

21   College of Surgeons of East, Central and Southern Africa. (2017). Training Curriculum. Fellowship in General Surgery–FCSgen (ECSA).[online] Available from http://www.cosecsa.org/sites/default/files/FCS%20GS%20curriculum%20Final.pdf. [Last accessed November, 2020].

22   Score® Inc. (2019-2020). Curriculum Outline for General Surgery. Surgical council on Resident Education. American Board of Surgery. [online] Available from https://www.absurgery.org/default.jsp?scre_booklet. [Last accessed November, 2020].

23   Royal College of Physicians and Surgeons of Canada. (2020). General Surgery Competencies. [online] Available from http://www.royalcollege.ca/rcsite/ibd-search-e?N=10000033+10000034+4294967081. [Last accessed November, 2020].

24   Royal College of Physicians and Surgeons of Canada. (2020). Orthopaedic Surgery Competencies. [online] Available from http://www.royalcollege.ca/rcsite/ibd-search-e?N=10000033+10000034+4294967074. [Last accessed November, 2020].

25   Royal Australian and New Zealand College of Ophthalmologists. (2014). Clinical Curriculum Performance Standards2014. [online] Available from https://ranzco.edu/wp-content/uploads/2019/06/VTP-Clinical-Curriculum-Performance-Standards-compendium.pdf. [Last accessed November, 2020].

26   College of Surgeons of Hong Kong. (2018). Training Program. [online] Available from https://cshk.org/site/CSHK/upload/mw_data/file/mw_data_5866_5be3b3a8d10a1.pdf. [Last accessed November, 2020].

27   College of Physicians and Surgeons Pakistan. Clinical Fellowship Examination in Surgery. Instructions to Candidates. [online] Available from https://www.cpsp.edu.pk/files/guidelines/clinical/FCPS-IIA/Surgery.pdf. [Last accessed November, 2020].

28   Scientific Council of The Israeli Medical Association. Chapter 3 Residency. [online] Available from https://www.ima.org.il/internesnew/viewcategory.aspx?categoryid=7449. [Last accessed November, 2020].

29   Ibrahim AM, Dimick JB. What metrics accurately reflect surgical quality? Ann Rev Med. 2018;69:481–491.

30   Chaudhry A, Winters Z. Breast Reconstruction: How do we Measure and Define Patient's Quality of Life and Satisfaction? Recent Advances in Surgery 35. New Delhi: Jaypee Brothers Medical Publishers (P) Ltd.; 2013. pp. 45–57.

31   Robert G, Cornwell J, Black N. Friends and family test should no longer be mandatory. BMJ. 2018;360:k367.

32   Kmietowicz Z. Friends and family test "unfit" for comparing NHS services, finds research. BMJ 2014; 348:g4355.

33   Davis R. How the friends and family test is conveyed to the public should be reconsidered. BMJ 2013; 347:f5158.

34   King AJ, Eyre T, Bruce D. Family and friends test is inappropriate for patients with cancer. BMJ 2013; 346:f3553.

35   Shanafelt TD, Balch CM, Bechamps G, et al. Burnout and medical errors among American surgeons. Ann Surg 2010; 251:995–1000.

36   Pulcrano M, Evans SR, Sosin M. Quality of life and burnout rates across surgical specialties: a systematic review. JAMA Surg 2016; 151:970–978.

37   Balch CM, Shanafelt T. Combating stress and burnout in surgical practice: a review. Adv Surg 2010; 44:29–47.

38   Saltus E. Oscar Wilde: An idler's impression. Chicago: Brothers of the Book; 2017. pp. 20.

Section 3

Transplant surgery

Chapter 6

Organ donation: ethical issues of consent and organ trade and strategies to increase donor numbers

Michael Stephens, Adnan Sharif

INTRODUCTION

Most people consider organ donation for the purpose of transplantation, an unproblematic good, but it can be an emotive and ethically challenging topic. The shortage of solid organ availability means that an unacceptable proportion of patients will die before a suitable organ is identified. This gap between supply and demand causes considerable morbidity, mortality, and economic pressure from healthcare costs and lost citizen productivity. Unfortunately, it also provides opportunity for those willing to exploit both desperate individuals in need of an organ transplant and other vulnerable members of our society. This chapter explores some of the ethical challenges around organ donation supply and strategies to increase organ donor numbers in an ethically acceptable way.

ILLEGAL ORGAN TRADE

Low supply and high demand provide a dangerous environment for illegal organ trading to flourish. The most up-to-date Global Observatory on Donation and Transplantation report estimates 139,024 solid organ transplants were performed globally in 2017 (http://www.transplant-observatory.org).While global organ donation and transplantation activity has been steadily increasing over years, this is still not sufficient to meet the demand for organs to support all transplantation needs internationally. Fuelled by the growing disparity between supply and demand for organs, scarcity can encourage some desperate individuals with end-stage organ failure to bypass the system and seek organs through illegal and/or unethical channels by engaging in organ trading.

Estimating global illegal activity with trading of organs is difficult due to the clandestine nature of the activity. The World Health Organisation (WHO) previously estimated 10–15% of global transplant activity to be illegal [1], estimated by the nongovernmental organisation Global Financial Integrity to generate incomes exceeding one billion US dollars (https://gfintegrity.org). However, these are historical and speculative figures that lack any contemporary validation. In a critical appraisal of the published literature, Ambagtsheer and colleagues [2] found published reports of patients buying organs to be speculative and anecdotal: their purchases are more often assumed than determined.

The empirical data published in the literature does not appear to reflect a large number of patients buying organs at home or abroad. However, the clandestine nature of the practice means published scientific literature may represent an under-reporting of cases. More rigorous quantitative and qualitative research is clearly needed to enable a more reliable picture of the scale of this trade to be established.

What is organ trading?

It is important to clarify terminology when discussing trading of organs, as the term can encompass many aspects of practice. In the published literature, practices including 'organ trafficking', 'trafficking in persons for organ removal', 'organ sales' 'transplant commercialism' and 'transplant tourism' have all been classified as the trading of organs, although this broad definition can have negative implications for law and policy [3]. While there may be some overlap between these practices, they are all loosely described as examples of organ trafficking. However, conflating trafficking with trade as a whole can be counterproductive and can be a risk ignoring aspects of organ trade that are not related to measures tackling serious organised crime alone.

The declaration of Istanbul introduced a broad definition of what was to be defined as organ trafficking at its inception in 2008 and in a recent update [4].

'Organ trafficking is the recruitment, transport, transfer, harbouring, or receipt of living or deceased persons or their organs by means of the threat or use of force or other forms of coercion, of abduction, of fraud, of deception, of the abuse of power or of a position of vulnerability, or of the giving to, or the receiving by, a third party of payments or benefits to achieve the transfer of control over the potential donor, for the purpose of exploitation by the removal of organs for transplantation.'

At the same time, the declaration provides the following definition of transplant commercialism:

'Transplant commercialism is a policy or practice in which an organ is treated as a commodity, including by being bought or sold or used for material gain.'

While the declaration of Istanbul was a landmark statement for raising awareness of organ trafficking and transplant tourism, it lacks clarity with regards to distinguishing between trade and trafficking. For example, Iran has openly piloted a regulated system of living unrelated paid donor kidney transplantation since 1988 [5,6], which has received plaudits for its candid transparency with regards to successes and failures [7]. The Iranian experience contradicts the statement from the declaration of Istanbul that '*Organ donation should be a financially neutral act*' [8]. However, it iterates the importance of separating trade from trafficking.

Examples of organ trafficking and associated outcomes

According to the Draft Council of Europe Convention against Trafficking in Human Organs (http://www.coe.int), trafficking in human organs is any of the following activities when committed intentionally:

- The removal of human organs from living or deceased donors where the removal is performed without the free, informed and specific consent of the living or deceased donor, or, in the case of the deceased donor, without the removal being authorised under its domestic law
- The use of these organs for purposes of implantation or other purposes than implantation

- The preparation, preservation, storage, transportation, transfer, receipt, import, and export of these organs
- Aiding or abetting the commission of any of these criminal offences or the intentional attempt to commit any of these criminal offences
- The solicitation and recruitment of an organ donor or a recipient, where carried out for financial gain or comparable advantage for the person soliciting or recruiting, or for a third party
- The promising, offering, or giving by any person, directly or indirectly, of any undue advantage to healthcare professionals, its public officials or persons who direct or work for private sector entities, in any capacity, with a view to having a removal or implantation of a human organ performed or facilitated, where such removal or implantation is illicit as defined above
- The request or receipt by healthcare professionals, its public officials or persons who direct or work for private sector entities, in any capacity, of any undue advantage with a view to performing or facilitating the performance of a removal or implantation of a human organ, where such removal or implantation is illicit as defined above

Both the ethical and the legal challenges posed by various forms of transplant trafficking, there are also disadvantageous clinical consequences.

The post-transplant course for patients who travel abroad to purchase kidneys, defined as 'transplant tourists', has been shown to be inferior. For example, returnees to the United States [9] in a single-centre study had higher rates of rejection and infectious complications, compared to others who received their transplant at the same centre from domestically sourced kidneys. In the United Kingdom [10], a single-centre experience of 40 transplant tourists who travelled abroad for a kidney between 1996 and 2006 revealed inferior survival and postoperative infectious complications versus ethnically matched patients who remained on dialysis.

The majority of people who are transplant tourists are purchasing kidney transplants, with fewer cases of people travelling for livers, hearts, and lungs [2]. However, because the literature presents inconsistent terminology about what constitutes tourism or commercialism, it is not possible to distinguish those who travel for transplantation from those who travel to participate in transplant commercialism. While the majority of studies present patients as 'transplant tourists' who 'purchased organs' by undergoing 'commercial transplants' abroad, many do not define these terms and, in those that do, they are defined differently.

Forced organ harvesting from prisoners

While illegal organ trafficking can occur in a number of ways, forced organ harvesting from executed prisoners has represented one of the most controversial areas from an ethical perspective. Obtaining organs for transplantation from executed prisoners has been unequivocally denounced by international declarations [11] but has occurred in the People's Republic of China (PRC) over many years; at first denied but then confirmed. Under increasing international pressure [12], the PRC announced cessation of using organs from executed prisoners from January, 2015 [13] and establishment of ethical procurement of all organ donors. While this assertion has been challenged from some quarters [14,15], it has been acknowledged by others [16,17] as a genuine case of reform.

The claim from the PRC that forced organ harvesting from executed prisoners officially ceased in January 2015 has never been independently verified. Of note, the PRC has only ever admitted harvesting organs from judicially sentenced and executed criminal prisoners. Government officials from the PRC have always strenuously denied forced organ harvesting from prisoners of conscience killed for their organs. Recent investigations cast doubt on the veracity of Chinese reports of their organ donation and transplantation activity. Robertson and colleagues examined the availability, transparency, integrity, and consistency of official transplant data from the PRC [2]. Forensic statistical methods were used to test two central-level Chinese datasets [China Organ Transplant Response System (COTRS) and the Red Cross Society of China] for coherence and accuracy, with corroboration to provincial- and individual-level data where available. Their analysis exposed statistically improbable precise conformity of these data to a one-parameter quadratic mathematical formula, together with contradictory and implausible corroboration with regional/individual centre data. These results indicate human-directed manipulation of data rather than an accurate reflection of voluntary organ donations from individuals dying of natural causes.

The independent China Tribunal (https://chinatribunal.com), an international expert panel that investigated claims of forced organ harvesting in the PRC from prisoners of conscience, categorically reported in 2019 that crimes against humanity have occurred. They concluded with the statement:

'Forced organ harvesting has been committed for years throughout China on a significant scale and that Falun Gong practitioners have been one–and probably the main–source of organ supply. The concerted persecution and medical testing of the Uyghurs is more recent and it may be that evidence of forced organ harvesting of this group may emerge in due course. The Tribunal has had no evidence that the significant infrastructure associated with China's transplantation industry has been dismantled and absent a satisfactory explanation as to the source of readily available organs concludes that forced organ harvesting continues till today.'

Therefore, until the international community is suitably reassured, concern about the organ procurement process in the PRC is likely to remain a contentious issue for the global transplantation community.

STRATEGIES TO REDUCE THE ILLEGAL ORGAN TRADE

The best way to reduce organ trafficking or the illegal organ trade is to bridge the gap between supply and demand for legitimate organs. Therefore, any strategy that legally and ethically increases organ procurement and/or allograft survival should be strongly encouraged. A need for national self-sufficiency, a paradigm that involves governments taking national-level responsibility to fulfil the organ donation and transplantation needs of patients by accessing resources from within the country's population, is key to overcome illegal organ trade [18]. Other strategies to tackle the illegal organ trade include improved legislation to prohibit exploitation of vulnerable adults, clearly defining physician code of conduct, enhanced donor pools and regulation of transplant services and public health strategies to prevent end-stage organ failure in the first case.

Beyond measures to improve consent processes and educational awareness, more novel strategies can be explored. The Iranian model provides a compelling but controversial argument for converting an illegal commercial system of organ procurement into a single buyer government-regulated programme [19]. However, significant resistance remains in the transplantation community for such proposals to become reality [20].

Finally, on the question of the PRC, without independent verification it is difficult to assume organ procurement from executed prisoners in China has stopped. Transparent access to data is a basic requirement of audit and governance processes for organ donation and transplantation activity and openness to scrutiny should be a basic requirement, which will allow verification of claims from the PRC that unethical organ procurement from executed prisoners ceased in 2015. Any legitimate independent review would require:

- Open access to review organ donation processes and verify sources
- Review of transplantation facilities (military and civilian)
- The ability to probe data registries to crosscheck donation and transplantation activity numbers

Consistent pressure from international political and professional bodies is critical to allow such a review and to support the PRC to embrace ethical organ donor systems.

STRATEGIES TO INCREASE ORGAN DONOR NUMBERS

Healthcare systems vary around the world and it is too simplistic to suggest that a single approach to organ donation and transplantation is better or best, or that a single intervention will guarantee more organs being made available for transplantation. The number of both potential organ donors and potential recipients who would benefit from organs transplants may also vary considerably between countries [21]. However, there are very few, if any, healthcare systems which have established organ donation processes that provide sufficient solid organs for all those who could benefit from a transplant. Thresholds of ethical tolerance, society and cultural norms, and numbers of potential donors and recipient can vary considerably between countries, and this makes between country organ donation comparisons difficult to interpret. For example, the population of one country might consider it acceptable to place a cannula in the femoral artery of a citizen who has died and commence organ preservation before discussions with the family about organ donation, thereby opening the option of uncontrolled DCD (donation after circulatory death) donation (a type of organ donation where the donor has suffered an out of hospital cardiac arrest and attempts to resuscitate have been unsuccessful). This may be considered completely unacceptable in another country. Given these differences, it is not surprising that the evidence supporting organ donation strategies is not strong, often relying on expert opinion or observational studies only. There are also fundamental differences in the required processes for different types of organ donors; establishing a proficient system for living kidney donation is quite different from the requirements for an uncontrolled DCD liver donation. Sometimes these systems might inadvertently compete; strong live donor programmes could disincentivise deceased donor programmes and vice versa [22].

Perhaps, the logical way to consider possible strategies to increase organ donor numbers is to follow the pathway from donor identification through to transplanted recipient chronologically.

IDENTIFYING MORE SUITABLE DONORS

Most deceased organ donors are identified from an intensive care unit (ICU), usually after a catastrophic brain injury, which may have been caused by trauma, hypoxia, or an intra-cerebral vascular event. Facilitating an organ donation from ICU requires time and resources, and these are not always readily available. For many units, a potential organ donation will be an infrequent occurrence and therefore could be overlooked, and an individual clinician's views or experiences of donation can also affect this [23]. Implementing a standardised approach to donor screening across the whole healthcare system, and likewise to the family approach, will overcome this but can only be delivered with a centrally coordinated system [24]. Many of the countries which have achieved success in increasing deceased donation rates have done so by introducing centralised systems and then allocating organ donation champions or specialists into regions with dedicated time separated from any other activities [25]. Incentivising ICU for organ donation has also been considered but, in a process which relies heavily on the trust of the population in the healthcare system, this can add a perceived conflict of interest [23,24].

CONVERT MORE POTENTIAL DONORS INTO ACTUAL DONORS

Consent or authorisation for organ donation to proceed is one of the main barriers to converting potential donors into actual donors. Public attitude surveys consistently show high levels of support for organ donation and a willingness by citizens to allow themselves to be organ donors if the situation arose [26]. However, for many countries it is the minority who either opt-in during life, or who's family consent to donation proceeding after death. Public awareness campaigns can help this and utilising the 'nudge theory' is an effective version of this [27]. The concept of death and defining death is upsetting and not well understood at a population level, and organ donation campaigns ideally need to include explanations of these as part of their agenda [24]. The language used in these campaigns is important, as evidenced by the experience when Wales introduced a new publicity campaign during the implementation of opt-out legislation [28,29].

The question of whether an opt-out system (where citizens are assumed to authorise organ donation after their death unless they make a declaration to the contrary) or an opt-in system (where individuals need to actively declare their willingness to donate) is more effective, often dominates discussions on increasing organ donor numbers. The question has not been definitively answered, and given the complexity of organ donation processes, healthcare systems, wider society, and also the differences between countries, this is not surprising. The principle of why an opt-out system may be better is simple; the majority of people are in favour of organ donation and would allow their own organs to be used after their death but it is only the minority who ever opt-in [26]. Changing the starting point to one that is in line with the majority view but ensuring there is a robust method for those who have a different view to register their decision seems reasonable. However, proponents of the opt-in system will note it is not as simple as that. Opinions and decisions on organ donation are based on multiple and complex reasons. Medical mistrust and bodily integrity are factors in individuals' decision making for any organ donation system [26], but with an opt-out system there could also be concern or suspicion about state involvement which may cause some to reconsider.

One of the causes of concern when changing from opt-in to opt-out is that this could fundamentally alter the altruistic nature of organ donation and the 'gift' element that is often a powerful part of the decision-making. It should be noted, however, that the 'consent' given for opt-in is not what we would normally recognise as consent for medical procedures.

It would be problematic ethically to change from a system where patients have been fully counselled and then made a documented informed decision, but it is difficult to be reassured of this when an opt-in decision can be made in seconds during a renewal of a driving license.

One of the attractions of a robust opt-out system is the possibility to make legal requirements for public education which cannot be reversed as political whims change. There is evidence from Wales that the legally required public education associated with the legislative change resulted in an increased understanding and awareness of organ donation [29,30]. There have not been any studies comparing opt-out versus a legal requirement for a comparable level of public education, but such an analysis would be interesting. Although opt-out versus opt-in is probably the most studied aspect of the organ donation process, the published studies are mostly limited to between country comparisons and a small number of before and after analyses. These in general, but not invariably show higher rates of deceased organ donation in countries with opt-out systems, but none have been able to demonstrate causation with confidence [31,32]. Simply making comparisons between countries with opt-in and opt-out systems can be misleading. A good example of why can be seen by considering Spain, which is consistently the highest performing country in the world with deceased donor numbers. Spain has an opt-out system but there is no register either for opting in or opting out, rather clinicians rely on a discussion with the family to ascertain the deceased views. It is clear the successes achieved by Spain are not related to opt-out.

The experience of introducing an opt-out system in Wales provided some useful insights. The organ procurement system in the United Kingdom (UK) is delivered by the National Health Service (NHS) Blood and Transplant, who are responsible for all aspects of the donation process including donor identification, donor approach and consent. Wales is one of four major nations which make up the UK (together with England, Scotland and Northern Ireland), and responsibility for healthcare is devolved to each nation. In 2015, Wales moved to an opt-out system for organ donation whilst all other UK nations continued with the previous opt-in system. All other aspects of the organ donation pathway remained standardised, thus offering a unique opportunity to assess the impact of opt-out on consent rates and ultimately organ donor numbers. Concerns that the change in legislation may result in a major backlash with mass opt-outs proved unfounded [29], and opt-out rates have remained stable at approximately 6% of the population. About 3 years after implementing the opt-out system, the chance of consent for organ donation to proceed was double in Wales in comparison to England [30], with correspondingly higher rates of organ donors per million population (29 vs. 24), despite Wales starting with lower figures than England prior to the law change. Introducing such a major legislative change inevitably requires a large amount of promotion and it is not possible to know whether, this publicity is the reason for the increased consent rates. It could even be argued that it does not matter how it works so long as it does, but this may be answered in time as the publicity campaign is scaled back. Nevertheless, the experience from Wales demonstrates that introducing an opt-out system with the necessary increase in public information can result in increases in consent rates and organ donor numbers.

Careful analysis of the implementation of the law change in Wales shows that in the early stages, although there was not the feared backlash and mass opting-out, there were few positive changes, either practically or in consent and organ donation rates [29]. Following this, further education and training was implemented for the specialist teams delivering the family discussions, and the public education campaign was changed to emphasise the role of the family in decision-making, and the importance of citizens making 'decisions' on organ donation rather than 'wishes'. This approach is akin to the 'nudge theory' [27] and could be implemented without the requirement for opt-out.

We have already discussed how increasing deceased donor rates could affect living donor transplantation and vice versa, and some studies have demonstrated an association between countries with an opt-out system and lower rates of live donation [22]. It is therefore important that if any changes to consent legislation are being implemented, all aspects of the donation and transplant programme are considered. There is no practical reason why a country cannot have both a world-class deceased donor programme and also the same standard for their live donor programme.

Offering direct financial incentives to donate carries difficult ethical connotations and is illegal throughout the world, except in the Islamic Republic of Iran [22]. However, incentivising donor registration in other ways has been attempted with some success. In Israel, a system of granting priority on transplant lists for registered donors and the next of kin of those who have donated after death was introduced in 2010 and was associated with an increase in donor consent rates from 45 to 55% [33]. This approach encourages reciprocal altruism and increases the chance of organs being made available for those who have or are willing to contribute to the donor pool. Longer-term data will be interesting.

Direct financial incentives for live donation are even more problematic, as has already been discussed. However, removing financial disincentives such as loss of income during the recovery from surgery are ethically sound, and have been shown to increase live donor rates when implemented [34,35].

IMPROVE ORGAN UTILISATION

Practitioners in the field of organ donation and transplant have a responsibility to ensure the decision of organ donors to donate is utilised to the fullest potential. This involves both using as many organs as possible and also maximising the function and longevity of those organs. The organ allocation system has a role to play in this, allocating organs to recipients in a utilitarian manner to maximise the benefit to the whole, although this can also bring further ethical consequences as a fully utilitarian allocation system compromises on justice (where every potential recipient has an equal right to access) to some degree. One area where organ allocation can be maximised without ethical concern is the use of 'sharing schemes' for live donor programmes. Here live donor pairs, usually ones where direct donation between the pair is not possible, e.g. due to blood group compatibility, are linked with another pair or pairs to make compatible exchanges. In the simplest form, it involves two pairs (donor A gives to recipient B, donor B to recipient A) but this can be extended to multiple pairs or chains of donors, thereby creating live donor transplants that would otherwise not be achievable.

Increasing the number of organs utilised from each donor can also be achieved by using 'higher-risk' organs, or by using advanced organ preservation or regeneration processes. Higher-risk donors might include those who are at higher risk of transmitting disease such as blood-borne viruses or malignancy, or where there is concern regarding organ function. The use of organs from hepatitis C-positive donors has recently become a reality due to advances in direct-acting antivirals [36,37], and the transplant community has become much better at understanding the risk of transmission of malignancy from donor to recipient such that it is now common place for organs to be utilised from patients with treated cancer and transplanted into appropriately consented recipients. Organ preservation, transport and regeneration continue to advance. Techniques for procuring, transporting and then successfully transplanting hearts from DCD donors are particularly exciting, and there have been considerable advances in this area over recent years [38]. Novel approaches to the organ procurement procedure such as normothermic regional perfusion (NRP) have opened up the possibility of organ assessment and recovery in a way that has not previously been available. NRP is similar to extracorporeal membrane oxygenation (ECMO) where blood from the deceased donor is pumped through an extra-corporeal system, heated and oxygenated but confined to the abdominal organs rather than the whole body. This has been shown to produce better transplant outcomes and can convert organs that would otherwise have been discarded into good-quality organs [39].

MAXIMISE LONGEVITY OF TRANSPLANTED ORGANS

Making sure organs are allocated to the most appropriate recipient, whether that be the one most in need or the one where the organ will function best is an important aspect of organ donation programmes. It is also important that transplanted organs are supported to function for as long as possible and thereby ensure the recipient does not require a further transplant. Investing in maintaining transplanted organs should therefore be part of any strategy to improve organ donation (reducing the need). Likewise, reducing the incidence of preventable forms of organ failure through population-based health strategies will ultimately reduce the requirement for transplants and narrow the gap between supply and demand.

CONCLUSION

The illegal trade in organs exists primarily because there is a gap between the need for organ transplants and the number of available organs. The evidence base for improving organ donor numbers is lacking, but there are several strategies that have been shown to be successful. Any planned changes would ideally look to address all steps in the donation to transplant pathway; donor identification, donor authorisation, donor conversion, and organ utilisation. It is important for policymakers to not assume a single intervention such as moving to an opt-out system for consent will solve the organ shortage, but the successes of a variety of strategies demonstrates that improvements are possible.

Key points for clinical practice

- Despite many advances in organ donation over recent years, there remains a gap between supply and demand for transplant organs
- Organ trafficking is a dark reality of global transplantation and reinforces the need to promote national self-sufficiency
- The differences in healthcare structure, culture, and society between countries limit the utility of international comparisons on organ donation
- Increasing organ donation requires consideration of all steps of the donation pathway, and different approaches for deceased and live donation

REFERENCES

1. Shimazono Y. The state of the international organ trade: a provisional picture based on integration of available information. Bull World Health Organ 2007; 85:955–962.
2. Ambagtsheer F, de Jong J, Bramer WM, et al. On patients who purchase organ transplants abroad. Am J Transplant 2016; 16:2800–2815.
3. Columb S, Ambagtsheer F, Bos M, et al. Re-conceptualizing the organ trade: separating "trafficking" from "trade" and the implications for law and policy. Transpl Int 2017; 30:209–213.
4. The Declaration of Istanbul on organ trafficking and transplant tourism (2018 Edition). Transplantation 2019; 103:218–219.
5. Ghods AJ, Savaj S. Iranian model of paid and regulated living-unrelated kidney donation. Clin J Am Soc Nephrol 2006; 1:1136–1145.
6. Mahdavi-Mazdeh M. The Iranian model of living renal transplantation. Kidney Int 2012; 82:627–634.
7. Delmonico FL. The alternative Iranian model of living renal transplantation. Kidney Int 2012; 82:625–626.
8. Martin DE, Van Assche K, Dominguez-Gil B, et al. Strengthening global efforts to combat organ trafficking and transplant tourism: Implications of the 2018 edition of the Declaration of Istanbul. Transplant Direct. 2019; 5:e433.
9. Gill J, Madhira BR, Gjertson D, et al. Transplant tourism in the United States: a single-center experience. Clin J Am Soc Nephrol 2008; 3:1820–1828.
10. Krishnan N, Cockwell P, Devulapally P, et al. Organ trafficking for live donor kidney transplantation in Indoasians resident in the west midlands: high activity and poor outcomes. Transplantation 2010; 89:1456–1461.
11. Sharif A, Singh MF, Trey T, et al. Organ procurement from executed prisoners in China. Am J Transplant 2014; 14:2246–2252.
12. Delmonico F, Chapman J, Fung J, et al. Open letter to Xi Jinping, President of the People's Republic of China: China's fight against corruption in organ transplantation. Transplantation 2014; 97:795–796.
13. Huang JF, Zheng SS, Liu YF, et al. China organ donation and transplantation update: the Hangzhou Resolution. Hepatobiliary Pancreat Dis Int 2014; 13:122–124.
14. Trey T, Sharif A, Singh MF, et al. Organ transplantation in China: concerns remain. Lancet. 2015;385:854.
15. Trey T, Sharif A, Schwarz A, et al. Transplant medicine in China: Need for transparency and international scrutiny remains. Am J Transplant 2016; 16:3115–120.
16. Chapman JR. Organ transplantation in China. Transplantation 2015; 99:1312–1313.
17. O'Connell PJ, Ascher N, Delmonico FL. The Transplantation Society believes a policy of engagement will facilitate organ donation reform in China. Am J Transplant 2016; 16:3297–3298.
18. Delmonico FL, Dominguez-Gil B, Matesanz R, et al. A call for government accountability to achieve national self-sufficiency in organ donation and transplantation. Lancet 2011; 378:1414–1418.
19. Harris J, Erin C. An ethically defensible market in organs. BMJ 2002; 325:114–115.
20. Matas AJ, Adair A, Wigmore SJ. Paid organ donation. Ann R Coll Surg Engl 2011; 93:188–192.
21. Liyanage T, Ninomiya T, Jha V, et al. Worldwide access to treatment for end-stage kidney disease: a systematic review. Lancet 2015; 385:1975–1982.
22. Arshad A, Anderson B, Sharif A. Comparison of organ donation and transplantation rates between opt-out and opt-in systems. Kidney Int 2019; 95:1453–1460.
23. Hart JL, Kohn R, Halpern SD. Perceptions of organ donation after circulatory determination of death among critical care physicians and nurses: a national survey. Crit Care Med 2012; 40:2595–2600.
24. Becker F, Roberts KJ, Nadal M, et al. Optimizing organ donation: expert opinion from Austria, Germany, Spain and the U.K. Ann Transplant 2020; 25:e921727.
25. Matesanz R, Domínguez-Gil B, Coll E, et al. How Spain Reached 40 Deceased Organ Donors per Million Population. Am J Transplant 2017; 17:1447–1454.
26. Miller J, Currie S, McGregor LM, et al. 'It's like being conscripted, one volunteer is better than 10 pressed men': A qualitative study into the views of people who plan to opt-out of organ donation. Br J Health Psychol 2020; 25:257–254.
27. Sharif A, Moorlock G. Influencing relatives to respect donor autonomy: should we nudge families to consent to organ donation? Bioethics 2018; 32:155–163.
28. Noyes J, Mclaughlin L, Morgan K, et al. Process evaluation of specialist nurse implementation of a soft opt-out organ donation system in Wales. BMC Health Serv Res 2019; 19:414.
29. Noyes J, McLaughlin L, Morgan K, et al. Short-term impact of introducing a soft opt-out organ donation system in Wales: before and after study. BMJ Open 2019; 9:e025159.

30. Madden S, Collett D, Walton P, et al. The effect on consent rates for deceased organ donation in Wales after the introduction of an opt-out system. Anaesthesia 2020; 75:1146–1152.
31. Ahmad MU, Hanna A, Mohamed AZ, et al. A systematic review of opt-out versus opt-in consent on deceased organ donation and transplantation (2006-2016).World J Surg 2019; 43:3161–3171.
32. Rithalia A, McDaid C, Suekarran S, et al. Impact of presumed consent for organ donation on donation rates: a systematic review. BMJ 2009; 338:a3162.
33. Stoler A, Kessler JB, Ashkenazi T, et al. Incentivizing authorization for deceased organ donation with organ allocation priority: the first 5 years. Am J Transplant 2016; 16:2639–2645.
34. Delmonico FL, Martin D, Domínguez-Gil B, et al. Living and deceased organ donation should be financially neutral acts. Am J Transplant 2015; 15:1187–1191.
35. Fisher JS, Butt Z, Friedewald J, et al. Between Scylla and Charybdis: charting an ethical course for research into financial incentives for living kidney donation. Am J Transplant 2015; 15:1180–1186.
36. Salomon DR, Langnas AN, Reed AI, et al. AST/ASTS Workshop on increasing organ donation in the United States: Creating an "Arc of Change" from removing disincentives to testing incentives. Am J Transplant 2015; 15:1173–1179.
37. Sise ME, Goldberg DS, Kort JJ, et al. multicenter study to transplant hepatitis c-infected kidneys (mythic): an open-label study of combined glecaprevir and pibrentasvir to treat recipients of transplanted kidneys from deceased donors with hepatitis c virus infection. J Am Soc Nephrol 2020:ASN.2020050685.
38. Messer S, Page A, Axell R, et al. Outcome after heart transplantation from donation after circulatory-determined death donors. J Heart Lung Transplant 2017; 36:1311–1318.
39. Muller X, Mohkam K, Mueller M, et al. Hypothermic oxygenated perfusion versus normothermic regional perfusion in liver transplantation from controlled donation after circulatory death: first international comparative study. Ann Surg 2020; 272:751–758.

Section 4

Vascular surgery

Chapter 7

Long-term outcomes of endovascular abdominal aortic aneurysm repair

Ummul Contractor, Dafydd Locker, Richard White, Ian Williams

INTRODUCTION

An abdominal aortic aneurysm (AAA) is defined as a focal enlargement of the abdominal aorta such that the diameter is > 50% of the normal diameter [1] with the infra-renal aorta being the most common location. Initial population screening studies reported a prevalence of 4–8%, predominantly affecting men over 65 years of age [2]. Risk factors for developing AAAs include smoking, hypertension, family history, Caucasian ethnicity, gender, age and other sites of aneurysmal disease [3]. An AAA is up to 6 times more common in men than women but the risk of rupture, growth rates, and aneurysm-related mortality are significantly higher in women [4]. The natural history of aneurysmal disease is progressive enlargement over time, although the rate of growth varies. The risk factors which contribute to rupture include large aneurysm diameter, rapid expansion, smoking, hypertension, elevated peak wall stress, a history of cardiac or renal transplant, decreased forced expiratory volume, and female gender [5].

Surgery by open repair (OR) has been the traditional treatment for AAA, but over the last 30 years, endovascular aneurysm repair (EVAR) has been performed with a variety of novel devices. This chapter will briefly review the rationale and indications for AAA surgery, describe the history of EVAR procedures and trials and discuss the long-term outcomes of clinical trials comparing EVAR and OR for AAA.

RATIONALE AND INDICATIONS FOR ABDOMINAL AORTIC ANEURYSM SURGERY

Any intervention for AAA is based on considering the balance between the diameter of the aneurysm, risk of rupture and mortality rates for any procedure undertaken [6]. Threshold sizes for intervention have now been established based on risk of rupture from longitudinal population studies of smaller aneurysms [7]. A Cochrane review, which summarised outcomes from four trials, concluded that repair conferred little advantage for small AAA < 5.5 cm diameter [8]. Currently in the UK, male patients would be considered for intervention for AAA > 5.5 cm diameter or in those which have shown rapid growth (> 1 cm) over the period of a year [9]. Patients with symptomatic tender aneurysms are also considered for urgent intervention as they may be at risk of imminent rupture. The intervention threshold for women is around 5.2 cm AAA diameter [4]. Patients with small AAA (<5 cm diameter) should be on surveillance programmes undergoing regular ultrasounds to assess size.

Medical management has been shown to have little impact on the disease course of AAAs [10]. Systematic reviews investigating medical therapies focussing on modifying risk factors for aneurysmal and cardiovascular disease failed to show evidence of any significant reduction in aneurysm size with use of anti-hypertensives. There is evidence; however, statin therapy may slow growth rates of AAAs [11].

The practice of detecting and potentially intervening on AAA at a pre-symptomatic stage has existed for a number of years. In the UK, this was initially undertaken by screening programmes in Chichester and Gloucester. The premise of these programmes was to offer an ultrasound of the abdominal aorta to a defined group who might be at risk of developing an AAA. Although few AAAs of a size meriting intervention were identified, there were significant numbers of smaller aneurysms which required long-term follow-up. This led to the implementation of aneurysm screening programmes in many developed countries. Programmes in England, Wales and Scotland have reported a steady decline in the incidence of AAA over time [12], as well as an increase in the age of first presentation [9]. This is validated by similar data from other countries with ongoing screening programmes [13].

Patients who fit the criteria for intervention for their AAA were historically offered open repair (OR) of the AAA and this has been considered the gold standard of treatment. However, since the 1990s EVAR has become a treatment option embraced by many vascular units around the world [14].

HISTORY OF ENDOVASCULAR ANEURYSM REPAIR

Although OR has long been established as successful, definitive management for AAA, many patients were excluded due to existing co-morbidities which led to significant morbidity and mortality rates. During the 1980s, several groups explored catheter-based intra-arterial treatment approaches, with the first successful EVAR being reported in 1991 by Parodi [15]. EVAR offers a minimally invasive option without the need for a laparotomy and in particular avoids cross-clamping of the aorta. In some cases, EVAR requires only local anaesthesia and percutaneous access to perform.

The concept is to introduce a covered stent intra-luminally to exclude the aortic sac from the systemic blood pressure and thus reduce the risk of complications such as rupture.

The early grafts were assembled in the operating theatre prior to deployment and were fairly rudimentary. These devices were deployed entirely within the abdominal aorta [16]. It quickly became apparent that distal fixation could be better achieved by the use of a bifurcated graft extending into the iliac arteries. This also led to the development of modifications to treat AAAs such as the aorto-uni-iliac graft followed by an extra-anatomical bypass such as a femoro-femoral cross-over to perfuse the contralateral limb. These were soon superseded by commercially developed modular systems which typically consisted of three components, with a main graft located within the abdominal aorta and varying lengths of separate stent grafts extending into the iliac arteries. This required accurate measurement of lengths and diameters of the aorto-iliac vessels to ensure adequate sealing peri-operatively and ensuring good durability. In an important step forward, the Food and Drug Administration in the United States of America approved the wider use of endovascular aortic grafts in 1999.

ADVANCES IN ENDOVASCULAR ANEURYSM REPAIR TECHNOLOGY

Advances in endovascular technology in the last three decades have revolutionised EVAR. The increased use of EVAR meant that the number of patients over 85 years of age undergoing intervention significantly increased and, by 2003, OR was no longer the most common AAA intervention [16]. Due to technological advances, some current commercially available grafts are now in their fourth generation.

There has been a constant drive to improve existing grafts and replace older technology with newer grafts to improve usability, safety and increase the range of aneurysmal disease amenable to treatment [17].

Some of the areas of development for modern EVAR devices include decreasing device profiles to enable access and passage through narrower vessels and even percutaneous delivery (pEVAR). The move towards pEVAR avoids the need for open surgical exposure at the access sites, typically in the groins. Also, by using percutaneous closure devices to seal the arteriotomy site, EVAR has been provided as a day case in some units. This is in stark contrast to the prolonged hospital admissions traditionally seen with OR for AAA surgery.

Early EVAR devices were designed to treat infra-renal aneurysms with suitably long and straight infra-renal aortic necks and a distal landing zone within the abdominal aorta. However, this restricted their use to a small percentage of the aneurysm population. Recent advances allow for EVAR deployment in AAA with more hostile shorter necks with the use of new sealing methods [18] and preservation of vital organ vessels with the use of fenestrations and branched grafts. There is the option to have custom-built grafts to treat suprarenal aneurysms and preserve mesenteric and renal artery perfusion. These devices need to be designed and manufactured on an individual basis after careful assessment of the proximal landing zone and spatial morphology of the renal and mesenteric vessels. They can take many weeks to produce and are considerably more costly than the straightforward EVAR grafts for infra-renal AAA.

An increasing volume of work and more clinical experience, using an increasing array of devices and adjuncts, has resulted in improved operator skills. There have been several large trials to assess the outcomes of endovascular repair and monitor long-term progress.

ENDOVASCULAR ANEURYSM REPAIR TRIALS

Although EVAR stents have been produced commercially since the late 1990s, there was initially little evidence to compare their performance against OR. To address this issue, four major multicentre prospective randomised control trials (RCTs) comparing OR versus EVAR for elective AAA repair have been conducted to date. Follow-up data from the initial trials are now available, with over a decade of outcome data in some cases. There has also been a separate prospective randomised trial which looked at outcomes of ruptured AAA, comparing EVAR with OR.

Endovascular aneurysm repair 1 trial

The EVAR 1 trial was the first trial established and was funded by the Health Technology Assessment programme in the United Kingdom. This was a RCT, investigating outcomes of EVAR versus OR in patients who were deemed fit to undergo intervention to treat the

AAA. The initial patients were recruited on 1st September 1999 and the trial closed on 31st August, 2004. A total of 1,082 elective (non-emergency) patients were randomised to receive either EVAR (n = 543) or OR (n = 539). Inclusion criteria for the trial were patients aged at least 60 years with AAA of diameter at least 5.5 cm, who were medically fit enough for OR. Patients were recruited from 41 British hospitals. The patients were followed up for peri-operative and late death, graft-related complications, and re-interventions until September 2009 (for an average follow-up of 7 years). The primary outcome measure was all-cause mortality and EVAR 1 remains the largest RCT of EVAR versus OR [19].

Dutch randomised endovascular aneurysm management trial

The DREAM (Dutch Randomised Endovascular Aneurysm Management) multicentre trial commenced a year after the EVAR 1 trial and involved 28 centres from the Netherlands and Belgium. It followed a similar protocol to the EVAR 1 trial and included patients with an AAA of at least 5 cm in diameter, who were considered suitable candidates for either EVAR or OR. Patients undergoing emergency AAA repair, or with inflammatory AAA, anatomical variations, connective-tissue disease, a history of organ transplantations, or a life expectancy of < 2 years were all excluded from the trial. The outcome events analysed were operative (30-day) mortality and two composite end points of operative mortality with severe complications and operative mortality with moderate or severe complications. Between 2000 and 2003, 345 patients were successfully recruited and followed up [20].

Open versus endovascular trial

The OVER (Open versus Endovascular) trial was the first United States-based RCT with a similar study design to the DREAM and EVAR 1 trials. The inclusion criteria were men with an AAA over 5 cm (or > 4.5 cm with rapid enlargement) or an iliac aneurysm over 3 cm. Between 2002 and 2008, 881 male patients were recruited from 42 vascular centres. Primary study outcomes included procedure failure, secondary interventions, major morbidity and death [21].

The Anévrysme de l'aorte abdominale, Chirurgie versus Endoprosthèse trial

The ACE (Anévrysme de l'aorte abdominale, Chirurgie versus Endoprosthèse) trial, a multicentre RCT based in France, shared similar protocols with the three other trials, with patients randomly assigned to OR or EVAR. Between 2003 and 2008, 316 patients were recruited from 25 centres throughout France. Women were also included in this trial, with their size threshold adjusted to a minimum of 4.5 cm before being considered for intervention [22].

The immediate management of patients with rupture: open versus endovascular aneurysm repair trial

The IMPROVE Immediate Management of Patients with Rupture: Open Versus EVAR) trial [23] was designed as a multicentre RCT to assess outcomes of intervention in patients diagnosed with AAA rupture. 613 patients, with a clinical diagnosis of ruptured AAA from across 30 centres, were randomised to either EVAR or OR. Patients randomised to EVAR then underwent an emergency computed tomography (CT) scan after clinical assessment to determine suitability for EVAR. If they were found to be anatomically unsuitable for EVAR, OR was undertaken. The primary outcome was 30-day mortality. Secondary outcomes included 24-hour mortality, in-hospital mortality, costs of primary admission and re-interventions during the primary admission.

Other studies

Data from regional databases and retrospective observational studies has also been analysed. Of particular note is the data from the 2015 Medicare study comparing outcomes of OR with EVAR [24]. This was a retrospective propensity-matched cohort study, analysing data from over 75,000 patients.

Registry data

The EUROSTAR (EUROpean collaborators on STent graft techniques for abdominal Aortic Repair) database also provides a source of longer-term outcomes from endovascular repair [25]. EUROSTAR was independent of any commercial interest and aimed to provide scientifically reliable assessment of endovascular AAA grafting. The results of 2,016 patients from 98 European institutions were collected and analysed.

Another observational study from Australia also compared the two treatment modalities for initial, and up to 15-year survival [26]. Data from 1,340 patients undergoing elective AAA repair was analysed over a period of 24 years.

The endovascular aneurysm repair 2 trial

The EVAR 2 trial recruited concurrently with EVAR 1 and focused on patients who were considered unfit for open AAA repair but were candidates for EVAR. Patients were eligible if they were at least 60 years of age and with an AAA of at least 5.5 cm on CT. Participants were randomised to receive either EVAR or no intervention. The primary outcome was all-cause mortality. Other outcomes were aneurysm-related mortality and graft-related complications with re-interventions. A total of 404 patients were recruited from 33 different British hospitals and there were no significant differences between the two groups at any time point following the repair. However, there were significantly less aneurysm-related deaths in the endovascular group compared to the no intervention group [27]. On follow-up, the EVAR group was not associated with a lower rate of death from any cause at any time, as the majority of the patients had a limited life span due to associated co-morbidities. Hence those patients with an AAA with significant co-morbidities did not benefit from EVAR and it was not found to be cost-effective

Complications after endovascular aneurysm repair

Peri-operative and early post-operative EVAR complications are relatively uncommon due to the minimally invasive nature of the intervention and often relate to the access sites. Careful observation is required to identify the development of limb ischaemia due to limb occlusion of the device. The development of post-operative bleeding can be clinically obvious but retroperitoneal haematomas can occur which may not present with external bleeding from the puncture site. One clinical sign may be flexion of the affected hip due to psoas major spasm.

Longer-term concerns are the durability of the graft and development of leaks; therefore, surveillance is vital to identify any complications which may arise. Surveillance strategies vary widely between vascular centres but typically included CT, duplex ultrasound, plain abdominal X-ray films or a combination of these imaging modalities at regular intervals. Most centres in the UK perform a CT scan at 6 weeks which sets a reference point for any future surveillance pathway.

Endoleaks are specific post-EVAR complications which may present at any time and have been classified into five types as shown in **Table 7.1.**

Types 1 and 3 endoleaks are considered to be the most important as the aneurysm sac is exposed to systemic blood pressure with increased risk of rupture, and emergent treatment may be necessary. Type 2 endoleak is the most common and the treatment remains controversial as it is often undertaken in the context of sac size increase. Analysis of EUROSTAR findings suggests the risk of rupture occurring with type 2 endoleak to be no greater than without type 2 endoleak. Other complications which may become apparent on long-term surveillance imaging include graft limb thrombosis, strut fracture and migration which may progress to type 1 endoleak.

Table 7.1 Classification of endoleaks	
Type of endoleak	**Characteristics of endoleak**
Type 1	Failure of proximal or distal sealing zones (**Figure 7.1**)
Type 2	Perfusion from patent lumbar or inferior mesenteric arteries (**Figure 7.2**)
Type 3	Failure at stent overlap sites or fractures/defects in the graft itself (**Figure 7.3**)
Type 4	Graft porosity (invariably detected during procedure or early post-procedural period)
Type 5	Aortic sac expansion without a definitive cause

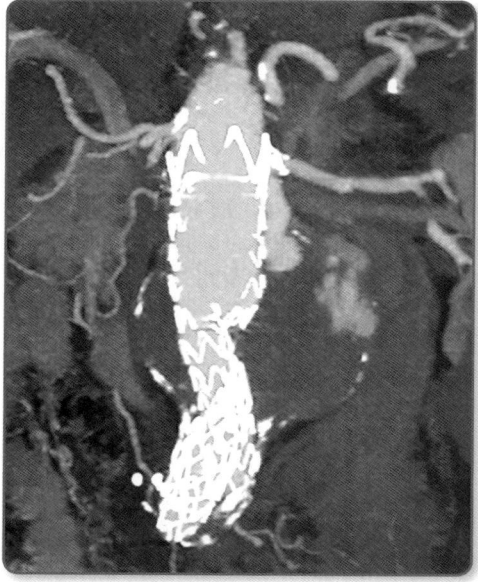

Figure 7.1 Large type 1 endoleak: The aneurysm sac now extends above the proximal graft markers, resulting in sac expansion and rupture.

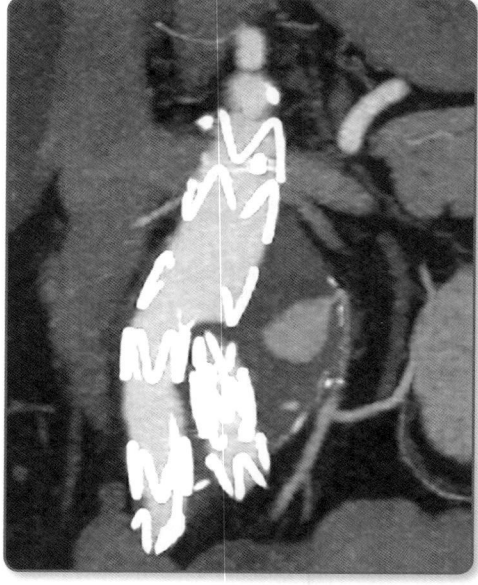

Figure 7.2 Type 2 endoleak with IMA as feeding vessel resulting in sac expansion.

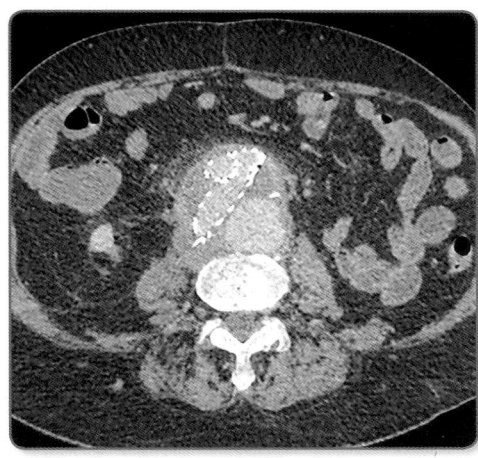

Figure 7.3 Disconnection of the left iliac limb is seen with large type 3 endoleak and significant increase in sac size.

OUTCOMES FROM CLINICAL TRIALS AND REGISTRIES

Early- and intermediate-term outcomes from endovascular aneurysm repair trials

The EVAR 1 was the first trial and has the longest follow-up to date. Baseline characteristics were similar between the two patient cohorts. All cause 30-day mortality results showed significantly lower peri-operative mortality for EVAR compared to OR (1.8 vs. 4.3%). This benefit of EVAR was maintained up to 6 months post-procedure with the EVAR group mortality approximately half that of the OR cohort (26/626 vs. 45/626). However by the end of 4-year follow-up this advantage was lost, with both all-cause mortality and aneurysm-related death higher in the EVAR group.

The DREAM trial, which had a similar study design to EVAR 1, showed similar 30-day outcomes. The combined rate of operative mortality and severe complications was higher in the OR (9.8%) group compared to EVAR (4.7%). At 6.4-year median follow-up, the principal finding was that for large aneurysms there was no significant difference in survival. Re-intervention rate was found to be significantly higher in the EVAR group at this time point.

The ACE trial, with a similar design protocol to EVAR 1 and DREAM, had a median follow-up of 3 years. Results from this trial at 1 year and 3 years showed no difference in the cumulative survival free of death or major events rates between OR and EVAR. In-hospital mortality, survival, and the percentage of minor complications were not statistically different. In the EVAR group, however, there was again a higher proportion of re-interventions with a trend toward a higher aneurysm-related mortality.

In the OVER trial, 30-day mortality was 0.5% after EVAR and 3% after OR. However, at 2-year follow-up both groups had similar mortality. Outcomes from the ACE trial showed no difference in short-term performance between EVAR and OR, with survival or major adverse events rates at 1-year follow-up was not significantly different.

A meta-analysis in 2013, using individual patient data from these four major trials, again showed similar outcomes, with the initial benefit conferred by EVAR lost by about 2–3 years, and a later surge in mortality in the EVAR group, resulting in similar mortality rates

Table 7.2 Comparison of the early outcomes of the four randomised prospective RCTs comparing EVAR to OR in patients undergoing elective intervention for AAA

	EVAR 1 (n=1252)	ACE (n=299)	DREAM (n=351)	OVER (n=881)
Age (mean)	74	69	70	70
Follow-up (years)	6	3.1	6	5.4
30-day mortality EVAR	1.8%	1.3%	1.2%	0.2%
30-day mortality OR	4.3%	0.7%	2.9%	1.9%
Re-intervention rates EVAR	5.1%	7.6%	8.5%	6.6%
Re-intervention rates OR	1.9%	2.5%	4.4%	4.6%

(AAA, abdominal aortic aneurysm; ACE, Anévrysme de l'aorte abdominale, Chirurgie versus Endoprosthèse; DREAM, Dutch Randomised Endovascular Aneurysm Management; EVAR, endovascular aneurysm repair; RCT, randomised controlled trial; OR, open repair; OVER, Open versus Endovascular)

in both groups (**Table 7.2**). Re-intervention rates remained consistently higher in the EVAR group in all four trials [28].

Results from the IMPROVE trial for management of ruptured AAAs showed no overall difference in 30-day mortality between OR and EVAR. Secondary outcomes of in-hospital mortality, number of re-interventions and overall cost remained similar. However, the length of critical care stay and total hospital stay was shorter for the EVAR group. Women were observed to have better outcomes after EVAR which may be of significance in clinical practice. 3-year follow-up data showed borderline benefit in survival for the EVAR group, with women still maintaining a benefit from EVAR. Open repair had longer hospital stays and higher initial complication rates compared to EVAR but health-related quality-of-life data (HRQoL) was equivalent at 3-year follow-up. A further publication reporting the 3-year results of the IMPROVE trial demonstrated a survival advantage for EVAR over open repair and evidence of cost effectiveness [29].

Results from the EUROSTAR registry show that complications post-EVAR are more common in patients with large aneurysms, advanced age, and in those where adjuvant procedures are required. In addition, compromise of either cardiac or general medical status has adverse effects on the risk of systemic complications. The experience of the operating team is an important factor, influencing device- and procedure-related complications. Data from the registry showed similar life expectancy in both groups [30].

Results from the Medicare retrospective data confirm the findings from the larger randomised trials, showing an increased risk of late rupture with the EVAR group [24]. However, it was noted that EVAR outcomes improved with time.

Results from other retrospective, smaller studies mentioned earlier also share similar results as the larger trials. An observational study from a single institution in Queensland, Australia [26] reported no differences in 5-year, 10-year, and 15-year survival between OR (n = 982; median follow-up 6·5 years) and EVAR (n = 358; median follow-up 4·0 years), but had incomplete patient reporting.

Longer-term outcomes of endovascular repair

The EVAR 1 trial is now in its second decade of data collection and remains the longest running trial on EVAR worldwide. The trial was initially funded for 4 years; however, further funding was secured to continue longer-term data collection.

Follow-up was undertaken until 30 June 2015 (mean 12.7 years; median 12.4 years; minimum 1.8 years; maximum, 15.8 years) for EVAR 1. Follow-up beyond 8 years showed an increase in mortality (all-cause and aneurysm-related) in the EVAR group. An early survival benefit of EVAR during the first 6 months was then lost, with similar mortality between the groups from 6 months to 8 years, but thereafter an increase in mortality in the EVAR group. Overall, there were 31 deaths from rupture after aneurysm repair in the EVAR group and five in the OR group. There was no evidence of a difference in cancer-related mortality between the groups overall; however, there was a suggestion of increase in cancer after 8-years follow-up in the EVAR group.

In total, there were 258 graft-related re-interventions performed in 165 patients in the EVAR group and 105 graft-related re-interventions performed in 74 patients in the OR group. The re-intervention rate was significantly higher in the EVAR group (including conversion to OR, repeat EVAR and treatment of graft infection) during every time period compared to OR. The relative difference in re-intervention rate between the groups was highest in the period 6 months to 4 years after randomisation.

The principal findings from the four major RCTs is that the initial peri-operative mortality rates are significantly higher for open AAA repair compared to EVAR (4.7% vs. 1.6%) [19]. However, the early benefit of EVAR diminishes by 4 years and there is evidence by 15 years there may be superior long-term survival rates for OR.

One possible reason for the late surge in the EVAR group mortality rates may be partly related to cancer deaths as the initial EVAR 1 follow-up protocol required annual CT scans for EVAR graft surveillance. Indeed, the need for long-term surveillance (with associated ionising radiation and contrast burdens) is an important consideration when making the initial decision between EVAR and OR.

Another consideration from the longer-term follow-up is that the number of re-interventions in the EVAR group remained significantly higher throughout the follow-up period. There is a potential for bias here as the EVAR group were followed up more vigilantly with annual scans, while the OR group saw a decline in frequency of follow-up imaging. Therefore, there is the possibility that further re-interventions were missed in the OR group due to a lack of post-operative imaging. Endovascular technology has progressed significantly over the two decades since the start of the EVAR 1 trial, with significant improvement in both devices and planning software. Thus, the device performance from those implanted in 1999 cannot be realistically compared to those currently available.

The cost effectiveness and health-related benefit of EVAR versus OR has been a subject of much debate [31]. The EVAR 1 trial collected HRQoL data in both groups and although there is a decline in scores in both, during the initial 6 months after intervention, those undergoing EVAR had a better HRQoL. After 6 months, there was no significant difference between the two groups and there was a decline in the HRQoL scores after every re-intervention. Therefore, the initial gain in the EVAR group due to shorter hospital stay, brief recovery period and lower operative mortality, is attenuated over the longer-term by increased re-interventions and an increase in mortality in this group. Lifetime costs are also higher for the EVAR group. The DREAM trial, concluded that EVAR was not cost-effective even after 1 year, whilst the OVER trial concluded that EVAR was effective and cost-effective at 2 years, but this was in a lower-risk group and did not take account of late mortality or re-interventions.

Five-year data from the ENGAGE registry [32], which followed up results from the next-generation endurant graft, showed promising 5-year outcomes in terms of freedom from aneurysm-related mortality, stable or decreased AAA sac diameter and less secondary endovascular procedures. However, these are results based on their own data collection and the performance of only one graft system.

One possible reason for the higher post-EVAR re-intervention may be poor adherence to the instructions for use (IFU). It is difficult to ascertain from the studies published whether failure of adherence to the IFU contributed to possible graft failure. This is potentially a major factor in the long-term follow-up of EVAR durability. There is no doubt that short infra-renal aortic necks are a source of failure for EVAR and more sophisticated devices have been produced in the form of branched or fenestrated EVAR. A meta-analysis has been performed concluding that short aortic necks (< 15 mm) and severe angulation (> 60°) are associated with a higher incidence of endoleaks and EVAR failure [33]. It has also been shown that over-sizing aortic grafts contributes to progressive aneurysm neck dilatation and thus the risk of proximal type 1 endoleak [34].

Current recommendations for endovascular aneurysm repair

Recently, both the European Society for Vascular Surgery (ESVS) and the National Institute of Clinical Excellence (NICE) have published recommendations regarding endovascular repair of AAA.

The ESVS recommends that patients with a 'reasonable' life expectancy and appropriate anatomy should be considered for an EVAR as the preferred treatment modality, with OR preferred for patients with a long life expectancy [35]. In patients with a ruptured AAA and suitable anatomy, EVAR should be the preferred modality.

The NICE guidelines, when initially published as a draft document, were met with controversy due to the recommendations which suggested that EVAR should not be considered for patients unfit for OR. This decision generated much debate as it was viewed as biased toward OR due to the better longer-term outcomes from trials. Subsequently, after a period of feedback from stakeholders and engagement, the full guidelines were published in 2020 [36]. These have now been modified to recommend the use of EVAR for patients who would not be suitable for OR. However, there remains an emphasis on consideration of OR as first-line treatment for AAAs.

Future directions for endovascular aneurysm repair

Surveillance techniques, to monitor the fixation of an endograft, are increasingly using non-invasive technologies such as duplex ultrasound, which reduces the need for ionising radiation. Over the long term, further dilatation of aortic wall can continue post-EVAR. This may result in either graft migration or development of endoleaks. Hence this necessitates rigorous post-operative surveillance to prevent sac expansion and rupture. Numerous commercial partners continue to develop smaller more flexible devices which address both patient individual anatomical features and aim to ease deployment and allow operators to use them effectively and follow IFU. The field of materials science is also a rich area for research in order to determine whether new materials can mitigate against stent fracture and displacement.

CONCLUSION

The incidence of AAA in developed countries seems to be decreasing, due partly to the introduction of screening programmes and better risk factor modification. Screened patients tend to be younger and fitter than symptomatic patients and therefore require surgery which confers a long-term benefit. The four RCTs comparing EVAR with OR showed an initial benefit of endovascular repair on 30-day survival. However, this benefit is later lost with potentially worse longer-term outcomes for patients undergoing EVAR. Therefore, clinicians need to be guided by anticipated life expectancy, aneurysm morphology and existing co-morbidities when deciding which treatment modality best suits individual patients.

Key points for clinical practice

- The incidence of AAA is declining in developed countries
- Endovascular AAA repair remains a viable option in patients medically unfit for open repair, but with reasonable life expectancy
- Advances in endovascular stent grafts now offer solutions for AAAs with unfavourable anatomy
- Open repair remains the "gold standard" based on long-term outcomes
- Endovascular AAA repair has been shown to be a better option in a ruptured aneurysm, especially for women
- Careful decision-making is important when considering OR versus EVAR based on patient age, life expectancy, aneurysm morphology, local expertise and outcomes

---

REFERENCES

1. Collin J, Araujo L, Walton J, et al. Oxford screening programme for abdominal aortic aneurysm in men aged 65 to 74 years. Lancet 1988; 2:613–615.
2. Ashton HA, Buxton MJ, Day NE, et al. The Multicentre Aneurysm Screening Study (MASS) into the effect of abdominal aortic aneurysm screening on mortality in men: a randomised controlled trial. Lancet 2002; 360:1531–1539.
3. Freestone T, Turner RJ, Coady A, et al. Inflammation and Matrix Metalloproteinases in the Enlarging Abdominal Aortic Aneurysm. Arterioscler Thromb Vasc Biol 1995; 15:1145–1151.
4. Hultgren R, Granath F, Swedenborg J. Different disease profiles for women and men with abdominal aortic aneurysms. Eur J Vasc Endovasc Surg 2007; 33:556–560.
5. Chaikof EL, Dalman RL, Eskandari MK, et al. The Society for Vascular Surgery practice guidelines on the care of patients with an abdominal aortic aneurysm. J Vasc Surg 2018; 67:2–77.e2.
6. Welch HG, Albertsen PC, Nease RF, et al. Estimating treatment benefits for the elderly: the effect of competing risks. Ann Intern Med 1996; 124:577–584.
7. Brown PM, Zelt DT, Sobolev B. The risk of rupture in untreated aneurysms: the impact of size, gender, and expansion rate. J Vasc Surg 2003; 37:280–284.
8. Ulug P, Powell JT, Martinez MA-M, et al. Surgery for small asymptomatic abdominal aortic aneurysms. Cochrane Database Syst Rev 2020.
9. Heather BP, Poskitt KR, Earnshaw JJ, et al. Population screening reduces mortality rate from aortic aneurysm in men. Br J Surg 2000; 87:750–753.
10. Golledge J, Norman PE. Current status of medical management for abdominal aortic aneurysm. Atherosclerosis 2011; 217:57–63.
11. Weiss N, Rodionov RN, Mahlmann A. Medical management of abdominal aortic aneurysms. VASA 2014; 43:415–421.
12. Norman PE, Jamrozik K, Lawrence-Brown MM, et al. Population based randomised controlled trial on impact of screening on mortality from abdominal aortic aneurysm. BMJ 2004; 329:1259.
13. Svensjö S, Björck M, Gürtelschmid M, et al. Low Prevalence of Abdominal aortic aneurysm among 65-year-old Swedish men indicates a change in the epidemiology of the disease. Circulation 2011; 124:1118–1123.

14. England A & McWilliams R. Endovascular Aortic Aneurysm Repair (EVAR). Ulster Med J 2013; 82:3–10.

15. Parodi JC, Palmaz JC, Barone HD. Transfemoral intraluminal graft implantation for abdominal aortic aneurysms. Ann Vasc Surg 1991; 5:491–499.

16. Schwarze ML, Shen Y, Hemmerich J, et al. Age-related trends in utilization and outcome of open and endovascular repair for abdominal aortic aneurysm in the United States, 2001-2006. J Vasc Surg 2009; 50:722–729.

17. Verzini F. (2016). Device developments in evar: what we learned from the past; what we need for the future vascular news. [online] Available from https://vascularnews.com/device-developments-in-evar-what-we-learned-from-the-past-what-we-need-for-the-future/. [Last accessed December, 2020].

18. Foteh M. Endoanchors advance treatment of aortic aaneurysms: experience in a community hospital. Endovascular Today 2016; 16–22.

19. EVAR trial participants. Endovascular aneurysm repair versus open repair in patients with abdominal aortic aneurysm (EVAR trial 1): randomised controlled trial. Lancet 2005; 365:2179–2186.

20. Prinssen M, Verhoeven ELG, Buth J, et al. A randomized trial comparing conventional and endovascular repair of abdominal aortic aneurysms. N Engl J Med 2004; 351:1607–1618.

21. Lederle FA, Freischlag JA, Kyriakides TC, et al. Outcomes following endovascular vs open repair of abdominal aortic aneurysm: a randomized trial. JAMA 2009; 302:1535–1542.

22. Becquemin JP, PilletJC, Lescalie F, et al. A randomized controlled trial of endovascular aneurysm repair versus open surgery for abdominal aortic aneurysms in low- to moderate-risk patients. J Vasc Surg 2011; 53:1167–1173

23. Investigators I trial. Endovascular or open repair strategy for ruptured abdominal aortic aneurysm: 30 day outcomes from IMPROVE randomised trial. BMJ 2014; 348:f7661.

24. Schermerhorn ML, Buck DB, O'Malley AJ, et al. Long-Term Outcomes of Abdominal Aortic Aneurysm in the Medicare Population. N Engl J Med 2015; 373:328–338.

25. Buth J. Endovascular repair of abdominal aortic aneurysms. Results from the EUROSTAR registry. EUROpean collaborators on Stent-graft Techniques for abdominal aortic aneurysm Repair. Semin Interv Cardiol 2000; 5:29–33.

26. Khashram M, Jenkins JS, Jenkins J, et al. Long-term outcomes and factors influencing late survival following elective abdominal aortic aneurysm repair: A 24-year experience. Vascular 2016; 24:115–125.

27. The United Kingdom EVAR Trial Investigators. Endovascular repair of aortic aneurysm in patients physically ineligible for open repair. N Engl J Med 2010; 362:1872–1880.

28. Powell JT, Sweeting MJ, Ulug P et al. Meta-analysis of individual-patient data from EVAR-1, DREAM, OVER and ACE trials comparing outcomes of endovascular or open repair for abdominal aortic aneurysm over 5 years. Br J Surg 2017; 104:166–178.

29. IMPROVE trial investigators. Comparative clinical effectiveness and cost effectiveness of endovascular strategy v open repair for ruptured abdominal aortic aneurysm: three year results of the IMPROVE randomised trial. BMJ 2017; 359:j4859.

30. Schermerhorn ML, Finlayson SRG, Fillinger MF, et al. Life expectancy after endovascular versus open abdominal aortic aneurysm repair: Results of a decision analysis model on the basis of data from EUROSTAR. J Vasc Surg 2002; 36:1112–1120.

31. Patel R, Powell JT, Sweeting MJ, et al. The UK EndoVascular Aneurysm Repair (EVAR) randomised controlled trials: long-term follow-up and cost-effectiveness analysis. Health Technol Assess Winch Engl 2018; 22:1–132.

32. Stokmans RA, Teijink JAW, Forbes TL, et al. Early results from the ENGAGE registry: real-world performance of the endurant stent graft for endovascular AAA repair in 1262 patients. Eur J Vasc Endovasc Surg 2012; 44:369–375.

33. Antoniou GA, Georgiadis GS, Antoniou SA, et al. A meta-analysis of outcomes of endovascular abdominal aortic aneurysm repair in patients with hostile and friendly neck anatomy. J Vasc Surg 2013; 57:527–538.

34. van Prehn J, Schlösser FJV, Muhs BE, et al. Oversizing of aortic stent grafts for abdominal aneurysm repair: a systematic review of the benefits and risks. Eur J Vasc Endovasc Surg 2009; 38:42–53.

35. Wanhainen A, Verzini F, Van Herzeele I, et al. Clinical practice guidelines on the management of abdominal aorto-iliac artery aneurysms. Eur J Vasc Endovasc Surg 2019; 57:8–93.

36. National Institute for Health and Care Excellence. (2020). Abdominal aortic aneurysm: diagnosis and management. [online] Available from https://www.nice.org.uk/guidance/NG156. [Last accessed December, 2020].

Section 5

Head and neck surgery

Chapter 8

Osteonecrosis of the jaw: An iatrogenic condition in the 21st century

Michael Fardy

INTRODUCTION

Osteonecrosis, also known as avascular necrosis or aseptic necrosis, is defined as the death of bone due to lack of blood supply. It is commonly seen in hip and knee joints but also occurs in the jaw, shoulders, hands, and feet. It often presents as pain and there is then an associated collapse with the development of degenerative arthritis.

The common causes are:

- Trauma, e.g. fractured neck of femur which results in avascular necrosis of the femoral head
- Prolonged use of high dose corticosteroid injections

Less common causes are:

- Blood disorders, e.g. sickle cell anaemia; systemic lupus erythematosus
- Radiation
- Medication, e.g. bisphosphonates

Osteonecrosis has differing clinical presentations depending upon cause and anatomical site and treatment is still a subject of both research and controversy.

HISTORY

Osteonecrosis is not a new disease. It was first recognised around 1860, as it was associated with environmental substances such as lead and white phosphorous used in matches and common medications available at that time such as mercury, arsenic or bismuth. During the 19th century, those who worked with white phosphorous, particularly in the matchstick industry, were reported to develop osteonecrosis of the mandible leading to loss of teeth and pathological fractures. It commonly occurred in those with poor gingival health and was known as Phossy jaw [1].

In modern times, the two main causes of osteonecrosis of the head and neck are:

1. Osteoradionecrosis (ORN)
2. Bisphosphonate related osteonecrosis of the jaw (BRONJ)

OSTEORADIONECROSIS

Osteoradionecrosis was first described by Regaud in 1922 [2] and in 1926 Ewing recognised the bone changes associated with radiation therapy and described them as 'radiation osteitis [3]'. The current definition of ORN is 'exposed irradiated bone that fails to heal over a period of 3 months, without evidence of tumour or recurrent tumour [4–6]'.

Although, surgery is the mainstay of treatment for head and neck cancers, adjuvant radiotherapy is recommended for stage 3 and 4 disease [7] and in cases where there are close or involved margins, or positive neck nodal disease. In the management of oropharyngeal cancer, the detection of human papillomavirus (HPV) has greatly altered its management. It has been reported that patients with HPV related oropharyngeal squamous cell carcinoma (SCC) have a better prognosis than HPV negative patients when treated with chemoradiotherapy [8]. The advantage of these oncological treatments in terms of organ preservation is obvious, but what must be borne in mind is the acute and long term effects associated with these protocols, in particular greater morbidity and reduced quality of life (QOL). Rogers et al [9]. noted that concurrent chemoradiotherapy is associated with considerable reduction in weight, mobility, and QOL [10].

As well as ORN (**Figure 8.1**), other life changing complications of radiotherapy include xerostomia, radiation caries, loss of taste, salivary dysfunction, oral mucositis which is extremely debilitating, as well as the potential for wound breakdown and skin loss (**Figure 8.2a** and **b**) after surgery in rehabilitating patients following ORN [10].

In the study by Jabbari et al [11]. QOL and xerostomia were compared between those patients who received intensity modulated radiotherapy (IMRT) and those who received standard radiotherapy and they found that QOL improved with time after IMRT [11]. These findings have also been supported by Ben-David et al [12]. Therefore, this new method of radiotherapy, may be the way forward to reduce some or all the complications of radiotherapy for head and neck and other cancers.

Comprehensive reviews of ORN have been published by Chronopoulos [13], Lyons [14], and Nadella [15] and a review of these articles is recommended.

Pathogenesis

The pathogenesis of ORN has been widely discussed and various theories have been proposed. Meyer [16] proposed that ORN was due to a combination of radiation, trauma, and infection. This theory was supported by experimental evidence demonstrating evidence of bacteria in tissues affected by ORN with microscopic evidence of thickening of arteriolar and arterial walls, loss of osteocytes and osteoblasts and the bony cavities containing inflammatory cells. This theory popularised the use of antibiotics with surgery to treat ORN.

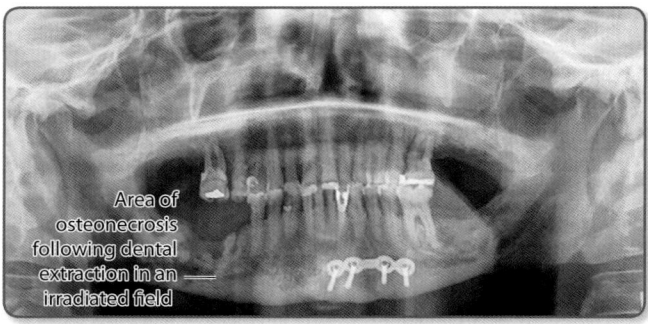

Figure 8.1 Osteoradionecrosis of jaw – postdental extraction.

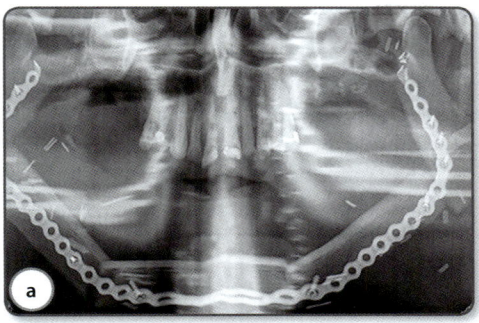
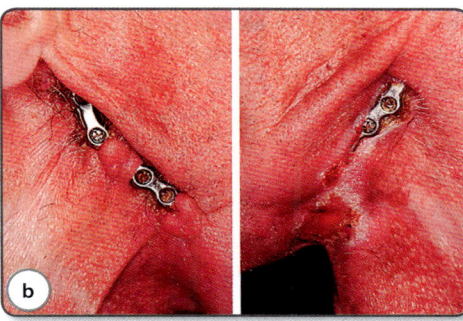

Figure 8.2 Skin loss after total mandibular reconstruction with fibular flap for treatment of osteoradionecrosis (ORN). (a) Radiological view of reconstruction; (b) Clinical photographs – bilateral jawline skin loss due to poor vascularity of skin, exposing reconstruction plates and predisposing to infection.

Following Meyer's theory, Marx [17] proposed a new theory to explain the pathophysiology of ORN – this was the 'hypoxic-hypocellular – hypovascular' theory. In looking at the possibility of confirming whether this was an infective process, the microbiology in ORN was noted to be different to that seen in osteomyelitis. In ORN, microbes detected were mainly surface contaminants, whereas in osteomyelitis *Staphylococcus* was the primary organism present. Marx concluded that ORN is not a primary infection of irradiated bone, but a complex metabolic deficiency of tissue, created by radiation induced cellular injury and then contaminated with micro-organisms from the local area.

More recently, a new theory has been put forward, namely 'radiation induced fibrosis [18]'. It has been proposed that the histopathology of ORN closely resembles that seen in the chronic healing of traumatic wounds [19]. According to this theory, the main event in the progression of ORN is the activation and dysregulation of fibroblastic activity which leads to atrophic tissue within a previously irradiated area [18]. A more extensive overview can be found in the review by Lyons [14].

It has been suggested that the mandible is more likely to be affected because the fibrosis causes the obliteration of the inferior alveolar artery, together with the failure of the facial artery to form a collateral supply [20].

Management

For the purpose of clinical management, ORN can be divided into two groups [21].
1. *Induced ORN*: This occurs when external factors are involved, e.g. dental extractions, dental implants, denture placement, and infection.
2. *Spontaneous ORN*: This was noted in over half of the patients in Patel's study despite excellent pre- and postradiotherapy dental care [21]. Addition of chemotherapy may also contribute to this condition.

The first priority of management is to try to prevent the occurrence of ORN. Therefore, regular dental visits are vital for patients undergoing radiotherapy to the jaw area, and close liaison with the head and neck team including the restorative consultant and hygienist are paramount.

Cases of ORN vary in their aetiology and severity and therefore staging has been proposed to rationalise the treatment plan. Numerous attempts to find an ideal classification have been based on clinical and radiological findings, disease progression, duration of bone exposure, imaging, and indication for treatment (reviewed by Chronopoulos) [13]. A recent classification by Notani et al [22]. is based on clinical findings. Cases are classified into three grades based on the extent of the ORN lesion:

- *Grade I*: ORN confined to the alveolar bone
- *Grade II*: ORN limited to the alveolar bone and/or the mandible above the level of the mandibular alveolar canal
- *Grade III*: ORN extends to the mandible below the level of the mandibular alveolar canal and a skin fistula and/ or a pathological fracture is present.

Conventional management of this condition currently includes both medical and surgical approaches.

Medical

It has been suggested that the treatment of choice for ORN is medical and includes drug treatments and hyperbaric oxygen.

Drug treatments

Several drugs have been proposed to reverse the changes in reactive oxygen species which produce radiation induced fibrosis and ultimately ORN.

Pentoxifylline is a methylxanthine derivative, used in vascular disease to manage intermittent claudication and works via an antitumour necrosis factor (TNF) effect to increase erythrocyte flexibility, dilate blood vessels, inhibit proliferation of human dermal fibroblasts, and stimulate production of extracellular matrix. Its use in the head and neck was first proposed by Futran et al [23]. in order to manage the problems of fibrosis and a comprehensive review of its use in ORN has been published [24]. It is used as a combination therapy with tocopherol in the treatment of ORN. Tocopherol (vitamin E) is a scavenger of reactive oxygen species which are generated during oxidative stress by protecting cell membranes against peroxidation of lipids and expression of procollagen genes. When these drugs are taken together, in a combination termed PENTO, they act synergistically as potent antifibrotic agents. However, Kahenasa reported that this combination was successful in healing superficial cases of radiation fibrosis but not cases of ORN [25]. In contrast, Patel et al [21]. reported that PENTO produced healing in 56% of these patients. Similar results were published by Robard, who added clodronate to the combination (PENTOCLO) producing healing in 59% [26]. However, the time to healing was considerably longer for the Patel group [237 days (62–1,080)] compared to the Robard study [82 days (32–266)].

Clodronate is a modern bisphosphonate which inhibits bone resorption by reducing the number and activity of osteoclasts. Delanin et al [27] found that a combination of clodronate and PENTO was beneficial in severe cases of radiation induced fibroatrophic processes inducing mandibular ORN, but there was the potential risk of medication induced osteonecrosis as it is a bisphosphonate.

Hyperbaric oxygen therapy

Oxygen is essential to restore the cohesion of hard and soft tissues in both normal tissue homeostasis and wound healing. It has been noted that all aspects of tissue repair– collagen synthesis, bone formation, matrix deposition for neoangiogenesis and leucocyte bactericidal activity are influenced by tissue oxygen tension [28–33].

It has been suggested that hyperbaric oxygen therapy (HBO) may be the only modality which can reverse the delayed radiation changes in tissues, by generating steep oxygen gradients between normal and irradiated tissue causing oxygen to diffuse into the affected areas [34].

Hyperbaric oxygen in the prevention of osteoradionecrosis: Hyperbaric oxygen has been proposed for the prevention of ORN by several groups including Mainous et al [35]. and Marx's team [36]. This randomised trial compared HBO with penicillin alone to prevent ORN after dental extraction and reported that the HBO group had a lower incidence of ORN [36].

In 2003, Sulaiman et al presented data from the Memorial Sloan Kettering Cancer Centre (MSKCC) reviewing 1,194 patients with a history of head and neck radiation who were subsequently treated in the dental service. Dental extractions were required in 187 and only 4 (2.14%) developed ORN. There were 7 who had extractions by professionals outside of MSKCC giving an overall incidence of ORN of 5.58%. Therefore, the results of the Marx paper [36] were not reproduced [37] and the use of HBO for the prevention of ORN remains unproven.

However, interest in this area continues and in 2019, Shaw published the results of a trial into the use of HBO – the Hyperbaric Oxygen for the Prevention of Osteoradionecrosis (HOPON) trial [38]. This was a prospective, multicentre, randomised controlled, phase III trial to assess the effectiveness of preventing ORN after surgical procedures in the irradiated mandible. The trial enrolled 144 patients and the data from 100 patients who had been treated for head and neck cancer and then required dental surgery were analysed. Primary outcome was development of ORN. The study concluded that the low incidence of ORN makes recommending HBO for dental extractions or implant placement in the irradiated mandible unnecessary.

Hyperbaric oxygen in the treatment of osteoradionecrosis: Hyperbaric oxygen has been used as a definitive treatment for ORN on an empirical basis in many units worldwide, but the evidence to support its use is again controversial [39-41]. In 2004, Annane published results of a prospective, multicentre, randomised placebo–controlled double blind trial [39]. This was conducted at 12 university hospitals where ambulatory adults with ORN were assigned to receive 30 HBO exposures preoperatively for 90 minutes or a placebo and 10 additional doses postoperatively. The primary outcome measure was 1 year recovery from ORN. Secondary end points included time to treatment failure, time to pain relief, 1 year mortality rate, and treatment safety. This trial enrolled 68 patients. At 1 year, 6/31 patients (19%) recovered in the HBO arm and 12/37 (32%) in the placebo group (p = 0.23). Time to treatment failure and time to pain relief, were similar in the two groups. The conclusion of this study was that patients with overt mandibular ORN did not benefit from HBO and the study was stopped prematurely due to the futility of the effectiveness of HBO [39].

In 2005, the Cochrane collaboration [42] published a review of the use of HBO therapy in relation to the late effects of radiation therapy. It was noted that apart from the trial published by Marx [43], which reported that HBO improves bony healing and maintains bony volume after nonvascularised reconstruction of hemimandibular defects in irradiated areas, no other trials were found to support its use.

Therefore, the management of ORN remains extremely challenging. There is conflicting evidence for the use of HBO as part of a preventative treatment plan, and there is no apparent advantage to the use of HBO for the active treatment of ORN. However, a recent trial protocol proposed by Bulsara [44] aims to conduct a prospective randomised pilot study comparing HBO to PENTO and clodronate for the management of early mandibular ORN. The results are eagerly anticipated, but what can be accepted is that further clinical trials are required to manage this very difficult and distressing complication of radiotherapy.

Surgery

Surgery plays a vital role in the management of ORN – either as primary treatment or when medical treatment has failed to resolve the situation. Where there is the need for bony reconstruction of the mandible, the only viable option is the utilisation of vascularised tissue since the use of nonvascularised bone grafts will fail due to the lack of adequate blood supply. The two sites mainly used as a source of vascularised bone are the fibula [45] and the iliac crest [46].

There have been major advances with the use of CadCam (computer aided design and computer aided manufacturing) technology, where everything is planned prior to the operating room - resection, bony reconstruction, formation of cutting guides and a preformed plate (**Figures 8.3a** to **f**). Using the technique of conformal design, a stronger alloy can be used with potentially a better fit. The preplanning allows significant surgical time to be saved and aesthetics are better predicted. The corresponding clinical/operative photographs are shown in **Figures 8.4a** to **f**. The important point to remember is the vital role of the dental technician who uses the 3D computed tomography (CT) to help plan the case in conjunction with the surgeon, supervising the construction of the cutting guides and final template. This emphasises the requirement of a team approach.

MEDICATION-RELATED OSTEONECROSIS OF JAW

Bisphosphonates are used widely in a variety of medical conditions including osteoporosis, Paget's disease, and ankylosing spondylitis. In oncology patients, bone pain and pathological fractures can be a very difficult problem to resolve. In particular, multiple myeloma can cause destruction which results in serious clinical issues. Bisphosphonates have an affinity for bone and are recognised as a first line agent for the treatment of patients with bony metastases, multiple myeloma and hypercalcaemia [47]. Unfortunately, bisphosphonate osteonecrosis was noted soon after its initial use and the first report appeared in 2003 by Marx [48].

The American Association of Oral and Maxillofacial Surgery (AAOMS) originally stated that patients had BRONJ if all three characteristics are present:

1. Current or previous treatment with bisphosphonates.
2. Exposed bone in the maxillofacial region for longer than 8 weeks.
3. No history of radiation therapy.

However, in 2014, AAOMS produced a position paper on osteonecrosis and recommended a name change to medication-related osteonecrosis of jaw (MRONJ), an example of which is shown in **Figure 8.5**. The paper centred on clinical findings and radiology, although using both criteria may overestimate the frequency [49]. The purpose of the position paper was to provide clinicians with-

- Risk estimates of developing MRONJ
- Comparisons of the risks and benefits of medications related to osteonecrosis to aid in treatment planning
- Assistance in the development of MRONJ prevention measures

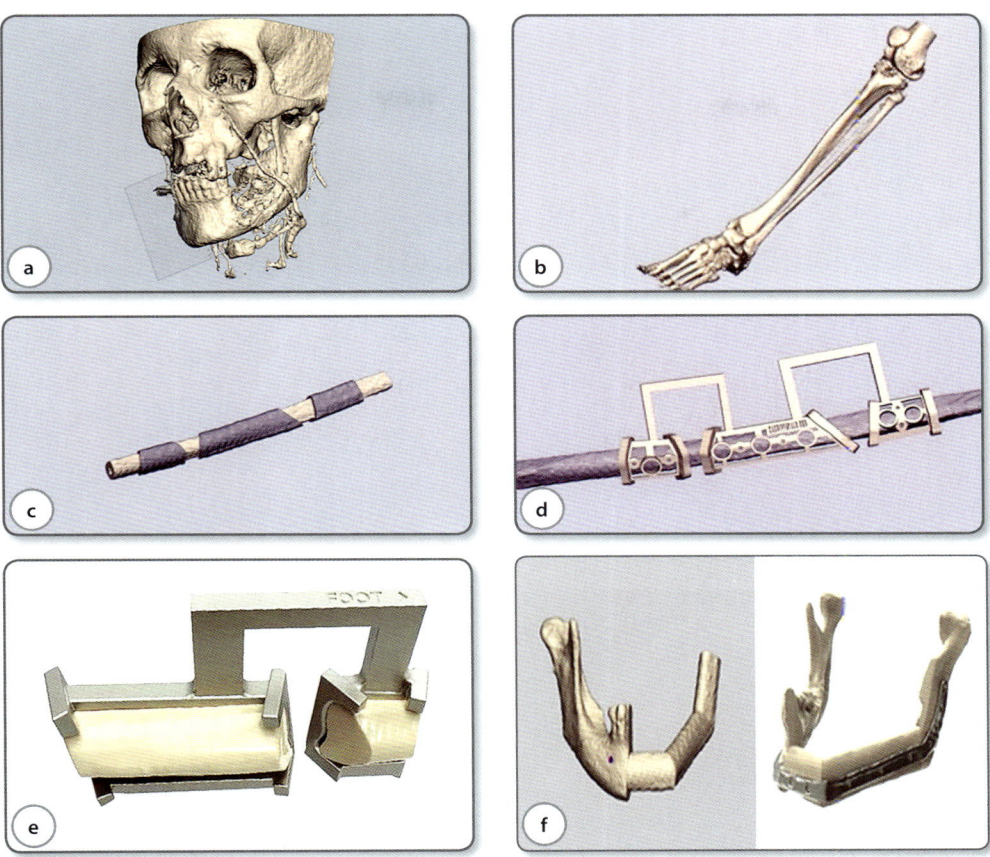

Figures 8.3a to f Computerised planning computer aided design and computer aided manufacturing (CadCam). (a) Reconstructed 3D CT scan demonstrating ORN in body of left mandible; (b) Reconstructed 3D CT scan demonstrating fibular anatomy; (c) Shape of cutting guide designed to produce accurate length of segments and angulated to good bony contact; (d) Design of cutting guide with screw holes which can then be sent electronically for milling; (e) Medial view showing the guide in place and the angulation of the cutting edge to allow good bony contact; (f) Fibular sections in place reconstructing the left body of the mandible. The titanium plate is also customised to the patient and adapted on the computer to the exact shape of the mandible.

Aetiology of medication-related osteonecrosis of jaw

It was originally thought that MRONJ was only related to bisphosphonates, but it is now clear that there are many other drugs which can cause this problem. The other main protagonists are denosumab, and the antiangiogenic inhibitors including:

- Antivascular endothelial growth factor (VEGF) monoclonal antibody (bevacizumab)
- Vascular endothelial growth factor decoy receptors or VEGF trap (aflibercept)
- Tyrosine kinase inhibitors (sorafenib, sunitinib, cabozantinib)
- Mammalian target of rapamycin (mTOR) inhibitors (everolimus)

In diseases which affect the remodelling of bone, blockade of receptor activator nuclear factor ligand–kB (RANKL) is essential. enosumab is a highly specific IgG2 monoclonal antibody to RANKL. The use of this drug has shown sustained reduction in bone turnover

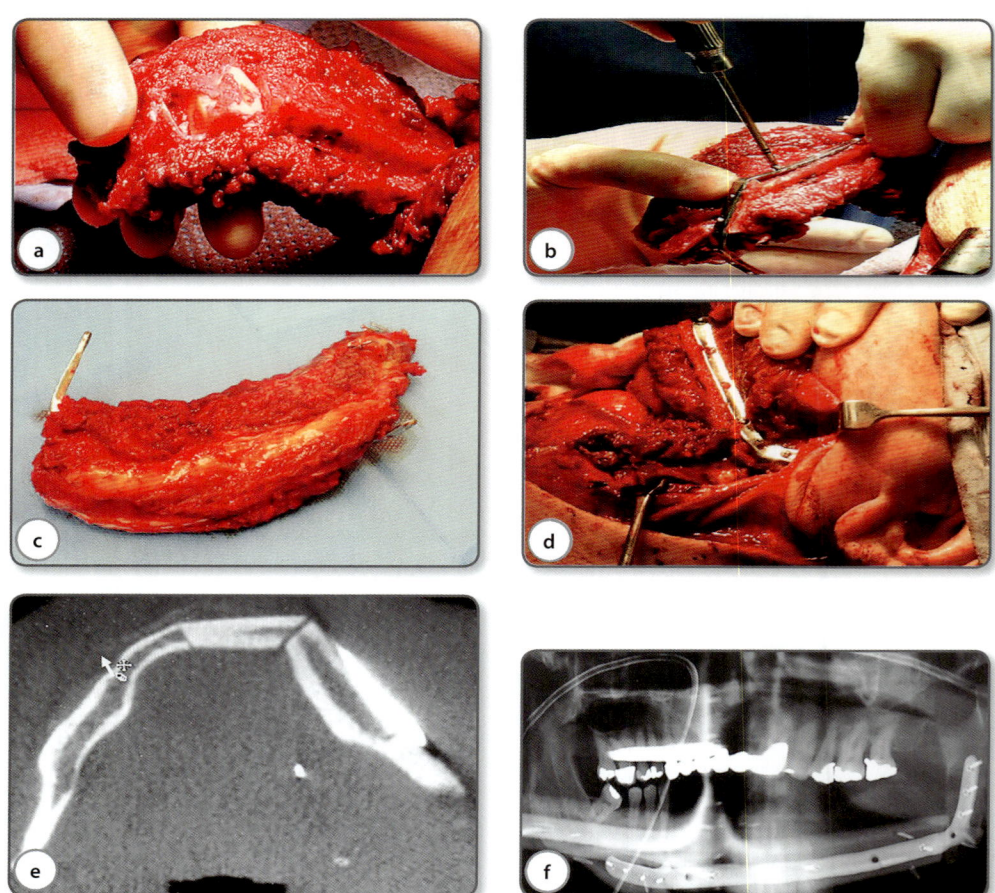

Figures 8.4a to f Clinical/operative photographs based on computerised plan from Figure 3. (a) Cuts made in fibular in situ—maintaining its vascularity; (b) Preformed plate secured onto fibula in situ; (c) Reformatted "mandible" with preformatted plate now disconnected and awaiting placement into defect; (d) Reconstructed mandible secured into defect with microvascular reconstruction to re-establish the vascular supply; (e) Axial computed tomography (CT) scan of mandible post-reconstruction, demonstrating accurate duplication of shape of mandible and good bony contact between fibular sections; (f) Orthopantomograph demonstrating plate in situ with left mandible having been reconstructed with fibula.

and an increase in mineral density and thus it appears to be superior to bisphosphonates in the management of osteoporosis. However, it now appears that there is a growing problem in relation to osteonecrosis with the use of denosumab and similar drugs [50]. When patients are on bisphosphonates it was hoped that suspension of the drug might improve the osteonecrosis, but unfortunately measurable levels may persist for up to 12 years after treatment has finished [51]. Therefore, little would be gained by stopping the drug, and more problems may occur in relation to the underlying bone condition [47,52]. The bioavailability of bisphosphonates after oral intake is poor compared to that after injection [53]. Likewise the incidence of osteonecrosis is significantly increased after intravenous compared to oral bisphosphonate administration [54]. It has been reported

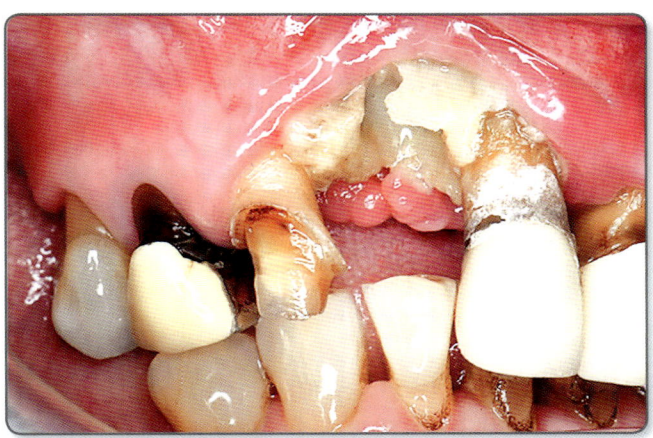

Figure 8.5 Clinical photograph of medication-related osteonecrosis of jaw (MRONJ).

that the risk of necrosis for those taking oral bisphosphonates and having a tooth extraction is 0.5%, but for those who have the drug intravenously the risk rises to 1.6–14.8% [55].

It has been proposed that the incidence of osteonecrosis is high in the jaws because alveolar bone turnover is roughly 5–10 times higher than that in the long bones [56].

Pathophysiology of medication-related osteonecrosis

Although, medications are the main cause, there are also local and systemic factors which can make the patient more susceptible to osteonecrosis. Local factors include inflammatory conditions of the jaw, dental procedures, and poor oral hygiene [57]. Systemic factors include corticosteroids, obesity, smoking, alcohol misuse, and medications as noted above [58,59]. Therefore, it is vitally important that these are considered when patients are prescribed these types of drugs.

Staging of medication-related osteonecrosis

The AAOMS have proposed a staging system which is based on clinical and radiological findings (**Table 8.1**) and its use will be outlined in the section on treatment.

Treatment

The management of MRONJ remains controversial, but what does remain consistent is that it should be linked to the staging, as stated in the position paper by the AAOMS (**Table 8.1**). Ferlito et al presented a longitudinal observational non-controlled study of 94 patients with confirmed BRONJ [60]. Treatment was in two phases:

1. Supportive with antimicrobial mouth rinses, antibiotics, and anti-inflammatory steroids) to minimise infection and pain before the formation of a bony sequestrum
2. Surgical plus pharmacological treatment (sequestrectomy with antibiotic prophylaxis) after the sequestrum had developed

The results showed that the mean time to formation of sequestra was 8 months and, what was of interest, was that the mean time for men was 5 months compared to women at 9 months and this was deemed to be significant. The authors suggested that this approach permits removal of all necrotic bone and avoids damage to the healthy bone when surgery

Table 8.1 Staging and treatment strategies: Position paper of American Association of Oral and Maxillofacial Surgeons (AAOMS)

MRONJ[†] staging	Treatment strategies[‡]
At risk category: No apparent necrotic bone in patients who have been treated with either oral or IV bisphosphonates	• No treatment indicated • Patient education
Stage 0: No clinical evidence of necrotic bone, but nonspecific clinical findings, radiographic changes and symptoms Radiographic findings: • Alveolar bone loss or resorption not attributable to chronic periodontal disease • Changes to trabecular pattern – dense woven bone and persistence of unremodelled bone in extraction sockets • Regions of osteosclerosis involving the alveolar bone and/or the surrounding basilar bone • Thickening/obscuring of periodontal ligament (thickening of the lamina dura and decreased size of the periodontal ligament space)	• Systemic management, including the use of pain medication and antibiotics
Stage 1: Exposed and necrotic bone, or fistulae that probes to bone, in patients who are asymptomatic and have no evidence of infection. These patients may also present with radiographic findings mentioned for stage 0 which are localised to the alveolar bone region	• Antibacterial mouth rinse • Clinical follow-up on a quarterly basis • Patient education and review of indications for continued bisphosphonate therapy
Stage 2: Exposed and necrotic bone, or fistulae that probes to bone, associated with infection as evidenced by pain and erythema in the region of the exposed bone with or without purulent drainage These patients may also present with radiographic findings mentioned for stage 0 which are localised to the alveolar bone region	• Symptomatic treatment with oral antibiotics • Oral antibacterial mouth rinse • Pain control • Debridement to relieve soft tissue irritation and infection control
Stage 3: Exposed and necrotic bone or a fistula that probes to bone in patients with pain, infection, and one or more of the following: Exposed and necrotic bone extending beyond the region of alveolar bone, (i.e. inferior border and ramus in the mandible, maxillary sinus and zygoma in the maxilla) resulting in pathologic fracture, extraoral fistula, oral antral/oral nasal communication, or osteolysis extending to the inferior border of the mandible of sinus floor	• Antibacterial mouth rinse • Antibiotic therapy and pain control • Surgical debridement/resection for longer term palliation of infection and pain

† Exposed or probable bone in the maxillofacial region without resolution for greater than 8 weeks in patients treated with an antiresorptive and/or an antiangiogenic agent who have not received radiation therapy to the jaws.
‡ Regardless of the disease stage, mobile segments of bony sequestrum should be removed without exposing uninvolved bone. The extraction of symptomatic teeth within exposed, necrotic bone should be considered since it is unlikely that the extraction will exacerbate the established necrotic process.
(MRONJ, medication-related osteonecrosis of the jaw; IV, intravenous)

is used and does not result in recurrences [60]. The limitations of this study were its size and lack of a control group due to ethical problems as debridement may induce further need for surgery. Therefore, these results should be interpreted with caution.

In the 2014, position paper by the AAOMS [49] the proposed measures are:

- *Stage 1:* Chlorhexidine mouthwash
- *Stage 2:* Judicious use of oral antibiotics, antibacterial mouthwash, pain control, minimal debridement (including sequestrectomy) to relieve soft tissue irritation and control of sources of infection

- *Stage 3:* More extensive surgery including debridement and formal resection for longer term palliation and pain control ± reconstruction including free tissue transfer

Coropciuc et al [61]. used these recommendations in a retrospective cohort study of patients with cancer who had been diagnosed with MRONJ after treatment with oral and intravenous bisphosphonates. The results supported this strategy especially regarding stage 3 MRONJ where conservative treatment had failed. The series emphasised that all patients required a multidisciplinary approach and the role of the consultant in restorative dentistry, general dental practitioner, and dental hygienist/therapist were mandatory. Teeth should be monitored closely and restored to the highest level.

McLeod et al [62]. produced an excellent literature review of United Kingdom and international management policies. This group reviewed all published guidelines to compare the conflicting advice from various national and international societies. Their conclusion was supportive of the conservative approach but recommended that high quality trials are required to answer the uncertainties.

Novel treatments

A number of novel treatment and emerging technologies have been proposed for the treatment of BRONJ/MRONJ:

- *Leucocyte-rich and platelet-rich fibrin (L-PRF) for the treatment of BRONJ*: A single group study of 34 patients showed complete resolution in 26 (77%), delayed resolution in 6 (18%) and no resolution in 2 (6%) [63]. This study was promising but larger randomised prospective trials are needed to confirm the findings
- *Laser stimulation using neodymium-doped yttrium aluminum garnet (Nd: YAG)* [64]: This seemed an interesting concept but the numbers in the series were low and a larger study is needed
- *Piezosurgical resection* [65]: A small case series was published which demonstrated that the use of piezosurgery to remove the necrotic mandible resulted in complete mucosal healing after only 3 weeks, but again the numbers were small and so further studies are recommended
- *Parathyroid hormone* [66]: The study was small and further studies are required
- *Bone morphogenic protein* [67]: The study was small and further studies are required

CONCLUSION

It can be seen that osteonecrosis, be it radiotherapy induced ORN or medication induced osteonecrosis (MRONJ), is a clinical problem with profound consequences which have a major impact on QOL. It is essential therefore that every effort is made to ensure that the management of these problems is evidence based and that the patient is fully informed of the risks and benefits of proposed treatment through the informed consent process. It is crucial that the patient is treated based on the clinical symptoms and not on the radiology alone, since severe radiological ORN may produce few, if any, symptoms (**Figure 8.6**).

It is vital that the patient understands that sometimes surgery may not be completely successful, and that complications may far outweigh the original problem. For example, if free tissue transfer is undertaken to reconstruct a defect and it fails, the resulting outcome can best be described as disastrous.

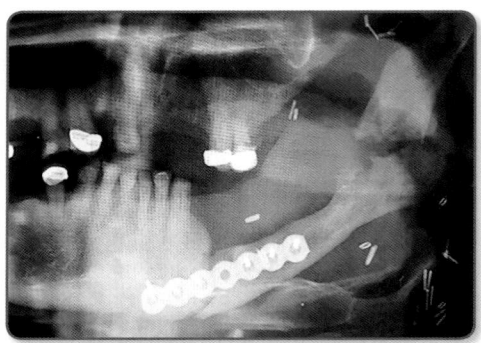

Figure 8.6 Radiograph of asymptomatic osteoradionecrosis (ORN) showing marked bone loss at the angle of left mandible and pathological fracture. Patient was pain free and treated conservatively.

Key points for clinical practice

- Prevention of ORN/MRONJ is better than cure
- Multidisciplinary approach to the problems of ORN/MRONJ is essential
- It is essential to take a full medical history including drug history especially, if bisphosphonates have been prescribed in last 20 years
- Patients should be fully informed of both the benefits and risks of treatment options
- Large clinical trials to assess management options in ORN/MRNOJ are required

ACKNOWLEDGEMENTS

Patients and photographers at Maxillofacial/Head and Neck Unit of Cardiff and Vale University Health Board for clinical photographs Mr Roger Maggs, Head of Laboratory Services at the University Dental Hospital, Cardiff for permission to use the pictures of Cadcam.

REFERENCES

1. Anonymous. Necrosis of the lower jaw in makers of Lucifer matches. Am J Dent Sci 1867; 1:96–97.
2. Regaud C. Sur la sensibilitie du tissu osseux normal vis-a- vis des rayons X et gamma et sur la mecanisme de l'osteoradionecrose. CR Soc Boil 1922; 87:629–932.
3. Ewing J. Radiation Osteitis. Acta Radiol 1926; 6:399–412.
4. Marx RE. Osteoradionecrosis: a new concept of its pathophysiology. J Oral Maxillofac Surg 1983; 41:283–288.
5. Marx RE, Johnson RP. Studies in the radiobiology of osteonecrosis and their clinical significance. Oral Surg Oral Med Oral Pathol 1987; 64:379–390.
6. Teng MS, Futran ND. Osteradionecrosis of the mandible. Curr Opin Otolaryngol Head Neck Surg 2005; 13:217–221.
7. Huang SH, O'Sullivan B. Overview of the 8th edition TNM classification for Head and Neck cancer. Curr Treat Options Oncol 2017; 18:40.
8. De Felice F, Tombolini V, Valentini V, et al. Advances in the Management of HPV-Related Oropharyngeal Cancer. J Oncol 2019; 2019:9173729.
9. Rogers SN, Travers A, Lowe D, et al. Importance of activity and recreation for the quality of life of patients treated for cancer of the head and neck. Br J Oral Maxillofac Surg 2019; 57:125–134.

10. Rosenthal DI, Mendoza TR, Fuller CD, et al. Patterns of symptom burden during radiotherapy or concurrent chemoradiotherapy for head and neck cancer: a prospective analysis using the University of Texas MD Anderson Cancer Center Symptom Inventory-Head and Neck Module. Cancer 2014; 120:1975–1984.
11. Jabbari S, Hyungin MK, Feng M, et al. Matched case-control study of Quality of life and Xerostomia after Intensity-Modulated Radiotherapy or Standard radiotherapy for Head and Neck cancer: initial report. Int J Radiat Oncology Biol Phys 2005; 63:725–731.
12. Ben-David MA, Diamante M, Radawski JD, et al. Lack of Osteoradionecrosis of the mandible after intensity modulated radiotherapy for head and neck cancer: likely contributions of both dental care and improved dose distributions. Int J Radiat Oncol Biol Phys 2007; 68:396–402.
13. Chronopoulos A, Zarra T, Ehrenfeld M, et al. Osteoradionecrosis of the jaws: definition, epidemiology, staging and clinical findings. A concise review. Int Dent J 2018; 68:22–30.
14. Lyons A, Ghazali N. Osteoradionecrosis of the jaw: current understanding of its pathophysiology and treatment. Br J Oral Maxillofac Surg 2008; 46:653–660.
15. Nadella KR, Kodali RM, Guttikonda LK, et al. Osteoradionecrosis of the jaws: clinico–therapeutic management: a literature review and update. J Maxillofac Oral Surg 2015; 14:891–901.
16. Meyer I. Infectious diseases of jaws. J Oral Surg 1970; 28:17–26.
17. Marx RE. A new concept in the treatment of osteoradionecrosis. J Oral Maxillofac Surg 1983; 41:351–357.
18. Delanian S, Lefaix JL. The radiation-induced fibroatrophic process: therapeutic perspective via the antioxidant pathway. Radiother Oncol 2004; 73:119–131.
19. Vozenin-Brotons MC, Milliat F, Sabourin JC, et al. Fibrogenic signals in patients with radiation enteritis are associated with increased connective tissue growth factor expression. Int J Radiat Oncol Biol Phys 2003; 56:561–572.
20. Delanian S, Baillet F, Huart J, et al. Successful treatment of radiation- induced fibrosis using liposomal Cu/Zn superoxide dismutase: clinical trial. Radiother Oncol 1994; 32:12–20.
21. Patel V, Gadiwalla, Sassoon I, et al. Use of Pentoxifylline and tocopherol in the management of osteoradionecrosis. Br J Oral Maxillofac Surg 2016; 54:342–345.
22. Notani K, Yamazaki Y, Kitada H, et al. Management of mandibular osteoradionecrosis corresponding to the severity of osteoradionecrosis and the method of radiotherapy. Head Neck 2003; 25:181–186.
23. Futran N, Trotti A, Gwede C. Pentoxifylline in the treatment of radiation related soft tissue injury: preliminary observations. Laryngoscope 1997; 107:391–395.
24. Lyons AJ, Brennan PA. Pentoxifylline–a review of its use in osteoradionecrosis. Br J Oral Maxillofac Surg 2017; 55:230–234.
25. Kahenasa N, Sung EC, Nabili V, et al. Resolution of pain and complete healing of mandibular osteoradionecrosis using pentoxifylline and tocopherol: a case report. Oral Surg Oral Med Oral Pathol Oral Radiol 2012; 113:e18–e23.
26. Robard L, Louis MY, Blanchard D, et al. Medical management of osteoradionecrosis of the mandible by PENTOCLO: preliminary results. Eur Ann Otorhinolaryngol Head and Neck Dis 2014; 131:333–338.
27. Delanian S, Chatel C, Porcher R, et al. Complete restoration of refractory mandibular osteoradionecrosis by prolonged treatment with pentoxifylline-tocophenol-clodronate combination (PENTOCLO): a phase II trial. Int J Radiat Oncol Biol Phys 2011; 80:832–839.
28. Niinikoski J, Hunt TK. Oxygen tensions in healing bone. Surg Gynecol Obstet 1972; 134:746–750.
29. Hunt TK, Pai MP. The effect of varying ambient oxygen tensions on wound metabolism and collagen synthesis. Surg Gynecol Obstet 1972; 135:561–567.
30. Hunt TK, Linsey M, Grislis H, et al. The effect of differing ambient oxygen tensions on wound infection. Ann Surg 1975; 181:35–39.
31. Knighton DR, Silver IA, Hunt TK. Regulation of wound healing angiogenesis–effect of oxygen gradients and inspired oxygen concentration. Surgery 1981; 90:262–270.
32. Knighton DR, Halliday B, Hunt TK. Oxygen as an antibiotic. A comparison of the effects of inspired oxygen concentration and antibiotic administration on in vivo bacterial clearance. Arch Surg 1986; 121:191–195.
33. Hunt TK. The physiology of wound healing. Ann Emerg Med 1988; 17:1265–1273.
34. Shefield PJ. Tissue oxygen measurements. In: Davis JC, Hunt TK, (Eds). Problem Wounds–The Role of Oxygen. Philadelphia: PA, Elsevier 1988. pp. 17–52.
35. Mainous EG, Boyne PJ, Hart GB. Elimination of sequestrum and healing. of osteoradionecrosis of the mandible after hyperbaric oxygen therapy: report of case. J Oral Surg 1973; 31:336–339.
36. Marx RE, Johnson RP, Kline SN. Prevention of osteoradionecrosis: a randomized prospective clinical trial of hyperbaric oxygen versus penicillin. J Am Dent Assoc 1985; 111:49–54.

37. Sulaiman F, Huryn J, Zlotolow IM. Dental extractions in the irradiated head and neck patient: a retrospective analysis of Memorial Sloan-Kettering Cancer Center protocols, criteria, and end results. J Oral Maxillofac Surg 2003; 61:1123–1131.
38. Shaw RJ, Butterworth CJ, Silcocks P, et al. HOPON (Hyperbaric Oxygen for the prevention of Osteoradionecrosis): a randomized controlled trial of hyperbaric oxygen to prevent osteoradionecrosis of the irradiated mandible after dentoalveolar surgery. Int J Radiat Oncol Biol Phys 2019; 104:530–539.
39. Annane D, Depondt J, Aubert P, et al. Hyperbaric oxygen therapy for radionecrosis of the jaw—a randomized, placebo-controled, double-blind trial from the ORN96 study group. J Clin Oncol 2004; 22:4893–4900.
40. Bessereau J, Annane D. Treatment of osteoradionecrosis of the jaw: the case against the use of hyperbaric oxygen. J Oral Maxillofac Surg 2010; 68:1907–1910.
41. Pitak-Arnnop P, Hemprich A, Dhanuthai K, et al. A systematic review in 2008 did not show value of hyperbaric oxygen therapy for osteoradionecrosis. J Oral Maxillofac Surg 2010; 68:2644–2645.
42. Bennett MH, Feldmeier J, Hampson N, et al. Hyperbaric oxygen therapy for late radiation tissue injury. Cochrane Database Syst Rev 2005; 20:CD005005.
43. Marx R. Bony reconstruction of the jaw. In: Kindwall EP, Whelan HT, (Eds). Hyperbaric medicine practice, 2nd edition. Flagstaff: Best Publishing 1999. pp. 460–463.
44. Bulsara VM, Bulsara MK, Lewis E. Protocol for prospective randomised assessor–blinded study comparing hyperbaric oxygen therapy with PENtoxifylline ± Tocopherol ± CLOdronate for the management of early osteoradionecrosis of the mandible. BMJ Open 2019; 9:e 026662.
45. Hidalgo D. Fibula free flap: a new method of mandible reconstruction. Plast Reconstr Surg. 1989;84:71-9.
46. Brown JS, Lowe D, Kanatas A, Schache A. Mandibular reconstruction with vascularised bone flaps: a systematic review over 25 years. Br J Oral Maxillofac Surg 2017; 55:113–126.
47. Badros A, Weikel D, Salama A, et al. Osteonecrosis of the jaw in multiple myeloma patients: clinical features and risk factors. J Clin Oncol 2006; 24:945–952.
48. Marx RE. Pamidronate (Aredia) and zoledronate (Zometa) induced avascular necrosis of the jaws: a growing epidemic. J Oral Maxillofac Surg 2003; 61:1115–1117.
49. Ruggiero SL, Dodson TB, Fantasia J, et al. American Association of Oral and maxillofacial surgeons position paper on medication-related osteonecrosis of the jaw--2014 Update. J Oral Maxillofac Surg 2014;72:1938–1956.
50. Taylor KH, Middlefell L, Mizen KD. Osteonecrosis of the jaws induced by anti-RANK ligand therapy. Br J Oral Maxillofac Surg 2010; 48:221–223.
51. Ruggiero SL, Fantasia J, Carlson E. Bisphosphonate-related osteonecrosis of the jaw: background and guidelines for diagnosis, staging and management. Oral Surg Oral Med Oral Pathol Oral Radiol Endod 2006; 102:433–441.
52. Gallego L, Junquera L. Consequence of therapy discontinuation in bisphosphonate–associated osteonecrosis of the jaws. Br J Oral Maxillofac Surg 2009; 47:67–68.
53. Vasikaran SD. Bisphosphonates: and overview with special reference to alendronate. Ann Clin Biochem 2001; 38:608–623.
54. Jarnbring F, Kashani A, Björk A, et al. Role of intravenous dosage regimens of bisphosphonates in relation to other aetiological factors in the development of osteonecrosis of the jaws in patients with myeloma. Br J Oral Maxillofac Surg 2015; 53:1007–1011.
55. Yamazaki T, Yamori M, Ishizaki T, et al. Increased incidence of osteonecrosis of the jaw after tooth extraction in patients treated with bisphosphonates: a cohort study. Int J Oral Maxillofac Surg 2012; 41:1397–1403.
56. Marx RE, Sawatari Y, Fortin M, et al. Bisphosphonate-induced exposed bone (osteonecrosis/osteopetrosis) of the jaws: risk factors, recognition, prevention, and treatment. J Oral Maxillofac Surg 2005; 63:1567–1575.
57. Sedghizadeh PP, Kumar SK, Gorur A, et al. Identification of microbial biofilms in osteonecrosis of the jaws secondary to bisphosphonate therapy. J Oral Maxillofac Surg 2008; 66:767–775.
58. Khamaisi M, Regev E, Yarom N, et al. Possible association between diabetes and bisphosphonate–related jaw osteonecrosis. J Clin Endocrinol Metab 2007; 92:1172–1175.
59. Wessel JH, Dodson TB, Zavras AI. Zoledronate, smoking and obesity are strong risk factors for osteonecrosis of the jaw: a case control study. J Oral Maxillofac Surg 2008; 66:625–631.
60. Ferlito S, Puzzo S, Palermo F, et al. Treatment of bisphosphonate- related osteonecrosis of the jaws: presentation of a protocol and an observational longitudinal study of an Italian series of cases. Br J Oral Maxillofac Surg 2012; 50:425–429.

61. Coropciuc RG, Grisar K, Aerden T, et al. Medication-related osteonecrosis of the jaw in oncological patients with skeletal metastases: conservative treatment is effective up to stage 2. Br J Oral Maxillofac Surg 2017; 55:787–792.
62. McLeod NM, Patel V, Kusanale A, et al. Bisphosphonate osteonecrosis of the jaw: a literature review of UK policies versus international policies on the management of bisphosphonate osteonecrosis of the jaw. Br J Oral Maxillofac Surg 2011; 49:335–342.
63. Kim JW, Kim SJ, Kim MR. Leucocyte-rich and platelet-rich fibrin (L-PRF) for the treatment of bisphosphonate-related osteonecrosis of the jaw: a prospective feasibility study. Br J Oral Maxillofac Surg 2014; 52:854–859.
64. Vescovi P, Merigo E, Meleti M, et al. Nd:YAG laser biostimulation of bisphosphonate-associated necrosis of the jawbone with and without surgical treatment. Br J Oral Maxillofac Surg 2007; 45:628–632.
65. Mathias Duarte LF, dos Reis HB, Tucci R, et al. Bisphosphonate related osteonecrosis of the jaws–promising early piezosurgical resection case series. Spec Care Dentist 2014; 34:77–83.
66. Bashutski JD, Eber RM, Kinney JS, et al. Teriparatide and osseous regeneration in the oral cavity. N Engl J ed 2010; 363:2396–2405.
67. Gerard DA, Carlson ER, Gotcher JE, et al. Early inhibitory effects of zoledronic acid in tooth extraction sockets in dogs are negated by recombinant human bone morphogenetic protein. J Oral Maxillofac Surg 2014; 72:61–66.

Chapter 9

Minimally invasive thyroidectomy

Aarathi Vijayashankar, Akshay Anand, Abhinav Arun Sonkar

INTRODUCTION

Thyroid surgery has an illustrious history and, whenever surgeons assume that the quest for a perfect operation is over, a new technique emerges in the surgical community. What began in Europe, as a dangerously bloody undertaking in the time of Billroth, is now one of the safest and most commonly performed surgical procedures. Kocher (**Figure 9.1**), a pupil of Billroth, pioneered the technique of open thyroidectomy in 1909 [1]. The successful era of thyroid surgery only occurred due to advancements in anaesthesia [2], asepsis [3] and haemostasis [4]. After more than a century, the focus of thyroid surgery has now seen a shift to minimally invasive, scar-less techniques for better aesthetic outcome and preservation of physiology.

The late 19th century saw the development of thyroidectomy into a safe procedure with < 1% mortality in the hands of Theodor Kocher. After trying vertical, midline and lateral incisions, he settled for a 7–10 cm long low collar transverse incision for best cosmetic results. The keys to his success were precise surgical technique and asepsis. He introduced suture ligation of arteries and veins along with identification and isolation of the laryngeal nerves [5]. Apart from bleeding and infection, other recognised complications of thyroidectomy were hypothyroidism, recurrent laryngeal nerve (RLN) injury leading to hoarseness, external laryngeal nerve (ELN) injury causing voice fatigue and hypocalcaemia due to hypoparathyroidism. By the early 20th century, identification and preservation of the nerves and parathyroid glands had become a mandatory step in the procedure in

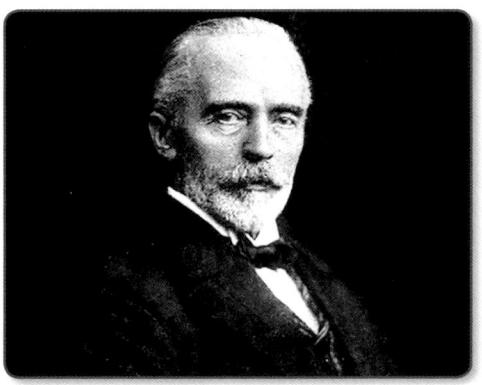

Figure 9.1 Theodor Kocher (1841–1917) 'Father of Thyroid Surgery'.

many centres. However, a clinical and philosophical debate between routine and selective identification still continues [6].

ORIGIN OF MINIMALLY INVASIVE THYROID SURGERY

Recent decades have seen the frontiers of thyroidectomy focus on the cosmetic and physiological impact of open surgery. Although, endoscopy was already in use in visceral surgery, its introduction into head and neck surgery occurred much later due to perceived anatomical constraints of a narrow operative field. Interest in minimally invasive endocrine surgery in the neck was sparked after 1996, when Gagner published his preliminary work on endoscopic parathyroid excision. Parathyroid adenomas were ideal for minimal access surgery due to their mostly benign nature and limited size [7]. The following year, Huscher performed the first completely endoscopic right thyroid lobectomy [8]. While minimally invasive thyroid surgery (MITS) causes lesser tissue trauma, offers better cosmetic satisfaction and reduced pain, conventional surgery has a shorter operative time, wider applicability and lower cost. Although, the magnified and illuminated view of the operative field gives a logistical advantage to the operating surgeon, the acceptance of MITS worldwide has remained weak. The reasons include a long learning curve, high cost, limited applicability, long operative times and, most importantly, the absence of a single universal standardised technique [9].

Currently, there is no consensus on definite criteria for suitability of a patient for MITS. However, it goes without saying that MITS needs very careful patient selection and should be limited to low risk malignancies. Some general indications [10] include:

- Benign nodules <3.5 cm, malignant lesions <2 cm, volume <30 mL
- Rearranged during transfection (RET) mutation carriers with normal basal calcitonin levels
- Absence of clinical nodal involvement
- No previous history of neck surgery, irradiation or thyroiditis

Although conventional surgery remains the preferred method for advanced malignancy and large benign goitres, some surgeons, especially from Asia, apply MITS to thyroid glands up to 10 cm size or 100 mL, muscle-invasive disease, irradiated necks and enlarged cervical lymphadenopathy [11,12].

TYPES OF MINIMALLY INVASIVE THYROID SURGERY

Minimally invasive thyroid surgery can be of three types:
1. Minimally invasive video-assisted thyroidectomy (MIVAT)
2. Minimally invasive non-endoscopic thyroidectomy (MINET)
3. Completely endoscopic techniques

The approach can be trans cervical or remote access, with or without gas insufflation. The most commonly used remote access approach is transaxillary. Each approach can be achieved by using the conventional endoscope or the robot. These permutations result in several combinations of techniques which are summarised in the rest of this chapter.

Cervical approaches

Early MITS were totally endoscopic surgeries via anterior or lateral cervical approaches, depending upon port placement [8]. Closed endoscopic techniques maintain the working space with gas insufflation using carbon dioxide (CO_2). Gas insufflation, however, was associated with several complications including subcutaneous emphysema, pneumomediastinum, gas embolism and vascular injury [13]. In order to reduce these complications, a procedure of MIVAT which used external retraction to create the operative space was developed in 1998 by Dr Paul Miccoli. MIVAT is currently the most established of all types of MITS. It includes a gasless procedure in three parts, starting with an open approach, followed by the use of the endoscope, finishing in an open fashion. A 1.5 cm central access is gained 2 cm above the sternal notch in the neck (**Figure 9.2**). The strap muscles are divided for a short distance in the midline, retracted with external instruments and the thyroid lobe is bluntly dissected away. A 30-degree, 5 mm or 7 mm wide endoscope is then inserted through the incision (**Figure 9.3**), deep to the strap muscles. The thyrotracheal groove is dissected and the superior pedicle ligated under endoscopic vision, staying clear of the external branch of the superior laryngeal nerve (EBSLN). Subsequently, the thyroid lobe is retracted medially and the RLN identified along with the parathyroid glands which are preserved. Once freed, the lobe can be extracted by rotating the upper pole [11,14].

Minimally invasive non-endoscopic thyroidectomies have also become popular as small incision open techniques because they produce similar advantages to MIVAT, without the need for expensive endoscopic equipment. Performed via a small skin crease incision high at the level of the superior pole, MINET gives direct exposure of the superior pedicle, allowing the laryngeal nerves to be easily visualised and preserved. This procedure is also less expensive and easier to learn [15].

Whilst MIVAT and MINET are clearly beneficial from a cosmetic standpoint, they still gave the patient a visible scar on the neck. Thus arose the demand for incisions at distant and less visible sites. With the advent of energy devices, formal ligation of the vascular pedicles also became no longer necessary. This allowed relocation of incisions to remote areas, circumventing scarring in the neck. The first report of its kind was published 3 years after the first MIVAT publication. Since then, remote access approaches have become more widely practiced and the American Thyroid Association (ATA) released a statement supporting remote access surgery in adequately motivated patients [18].

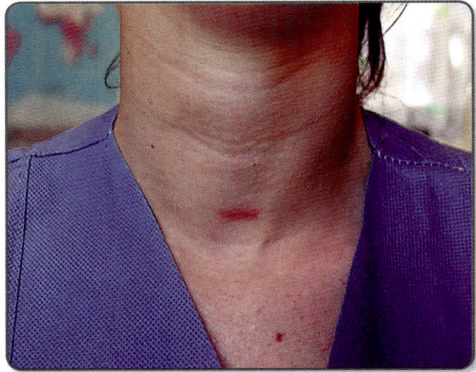

Figure 9.2 Surgical scar after minimally invasive video-assisted thyroidectomy [16].

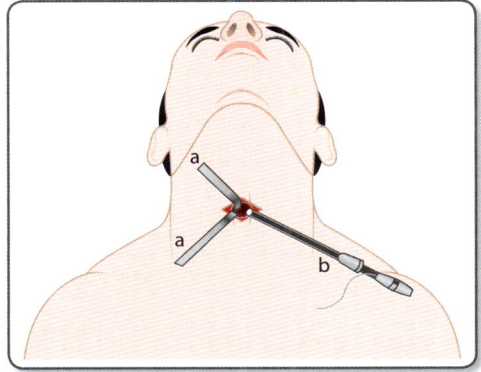

Figure 9.3 Schematic representation of retractors (a) and endoscope (b).

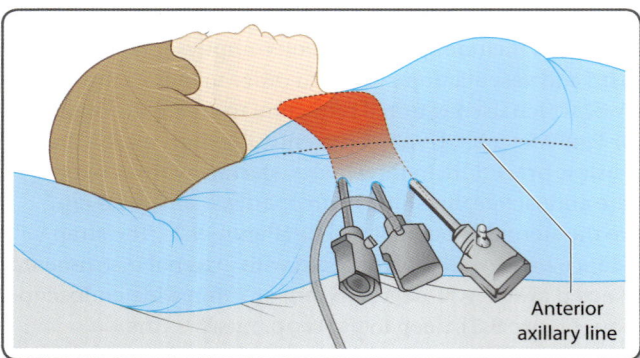

Figure 9.4 Diagrammatic representation of transaxillary approach [17].

Closed endoscopic transaxillary approach (Figure 9.4)

Initial experience in remote access surgery came from Ikeda who described a transaxillary approach [19]. He reported excellent cosmesis and negligible sensory disruption in the axilla. The method includes placement of a 10 mm zero-degree scope through the axilla along with two 5 mm working ports under low-pressure (<10 mmHg) gas insufflation. The neck is entered through the natural split between the two heads of the sternocleidomastoid (SCM). The strap muscles are retracted away from the gland. Energy devices are used to ligate and divide vessels close to the thyroid. A drain may be placed temporarily. The main advantage of this technique is its truly minimal invasive nature with a remote incision causing minimal disruption. It is ideal for unilateral benign or early stage disease.

Gasless transaxillary robotic approach

Practiced mainly in South Korea over the past decade, this technique is their standard approach for most thyroid pathology (**Figure 9.5a** and **b**). However, worldwide, it is attempted specifically in patients with a significant tendency for keloid formation. Initially, the technique resembled closed endoscopic thyroidectomy using two separate incisions, one in the axilla and another in the anterior chest wall. With sufficient experience, the anterior chest wall incision was omitted and the procedure is now being applied to more advanced malignancy. It starts with a 6–7 cm incision lateral to the pectoralis, parallel to its lateral border. A working tunnel is created through this incision subcutaneously up to the SCM. The space is kept open with a table-fixed deep retractor developed by Dr WY Chung. Operative instruments including the endoscope are inserted through holes in a table-mounted stable metallic platform. The steps are otherwise similar to the closed transaxillary approach [22]. Despite its popularity and excellent results in South Korea, worldwide acceptance has been limited. The procedure is not only expensive but also time-consuming and more invasive due to wide dissection from the axilla. Most surgeons also found the anatomy unconventional and difficult to follow due to access from one side of the body. This also made contralateral dissection more difficult [23].

Bilateral axillo-breast approach

In order to increase the familiarity and symmetry of remote endoscopic surgery, surgeons began to experiment with bilateral approaches along with midline exposure, much like the exposure in conventional thyroidectomy (CT). Bilateral axillo-breast approach (BABA)

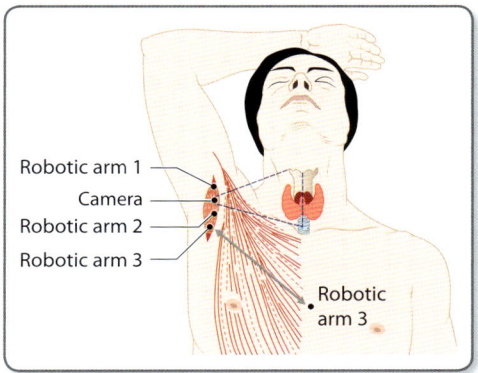

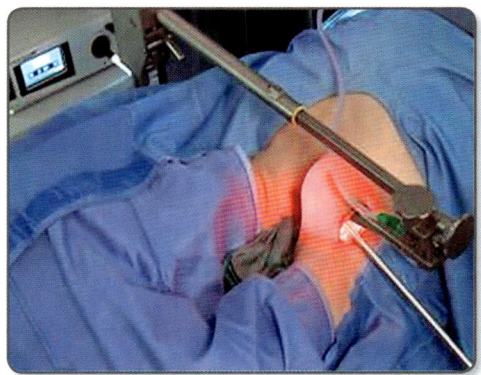

Figure 9.5a Landmarks of gasless transaxillary robotic approach, also showing auxiliary chest access.

Figure 9.5b Deep Chung retractor in place, maintaining operative space [20].

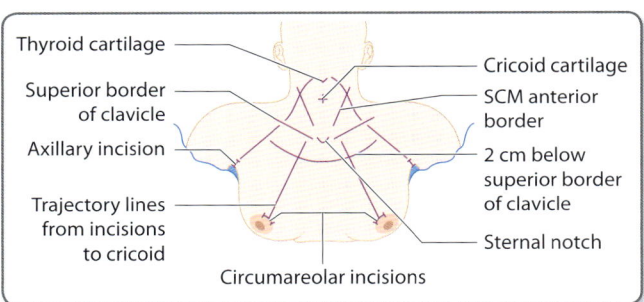

Figure 9.6 Landmarks of bilateral axillo-breast approach (BABA) [21]. (SCM, sternocleidomastoid)

was developed in 2004 as a four port technique through small incisions in both axillae and breasts (**Figure 9.6**). The subplatysmal neck and the subcutaneous anterior chest wall are injected with adrenaline: Saline (1:2,00,000) to achieve a bloodless plane. Along with bilateral axillary ports, two working ports are inserted at the superomedial margin of the areola. Blunt dissection is used to create the track to the cervical field. BABA may be done via closed endoscopic or robotic methods. Comparison of the surgical outcome of BABA and conventional surgery showed that the completeness of thyroidectomy in both approaches was similar. However, BABA showed a higher rate of transient vocal cord palsy (25.2% vs. 2.5%) while permanent damage was negligible [24].

Natural orifice transluminal endoscopic surgery

The latest and most promising in the series of MITS is natural orifice transluminal endoscopic surgery (NOTES). It is a closed endoscopic method of surgery that uses natural orifices in the body for trocar access [25]. Its application in thyroid surgery has sparked recent interest among surgeons as an absolutely scar free, 'microinvasive' method which limits postoperative swallowing disorders and avoids keloid formation. In 2010, Wilhelm and Metzig reported the first successful human series of totally transoral endoscopic thyroidectomies. The transoral technique of endoscopic neck surgery commenced with cadaveric studies in 2008, and initially was done via sublingual access alone [26]. Due to restricted triangulation, a combined sublingual and bivestibular approach was subsequently developed [27]. A sublingual trocar is used to enter the subplatysmal plane and CO_2 insufflated. Bilateral 5 mm working ports enter through the vestibule into the created space. Sublingual access has long been criticised for its difficulty and has now become unpopular. In 2013, Nakajo published his preliminary work on an exclusively vestibular approach, which documented no mental nerve injury but temporary sensory disturbances around the chin. In 2018, Anuwong published the largest retrospective series of this technique in 422 patients. Apart from longer operating time, the study showed few complications and satisfactory outcomes, to the extent of declaring exclusively vestibular approaches to the thyroid no longer experimental [28,29]. While the incidences of hypoparathyroidism and nerve injury are similar to CT, mental nerve injury has been a unique complication attributed to this technique. The procedure is now commonly termed transoral endoscopic thyroidectomy vestibular approach (TOETVA) (**Figures 9.7** and **9.8**).

Other techniques

While the above-mentioned techniques are the most commonly used forms of MITS, other nonmainstream methods also exist. Video-assisted neck surgery (VANS) is the first closed endoscopic method that did not utilise gas insufflation for maintaining the operative space. It used anterior neck subcentimetre incisions to retract the skin using Kirschner wires while access for dissection was through trocars on the anterior chest wall [32]. Another technique, the breast approach, as described by Ohgami in 2000, uses bilateral breast incisions with a parasternal port. While the breast scars became inconspicuous after several weeks, the parasternal wound often left a disfiguring scar [33]. To overcome this pitfall, Shimazu developed the axillo-bilateral-breast approach (ABBA) and utilised a well-hidden ipsilateral axillary access instead [34]. To address the issue of extensive dissection in robotic transaxillary thyroidectomy, Terris assessed the feasibility of a less invasive postauricular occipital approach, in a case series of 14 patients [35]. As the incision was closer to the thyroid, the dissection was considered less extensive.

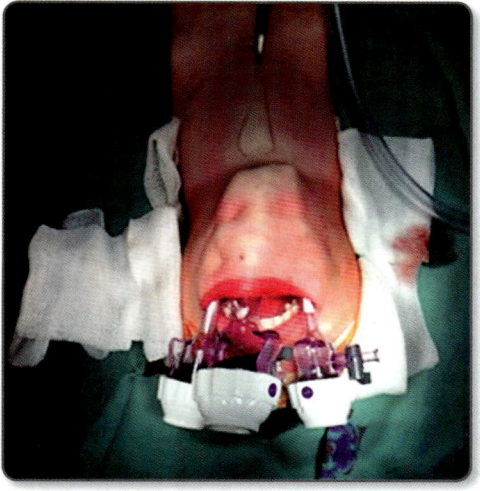

Figure 9.7 Transoral endoscopic thyroidectomy vestibular approach (TOETVA) approach [30].

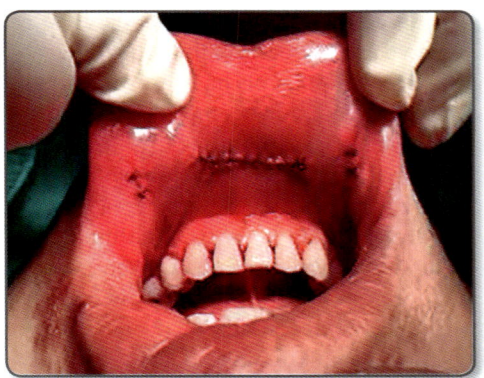

Figure 9.8 Vestibular incisions after closure [31].

Confirmatory evidence on the safety of many of the above techniques is awaited, which has restricted their uptake more widely.

Adjuncts of minimally invasive thyroid surgery

While Spencer's haemostatic forceps [4] and Lahey's insistence on routine identification of laryngeal nerves [36] changed the face of CT, two inventions have served MITS similarly - intraoperative nerve monitoring (IONM) and new energy devices.

Intraoperative nerve monitoring

The reported incidence of laryngeal nerve palsies following thyroid surgery varies in the literature as there is no single method of identification and reporting that is universally accurate or routinely used. The incidence of temporary RLN palsy ranges between 1.4 and 38% in various studies [37]. While visual identification during surgery is considered the gold standard for preservation of the laryngeal nerves, IONM is gaining wide acceptance since the advent of MITS. Open surgery allows laryngeal palpation for identification of the RLN, a luxury that MITS does not give. Nonetheless, IONM is not a replacement for surgical finesse or knowledge of anatomy. IONM includes simultaneous stimulation of RLN and electromyographical assessment of vocal cord response during surgery. The stimulation of the nerve is used to map out its trajectory. Dionigi prospectively studied video-assisted thyroidectomy with and without the use of IONM. While the incidence of temporary RLN injury in the IONM group was 2.7% versus 8.3% in the non-IONM group, there was no permanent injury [38]. Similar tracking of the EBSLN can also be done but the interest in it is not as great, since damage is not as debilitating as that of the RLN. Although, IONM can be used to track the laryngeal nerves and their function, it is probably most important in deciding on contralateral surgery when the signal is lost on the ipsilateral side.

Energy devices in thyroid surgery

While suture ligation was the gold standard for obtaining haemostasis in CT, many energy devices have come into use and have proven to be as safe. An ultrasonic shear was used to simultaneously cut and coagulate vessels in thyroid surgery for the first time in 1999. Voutilainen showed that ultrasonic dissection reduced operating time significantly without increasing complications in a reliable prospective randomised trial in 2000 [39]. Other benefits include reduced blood loss, reduced postoperative pain, decreased incidence of hypoparathyroidism and improved cosmetic satisfaction due to less tissue charring. While most studies since then have able to recreate these results, there have been occasional reports of increased nerve palsy [40]. This has unfortunately kept the debate on their benefits alive. More recently, Kiriakapoulos demonstrated equal safety with another device that operated on the principles of diathermy [41]. As the peak temperature achieved by this bipolar vessel sealer is lower than that of the ultrasonic shear, lateral thermic spread and damage in bipolar sealer is theoretically lower (70–90°C vs. 200°C). Both devices are disposable and might increase operative costs, but this is balanced by an unequivocal advantage of reduced operative time. Despite proven safety, some surgeons still fear an unidentified collateral injury to adjacent structures including the parathyroid glands and the laryngeal nerves. The apprehension may be overcome by careful dissection near Berry's ligament, leaving behind a small remnant, or by using only sutures and clips near the nerve.

ANALYSIS OF OUTCOME

What Huscher [8] began as an experiment in 1997 has seen an exponential increase over the last two decades into a plethora of different techniques, each of them shows almost comparable efficacy, safety and radicality. Linos performed a literature review of MITS since its inception and has found over 20 different techniques described [15]. Apart from providing superior cosmesis, several studies have shown that MITS improves hospital stay and reduces postoperative pain, especially in the first 24 hours [42]. While acceptance of endoscopy worldwide has been slow but steadily progressive, the exorbitant cost of the robot has limited its use not only in developing nations, but also developed western countries. Robotic remote access surgery is associated with longer operating times and extensive tissue dissection. These financial and technical factors contributed to the 2011 withdrawal of support for robotic thyroidectomy by the United States Food and Drug Administration.

    With the advent of MITS, concern was raised regarding the issue of the completeness of surgical excision. While the wristed instruments of a robot improved surgical dexterity, the design of most endoscopes carries the potential risk of incomplete resection at difficult areas due to limited access. While the incidences of hypoparathyroidism and nerve injury in CT and MITS are considered similar, the potential harm of energy devices around these critical structures might compromise radicality in either of the techniques. Hence, the debate comparing the oncological safety of various MITS techniques to CT continues. While confirmatory studies on most scarless techniques are awaited, there is level 1 evidence for MIVAT [43,44]. The 2015 ATA guidelines have also begun to encourage lobectomies for low risk malignancies which has improved the confidence of surgeons to take up MITS [45]. At present MIVAT has managed to find the optimum middle ground between the bipolar techniques of CT or totally endoscopic procedures. It is also the ideal minimally invasive option for a low volume surgeon with affordable costs and acceptable operative time compared to CT, with the added advantage of better patient satisfaction [46]. Currently, MIVAT is the most acceptable and widespread technique of MITS across the world.

    Any minimally invasive surgery is associated with a learning curve. While it would be easy to assume that robotic surgeries would have a steeper learning curve than routine endoscopy, a large multicentre trial on robotic thyroidectomy in Korea has shown that ergonomics of the robot allowed surgeons to attain proficiency sooner than routine endoscopic methods (40–50 operations vs. 55–60 operations) [47]. MIVAT was considered one of the easier operations to master with the shortest learning curve of 30 operations [48]. However in 2018, Razavi published a case series of 30 patients who underwent TOETVA and showed that the procedure had a learning curve of only 11 cases [49].

The most striking pitfall of any MITS has been its restricted selection criteria, as previously described. It is not feasible as a surgical option in large volume endemic goitres. While most MITS have restricted themselves to these criteria, ambitious authors have attempted to push the limits in TOETVA by removing goitres up to 10 cm, such as in Grave's disease, by endoscopically scoring the thyroid capsule and squeezing the specimen through the trocar site. However, the risk of occult malignancy in these thyroids is unknown and this technique is not advisable [50]. Hence, in unequivocally proven cases of carcinoma, the upper limit of specimen size is kept to 2 cm. The only type of MITS so far that allows large tumour removal is the gasless transaxillary robotic thyroidectomy practiced almost exclusively in Korea.

CONCLUSION

From safe to scar-free, thyroid surgery has progressed a long way in two decades. As beneficial as MITS might seem compared to CT, the true superiority of any particular procedure is not yet proven. The perseverance of the East Asians has garnered rewards in the fields of robotic surgery and NOTES. However, only time will tell if the West and the rest of the world will become accepting of their innovation as most of the reported studies are case series or retrospective studies. While well designed clinical trials are becoming available for methods other than MIVAT, the study population is still limited in number and may not be adequate to provide unequivocal proof of superiority [51,52]. At present MITS cannot truly replace conventional surgery as the standard of care for all patients requiring thyroidectomy but remains an exciting area of surgical development and research.

Key points for clinical practice

- Minimally invasive thyroid surgery (MITS) has comparable efficacy and safety to CT
- Minimally invasive video-assisted thyroidectomy (MIVAT) has been the minimally invasive procedure of the last decade
- Transoral endoscopic thyroidectomy vestibular approach (TOETVA) is an emerging technique which is gaining increased acceptance, despite the unique complication of mental nerve injury
- Natural orifice transluminal endoscopic surgery (NOTES) is a microinvasive, scar-free method of surgery
- NOTES thyroidectomy has similar outcome and complication as CT
- MITS may be viewed as a potential standard of care for thyroid surgery in the future

---

REFERENCES

1. Tröhler U. Emil Theodor Kocher (1841–1917). J R Soc Med 2014; 107:376–377.
2. Chaturvedi R, Gogna RL. Ether day: an intriguing history. Med J Armed Forces India 2011; 67:306–308.
3. Osborn GG. Joseph Lister and the origins of antisepsis. J Med Humanit Bioeth 1986; 7:91–105.

4. Sarkar S, Banerjee S, Sarkar R, et al. A Review on the History of "Thyroid Surgery". Indian J Surg 2016; 78:32–36.
5. The James Lind Library. Kocher T (1883). [online] Available from http://www.jameslindlibrary.org/kocher-t-1883/ [Last accessed November, 2020].
6. Chang YK, Lang BHH. To identify or not to identify parathyroid glands during total thyroidectomy. Gland Surg 2017; 6:S20–S29.
7. Gagner M. Endoscopic subtotal parathyroidectomy in patients with primary hyperparathyroidism. Br J Surg 1996; 83:875.
8. Hüscher CS, Chiodini S, Napolitano C, et al. Endoscopic right thyroid lobectomy. Surg Endosc 1997;11:877.
9. Miccoli P, Berti P, Raffaelli M, et al. Comparison between minimally invasive video-assisted thyroidectomy and conventional thyroidectomy: a prospective randomized study. Surgery 2001; 130:1039–1043.
10. Chen S, Zhao M, Qiu J. Transoral vestibule approach for thyroid disease: a systematic review. Eur Arch Otorhinolaryngol 2019; 276:297–304.
11. Miccoli P, Materazzi G. Minimally invasive, video-assisted thyroidectomy (MIVAT). Surg Clin North Am 2004; 84:735–741.
12. Radford PD, Ferguson MS, Magill JC, et al. Meta-analysis of minimally invasive video-assisted thyroidectomy. Laryngoscope 2011; 121:1675–1681.
13. Gottlieb A, Sprung J, Zheng XM, et al. Massive subcutaneous emphysema and severe hypercarbia in a patient during endoscopic transcervical parathyroidectomy using carbon dioxide insufflation. Anesth Analg 1997; 84:1154–1156.
14. Irawati N. Endoscopic Right Lobectomy Axillary-Breast Approach: a report of two cases. Int J Otolaryngol 2010; 2010:958764.
15. Linos D. Minimally invasive thyroidectomy: a comprehensive appraisal of existing techniques. Surgery 2011; 150:17–24.
16. Bakkar S, Miccoli P. Minimally invasive video-assisted thyroidectomy (MIVAT) in the era of minimal access thyroid surgery. J Minim Invasive Surg Sci 2017; 6:e42470.
17. Duncan TD, Ejeh IA, Speights F, et al. Endoscopic transaxillary near total thyroidectomy. J Soc Lap Surg 2006; 10:206–211.
18. Berber E, Bernet V, Fahey TJ, et al. American Thyroid Association Statement on Remote-Access Thyroid Surgery. Thyroid 2016; 26:331–337.
19. Ikeda Y, Takami H, Niimi M, et al. Endoscopic thyroidectomy by the axillary approach. Surg Endosc 2001; 15:1362–1364.
20. Kandil E, Abdelghai S, Noureldine SI, et al. Transaxillary gasless robotic thyroidectomy. Arch Otolaryngol Head Neck Surg 2012: 138:113–117.
21. Choi JY, Lee KE, Youn YK. Bilateral Axillo- Breast Approach (BABA) Endoscopic and Robotic Thyroid Surgery. In: D Linos, WY Chung, (Eds). Minimally invasive thyroidectomy. Berlin Heidelberg: Springer Publications; 2012. pp. 171.
22. Lee S, Ryu HR, Park JH, et al. Excellence in robotic thyroid surgery: a comparative study of robot-assisted versus conventional endoscopic thyroidectomy in papillary thyroid microcarcinoma patients. Ann Surg 2011; 253:1060–1066.
23. Yoon JH, Park CH, Chung WY. Gasless endoscopic thyroidectomy via an axillary approach: experience of 30 cases. Surg Laparosc Endosc Percutan Tech 2006; 16:226–231.
24. Chung YS, Choe JH, Kang KH, et al. Endoscopic thyroidectomy for thyroid malignancies: comparison with conventional open thyroidectomy. World J Surg 2007; 31:2307–2308.
25. Kalloo AN, Singh VK, Jagannath SB, et al. Flexible transgastric peritoneoscopy: a novel approach to diagnostic and therapeutic interventions in the peritoneal cavity. Gastrointest Endosc 2004; 60:114–117.
26. Witzel K, von Rahden BH, Kaminski C, et al. Transoral access for endoscopic thyroid resection. Surg Endosc 2008; 22:1871–1875.
27. Benhidjeb T, Wilhelm T, Harlaar J, et al. Natural orifice surgery on thyroid gland: totally transoral video-assisted thyroidectomy (TOVAT): report of first experimental results of a new surgical method. Surg Endosc 2009; 23:1119–1120.
28. Nakajo A, Arima H, Hirata M, et al. Trans-Oral Video-Assisted Neck Surgery (TOVANS). A new transoral technique of endoscopic thyroidectomy with gasless premandible approach. Surg Endosc 2013; 27:1105–1110.
29. Anuwong A, Ketwong K, Jitpratoom P, et al. Safety and Outcomes of the Transoral Endoscopic Thyroidectomy Vestibular Approach. JAMA Surg 2018; 153:21–27.
30. Le Q, Ngo D, Ngo Q. Transoral endoscopic thyroidectomy vestibular approach (TOETVA): A case report as new technique in thyroid surgery in Vietnam. Int J Surg Case Reports 2018; 50:60–63.

31. Anuwong A, Sasanakietkul T, Jitpratoom P, et al. Transoral endoscopic thyroidectomy vestivular approach (TOETVA): indications, techniques and results. Surg Endosc 2018; 32:456–465.
32. Shimizu K, Akira S, Tanaka S. Video-assisted neck surgery: endoscopic resection of benign thyroid tumor aiming at scarless surgery on the neck. J Surg Oncol 1998; 69:178–180.
33. Ohgami M, Ishii S, Arisawa Y, et al. Scarless endoscopic thyroidectomy: breast approach for better cosmesis. Surg Laparosc Endosc Percutan Tech 2000; 10:1–4
34. Shimazu K, Shiba E, Tamaki Y, et al. Endoscopic thyroid surgery through the axillo-bilateral-breast approach. Surg Laparosc Endosc Percutan Tech 2003; 13:196–201.
35. Terris DJ, Singer MC, Seybt MW. Robotic facelift thyroidectomy: II. Clinical feasibility and safety. Laryngoscope 2011; 121:1636–1641.
36. Lahey FH, Hoover WB. Injuries to the recurrent laryngeal nerve in thyroid operations: their management and avoidance. Ann Surg 1938; 108:545–562.
37. Jeannon JP, Orabi AA, Bruch GA, et al. Diagnosis of recurrent laryngeal nerve palsy after thyroidectomy: a systematic review. Int J Clin Pract 2009; 63:624–629.
38. Dionigi G, Boni L, Rovera F, et al. Neuromonitoring and video-assisted thyroidectomy: a prospective, randomized case-control evaluation. Surg Endosc 2009; 23:996–1003.
39. Voutilainen PE, Haglund CH. Ultrasonically Activated shears in thyroidectomies: a randomized trial. Ann Surg 2000; 231:322–328.
40. Marchesi M, Biffoni M, Cresti R, et al. [Ultrasonic scalpel in thyroid surgery]. Chir Ital 2003; 55:299–308.
41. Kiriakopoulos A, Dimitrios T, Dimitrios L. Use of a diathermy system in thyroid surgery. Arch Surg 2004; 139:997–1000.
42. Pisanu A, Podda M, Reccia I, et al. Systematic review with meta-analysis of prospective randomized trials comparing minimally invasive video-assisted thyroidectomy (MIVAT) and conventional thyroidectomy (CT). Langenbecks Arch Surg 2013; 398(8):1057–1068.
43. Miccoli P, Elisei R, Materazzi G, et al. Minimally invasive video-assisted thyroidectomy for papillary carcinoma: a prospective study of its completeness. Surgery 2002; 132:1070–1073.
44. Terris DJ, Angelos P, Steward DL, et al. Minimally invasive video-assisted thyroidectomy: a multi-institutional North American experience. Arch Otolaryngol Head Neck Surg 2008; 134:81–84.
45. Haugen BR, Alexander EK, Bible KC, et al. 2015 American Thyroid Association Management Guidelines for Adult Patients with Thyroid Nodules and Differentiated Thyroid Cancer: The American Thyroid Association Guidelines Task Force on Thyroid Nodules and Differentiated Thyroid Cancer. Thyroid 2016; 26:1–133.
46. Minimally Invasive Surgical Sciences. Minimally Invasive Video-Assisted Thyroidectomy (MIVAT) in the Era of Minimal Access Thyroid Surgery [online] Available from: http://minsurgery.com/en/articles/14026.html. [Last Accessed November, 2020].
47. Lee J, Yun JH, Nam KH, et al. The learning curve for robotic thyroidectomy: a multicenter study. Ann Surg Oncol 2011; 18:226–232.
48. Pons Y, Vérillaud B, Blancal JP, et al. Minimally invasive video-assisted thyroidectomy: learning curve in terms of mean operative time and conversion and complication rates. Head Neck 2013; 35:1078–1082.
49. Razavi CR, Vasiliou E, Tufano RP, et al. Learning Curve for transoral endoscopic thyroid lobectomy. Otolaryngol Head Neck Surg 2018; 159:625–629.
50. Anuwong A, Kim HY, Dionigi G. Transoral endoscopic thyroidectomy using vestibular approach: updates and evidences. Gland Surg 2017; 6:277–284.
51. Ren X, Dai Z, Sha H, et al. Comparative study of endoscopic thyroidectomy via a breast approach versus conventional open thyroidectomy in papillary thyroid microcarcinoma patients. Biomed Res 2017; 28.
52. Yang J, Wang C, Li J, et al. Complete Endoscopic Thyroidectomy via Oral Vestibular Approach Versus Areola Approach for Treatment of Thyroid Diseases. J Laparoendosc Adv Surg Tech A 2015; 25:470–476.

Section 6

Breast surgery

Chapter 10

Partial breast irradiation for cancer

Justina CJ Tai, Muneer Ahmed

INTRODUCTION

Radiotherapy is an established component of multimodal treatment for most breast cancers. This is following evidence that breast irradiation after breast-conserving surgery significantly reduces both locoregional recurrence rates and deaths due to breast cancer [1,2]. Long-term follow-up of seminal trials also demonstrated the equivalence of this regimen to modified radical mastectomy in terms of disease-free survival and overall survival [3].

The National Institute for Health and Care Excellence (NICE) 2018 guidelines [4] advocate the utility of adjuvant radiotherapy in multiple contexts: after breast-conserving therapy for patients with clear margins, as a 'breast boost' for patients with a higher risk of local recurrence, post-mastectomy, and for supraclavicular nodal areas in specific patient groups. While external beam whole-breast radiation therapy (WBRT) has been generally accepted as the conventional irradiation technique in breast cancer, recent years have seen the pursuit of more localised treatment (partial breast irradiation) and shorter treatment plans, in order to maximise the therapeutic ratio of radiotherapy and to increase convenience. This resulted in a shift towards accelerated partial breast irradiation (APBI). APBI is a combination of two approaches: (1) a reduction in the number of radiotherapy treatments (i.e., hypofractionated or accelerated radiotherapy) and (2) a reduction in volume of breast irradiated (i.e., partial breast irradiation).

In APBI, only the predetermined index quadrant receives irradiation. Various studies have demonstrated compelling benefits in using APBI among patients with early-stage breast cancer, and the body of evidence is growing as newer techniques for delivering more focused therapy regimens, are introduced. This chapter outlines the rationale for APBI and appraises the range of techniques that are available in clinical practice today.

RATIONALE

Relative toxicity of whole-breast radiation therapy

Given the excellent survival rates of breast cancer, attempts to maximise quality of life have been considered with great interest. The ranges of systemic therapies used in cancer management are already known to be associated with a number of complications. For instance, endocrine therapy involving selective oestrogen receptor modulators (SORMs) that also act as partial agonists in the endometrium, increase the risk of endometrial cancer, while cytotoxic drugs used in chemotherapy commonly result in anaemia and neutropenia, and in rare cases, may even lead to leukaemia. Irradiation to the whole breast, on the other hand, is associated with long-term side effects related to damage to residual normal breast tissue and overlying skin as well as damage caused by incidental irradiation to nearby structures like the heart, lungs, and oesophagus.

The association between whole-breast radiotherapy and subsequent major coronary events is well established. The risk of ischaemic heart disease is proportional to the mean dose of ionizing radiation to the heart; this increase in risk begins just a few years after radiotherapy and lasts at least 20 years [5]. It has been shown that patients who receive irradiation to the left breast (thus receiving a higher dose of incidental radiation to the heart) have significantly worse outcomes than those receiving radiotherapy to the right breast. This has implications of greater magnitude for patients with pre-existing cardiac risk factors. Although techniques such as prone breast radiotherapy and deep inspiration breath hold (DIBH) [6] have been beneficial in reducing radiation doses to the heart, the residue radiation remains clinically significant. This is where APBI proves instrumental in reducing radiation doses to the heart, especially in patients receiving treatment to the left breast [7].

With regards to the lungs, more grave complications include radiation-induced lung cancer, which has been shown to present > 10 years after radiotherapy. This is mainly relevant among smokers, who already have a significantly increased baseline risk of developing lung cancer. For smokers who have small, early-stage breast cancers, the absolute risks may outweigh the absolute benefits of adjuvant radiotherapy [8]. With APBI, individual treatment plans for at-risk patients may be arranged to prioritise lung sparing—this has shown favourable outcomes in terms of reducing both the risk of secondary lung cancer and cardiovascular toxicity [9].

Clinical outcomes: non-inferiority of partial irradiation compared to whole-breast irradiation

Non-inferiority trials are used in an attempt to display how a new, more conservative, treatment – in light of other benefits – may still be within an acceptable limit of 'inferiority' compared to the existing standard. Indeed, although it is sensible to expect that APBI is unlikely to be *more* effective than WBRT, it may still be considered as a suitable treatment alternative if the degree of its inferiority falls within a small, predetermined, margin.

Over 90% of local recurrences of cancer after breast-conserving surgery occur at, or in close proximity to, the original site of the operation. This means that while analyses of mastectomy specimens have found that the majority of additional cancer foci are found *outside* the index quadrant, the incidence of new breast cancers in other breast quadrants in the ipsilateral breast, remain similar to that of the contralateral breast [10,11]. A possible reason for this is that the local microenvironment may sometimes develop a tumour-promoting effect, perhaps due to the surgery (i.e., tumour seeding). This affirms the rationale towards using APBI, which offers more localised irradiation such that good control is preserved over the site that is most relevant despite the lower overall radiation dose.

A number of major clinical trials have since been conducted, comparing APBI to WBRT, with varying results due to the diversity of sample populations. Major multicentre trials conducted in the United Kingdom (UK IMPORT trial, 2017) [12] and in Canada, Australia, and New Zealand (RAPID, 2019) [13] found that APBI was non-inferior to WBRT. On the other hand, the NSABP B-39/RTOG 0413 2018 equivalence trial conducted in the United States concluded that APBI did not meet their equivalence criteria [14].

Meta-analyses have concluded that while APBI is associated with a small, statistically significant increase in local recurrence rates, other outcomes such as nodal or systemic recurrence, mortality rates, and overall survival were similar to that of WBRT [15,16]. Interestingly, studies which included only patients with low-risk characteristics saw comparable local recurrence rates between APBI and WBRT groups [17,18]. As expected, patients with larger tumours saw a lower degree of improvement in mortality and overall survival rates without recurrence. This is likely due to the fact that, even with APBI, more extensive radiation fields had to be used to account for larger tumours, thus diminishing the distinction in radiation field size between APBI and WBRT in the first place. This showed that there is, indeed, a specific population (i.e., patients with small, early stage, tumours) that may benefit optimally from APBI.

Quality of life

There has been an increasing emphasis on cosmesis in breast-conserving surgery, especially since satisfaction with cosmetic outcomes highly correlates with psychological morbidity [19]. Cosmetic outcomes after APBI have shown mixed results depending on the modality of APBI used. Initial reviews showed worse late radiation toxicity (e.g., subcutaneous fibrosis, telangiectasia, fat necrosis) with external beam APBI compared to WBRT [15]. However, many subsequent trials have shown very promising cosmetic outcomes, even with longer follow-up periods. This is likely to be due to the use of new techniques that have gained traction in the past few years, such as newer brachytherapy applicators, intensity-modulated radiotherapy (IMRT), as well as intraoperative radiotherapy (IORT) [20]. More research needs to be conducted with regard to cosmesis, especially with the emerging techniques that are quickly taking over the space.

Other significant outcomes affecting quality of life include fatigue, skin irritation, breast pain, and social functioning. Various studies have shown that women treated with APBI reported either similar or significantly better overall quality of life compared to those who had undergone WBRT [21–23]. APBI is generally well-tolerated, and even if temporary deterioration is experienced shortly after treatment, quality of life has been shown to return to baseline levels within 3 months [24].

Economics of cancer care: material and immaterial costs

The cost of treatment should never be a deterrent when presenting a more efficacious intervention to a patient. With this said, economic evaluation still has a place in medicine, especially when the clinical efficacy between two given interventions is deemed to be similar or only slightly different. In such cases, cost-minimisation strategies and cost-effectiveness need to be considered with great scrutiny [25]. Cancer care is incredibly complex in this regard because hidden costs permeate every aspect of the illness – this includes everything from managing side effects of treatment to potential disease progression or recurrence. Non-medical costs must also be taken into consideration, such as time lost travelling to additional hospital appointments, time taken off work, and childcare. Finally, in keeping with the recent emphasis on patient-centred care, it is paramount that non-material costs such as the psychological burden of repeated visits to the hospital, the perception of being a burden to family members, and general patient satisfaction must be taken into account since these can sometimes be the factors that matter most to patients.

Whole-breast radiation therapy is ordinarily delivered daily over up to 7 weeks following breast-conserving surgery. Regrettably, this treatment duration was found to be less than ideal for a significant proportion of patients. There are reports of rates of up to 50% of patients declining adjuvant WBRT following breast-conserving surgery, due to a range of reasons, one of them being geographical location [26,27]. Other studies have found that patients, for reasons related to the nuisance of attending daily treatment, have declined WBRT or even opted for mastectomy simply to avoid this daily treatment [28]. This has led to trials exploring the merit of hypofractionated radiotherapy, which considerably reduces the dose and duration of adjuvant radiotherapy. The FAST-Forward trial recently found hypofractionated radiotherapy over 1 week to be non-inferior to the standard 3-week treatment course, in terms of local control, although there was a trend towards higher late normal tissue effects with the 1-week course reaching statistical significance in the group receiving 27 Gy [29]. APBI is another, possibly more cost-effective [30,31], way to deliver shorter courses of radiotherapy. One form of APBI, IORT, even enables patients to receive all the radiotherapy treatment during the surgery itself. This means that the patient does not have to return to the hospital for further radiotherapy treatment post-operatively, allowing patients who would ordinarily forgo adjuvant radiotherapy (perhaps due to financial or time restraints) to receive their treatment in its entirety without compromising clinical outcomes.

Those treatments requiring fewer hospital visits will prove to be of additional value in the new coronavirus disease 2019 (COVID-19) pandemic, where exposure to COVID-19 should be avoided as far as possible, especially among vulnerable cancer patients. Regardless, it is likely that APBI will dominate treatment for patients with early-stage cancers who benefit equally from shorter or longer regimens.

RECENT TECHNIQUES

Brachytherapy

One of the pioneering APBI techniques is *multi-catheter interstitial brachytherapy* (MIB), which has been in use for decades and has been shown to be non-inferior to WBRT in terms of local recurrence, in the GEC-ESTRO trial [18]. In MIB, radioactive catheters are positioned within and around the lumpectomy cavity either free-hand or by using a template. Radiation is delivered either in the form of high, low, or pulsed dose rates. Once the radiation has been delivered, the non-permanent catheters are removed in a relatively painless process requiring no anaesthesia. MIB has been evaluated extensively and is not just an attractive option among the standard APBI target population, but also has been described as an excellent compromise for elderly patients, who may not be physiologically fit for WBRT but can be treated with even a single fraction of MIB, if the alternative is to have endocrine therapy alone [32,33].

A technique that has gained popularity in the United States is *intra-cavity balloon brachytherapy*. In this technique, applicators are positioned within the lumpectomy cavity with balloons that are inflated with water or saline, along with some contrast. The core of the catheter contains radioactive seeds which then deliver the radiation to the target site. Out of the newer balloon brachytherapy techniques, the *Xoft Axxent* electronic *brachytherapy* device [34] completely omits the use of radioisotopes through its use of miniaturised X-rays as a low-energy source. Apart from the undeniable benefit of not requiring shielding from radiation, its controller is portable, widening the scope for use in even outpatient clinics. However, neither technique has been evaluated within a randomised controlled trial and long-term outcomes are not known.

Non-invasive image-guided breast brachytherapy (NIBB) is also a newer technique allowing greater precision in delivering radiation to the tumour bed. It utilises breast compression and mammographic-like image guidance, and unlike all the other brachytherapy approaches, does not require any catheter placement. This completely non-invasive technique eliminates the risk of infection due to indwelling foreign objects. It may also be an attractive option for patients who are less tolerant towards the discomfort of having catheters placed in their breast. Research data is promising; NIBB is well-tolerated, associated with a low incidence of significant late toxicity, and results in favourable cosmetic outcomes [35,36].

Three-dimensional conformal radiotherapy and intensity-modulated radiotherapy

Traditional WBRT is typically carried out using the external beam approach, also known as external beam radiotherapy (EBRT). It is not a surprise, then, in the quest for a partial breast irradiation technique, researchers have come up with a modern approach using EBRT to target regions of the breast more selectively. The main merit of doing this is the fact that the process remains non-invasive. The process is also simpler and not as technically-challenging as brachytherapy.

The initial product that emerged was *three-dimensional conformal radiotherapy* (3D-CRT), which involves multiple beams of radiation being directed to the lumpectomy cavity in various different planes. 3D-CRT quickly garnered widespread use since many hospitals already utilised this technique for other cancers.

A newer EBRT technique which shortly succeeded 3D-CRT is *intensity-modulated radiotherapy*. IMRT is a more complex form of 3D-CRT which allows more precise modulation of radiation doses as it involves computerised inverse planning and permits non-uniform intensity of radiation beams. IMRT has been shown to result in favourable outcomes in terms of dosimetric analysis, while maintaining comparable or reduced toxicity and improved cosmesis [37,38]. It also allows more homogeneous dose distribution among larger-breasted women [39]. However, duration of treatment is still 3 weeks and IMRT suffers from the same drawbacks of EBRT related to late normal tissue effects.

Intraoperative radiation therapy

Intraoperative radiation therapy is unique in that irradiation occurs during the breast-conserving surgery itself. It allows very accurate delivery of radiation to the target site, since this occurs by direct visualisation of the lumpectomy cavity during surgery itself. IORT was evaluated for breast cancer treatment since the late 1990s [40]. The TARGIT-A randomised controlled trial of IORT, randomised its first patient in March 2000 and demonstrated non-inferiority against EBRT [41], with long-term follow-up [42]. IORT is also currently being explored for its use in colorectal cancer (CRC) [43], glioblastoma multiforme (GBM) [44], and head and neck cancers, with very promising results to date.

Since IORT is defined by the circumstance in which radiation is delivered (i.e., intraoperatively), and not by the irradiation technique used, there are a wide range of techniques that fall within the definition of IORT, some of which also fall under the categories mentioned previously. The most relevant IORT techniques are summarised in **Table 10.1**.

Overall, the evidence for IORT is very good. The obvious benefit is that a more accurately demarcated target area is irradiated during the surgery itself. Irradiation in this manner avoids inaccuracy caused by inconsistent displacement of breast tissue after surgery and misleading positional relation of breast scars from the actual lumpectomy site [50]. IORT may also prove beneficial in populations with breasts that are smaller in size, as it has been noted that EBRT techniques such as 3D-CRT have been unsuccessful at effectively targeting medial tumours without unnecessarily exposing the contralateral breast to additional radiation [51,52]. Another significant advantage is the fact that there is no time delay between resection of the tumour and the delivery of radiotherapy. This is significant because there is a statistically significant increase in local recurrence with

Table 10.1 Intraoperative radiation therapy (IORT) techniques	
Technique	**Major trials**
Low-energy X-rays (Intrabeam) A single dose of around 20 Gy of low-energy X-rays is delivered using a spherical applicator of a chosen size that is anchored to position in the lumpectomy cavity. Beyond the surface of the applicator, up to 6 Gy of radiation is delivered at a 1-cm depth. The treatment lasts for around 20–35 minutes	• *TARGIT-A* [41,42] There was a slightly higher rate of recurrence with IORT, but this was within the 2.5% non-inferiority margin. There was no significant difference in overall survival, local recurrence-free survival, mastectomy-free survival, distant disease-free survival, and breast cancer mortality. Mortality from other causes was significantly lower with IORT. IORT was also cheaper than EBRT • *TARGIT-B* [45] This ongoing trial explores the utility of IORT in delivering a tumour bed boost after breast-conserving surgery, in comparison to EBRT. The population being studied is patients under 45 years of age or those with a higher risk of cancer recurrence
Intraoperative electron radiotherapy (IOERT) (Lilac, Novac7, Mobetron) Electron radiation is delivered with a mobile linear accelerator at a uniform dose of around 10–25 Gy in a single fraction. The accelerators are able to deliver radiation at higher rates, so the procedure only lasts around 15–20 minutes	• *ELIOT* [46] There was a significantly higher rate of local recurrence with IOERT compared to EBRT, but this difference was within the 4.5% non-inferiority margin • *HIOB trial* [47] This is another ongoing trial investigating the use of IOERT tumour bed boost followed by hypofractionated whole-breast radiation therapy (WBRT). Preliminary results after a short/mid-term follow-up show excellent tolerance of the regimen. Cosmetic appearance was also well-preserved after 3 years
192Ir high-dose-rate (HDR) brachytherapy Iridium-192 (192Ir) is delivered via multiple catheters positioned using a flexible template applicator. Approximately, 18 Gy is delivered at a 1-cm depth, with the process taking around 20–40 minutes. Shielding is required, where only the patient remains in the shielded room during the delivery of treatment	• *Maranzano et al.* [48] and *Gaudet et al.* [49] HDR brachytherapy in women with early-stage breast cancer is associated with local control, survival rates, and cosmetic outcomes that are comparable to that in WBRT

delays in commencing radiotherapy [53]. This means that, with IORT, irradiation can occur before the tumour cells start to proliferate. There is considerable interest also in the role of IORT as a tumour bed breast boost, for which findings have been promising so far. Another possible application of IORT may include settings where nipple-sparing mastectomies are performed in order to preserve cosmetic outcomes; in such cases, IORT should be explored further as a possible option in order to maximise oncological outcomes [54,55].

To date, the British Association of Surgical Oncology (BASO) has produced guidelines for the practical management of breast cancer during the COVID-19 pandemic; these guidelines recommended that, where possible, targeted intraoperative radiotherapy (TARGIT-IORT) be offered to patients who are either suitable for breast conservation or patients who are considering mastectomy in order to avoid EBRT.

Among the IORT techniques listed above, Intrabeam˚ was found to be cheaper than EBRT, which may tip the balance in its favour. However, out of the above-listed techniques, only high-dose-rate (HDR) brachytherapy is routinely performed in conjunction with intraoperative image-guidance [i.e., computed tomography (CT) scan], which allows identification of errors in applicator positioning, dosimetric analysis to the target area and adjacent structures, and documentation of other actionable findings [56].

Given the meaningful benefits of IORT and its clinical non-inferiority to WBRT in low-risk patients, there has been an increase in the implementation of IORT around the world, especially following the publication of the American Society for Radiation Oncology (ASTRO) APBI guidelines and the TARGIT-A trial. In order to encourage widespread use of this APBI modality, further fine-tuning of patient selection criteria for IORT and greater awareness outside academic centres, are required.

CONCLUSION

The current paradigm in breast cancer treatment is to strive to deliver the 'minimum effective treatment' to patients, including hypofractionated or accelerated adjuvant radiotherapy and partial breast irradiation. APBI techniques should now be considered as an alternative to EBRT for selected patients, in line with published evidence. With some techniques such as IORT, the risk of local recurrence should be discussed with patients and considered along with evidence on breast cancer and non-breast cancer mortality and the great advantage of a single-fraction radiation treatment.

Key points for clinical practice

- The recent publication of numerous long-term studies have corroborated the preliminary findings supporting APBI and validated its use in lower risk, early-stage breast cancers
- Although APBI can be used as an exclusive modality of radiotherapy following breast-conserving surgery, there is also potential for its use in the context of a breast boost following whole-breast irradiation, or in addition to post-surgical EBRT
- Most systematic reviews to date have displayed heterogeneity in the APBI modalities used. It may be beneficial for comparisons to be made *between* different APBI modalities in order to delineate the specific settings in which some techniques may be better suited than others

REFERENCES

1. Early Breast Cancer Trialists' Collaborative Group, Darby S, McGale P, et al. Effect of radiotherapy after breast-conserving surgery on 10-year recurrence and 15-year breast cancer death: meta-analysis of individual patient data for 10,801 women in 17 randomised trials. Lancet 2011; 378:1707–1716.
2. Blamey RW, Bates T, Chetty U, et al. Radiotherapy or tamoxifen after conserving surgery for breast cancers of excellent prognosis: British Association of Surgical Oncology (BASO) II trial. Eur J Cancer 2013; 49:2294–2302.
3. Fisher B, Anderson S, Bryant J, et al. Twenty-year follow-up of a randomized trial comparing total mastectomy, lumpectomy, and lumpectomy plus irradiation for the treatment of invasive breast cancer. N Engl J Med 2002; 347:1233–1241.
4. NICE. Adjuvant therapy for early and locally advanced breast cancer 2018. [online] Available from https://www.nice.org.uk/guidance/ng101 [Last accessed January, 2021].
5. Darby SC, Ewertz M, McGale P, et al. Risk of ischemic heart disease in women after radiotherapy for breast cancer. N Engl J Med 2013; 368:987–998.
6. Bergom C, Currey A, Desai N, et al. Deep inspiration breath hold: techniques and advantages for cardiac sparing during breast cancer irradiation. Front Oncol 2018; 8:87.
7. Korzets Y, Fyles A, Shepshelovich D, et al. Toxicity and clinical outcomes of partial breast irradiation compared to whole breast irradiation for early-stage breast cancer: a systematic review and meta-analysis. Breast Cancer Res Treat 2019; 175:531–545.
8. Taylor C, Correa C, Duane FK, et al. Estimating the risks of breast cancer radiotherapy: evidence from modern radiation doses to the lungs and heart and from previous randomized trials. J Clin Oncol 2017; 35:1641–1649.
9. Hoekstra N, Habraken S, Swaak-Kragten A, et al. Reducing the risk of secondary lung cancer in treatment planning of accelerated partial breast irradiation. Front Oncol 2020; 10:1445.
10. Fisher ER, Anderson S, Redmond C, et al. Ipsilateral breast tumor recurrence and survival following lumpectomy and irradiation: pathological findings from NSABP protocol B-06. Semin Surg Oncol 1992;8:161–166.
11. Veronesi U, Luini A, Del Vecchio M, et al. Radiotherapy after breast-preserving surgery in women with localized cancer of the breast. N Engl J Med 1993; 328:1587–1591.
12. Coles CE, Griffin CL, Kirby AM, et al. Partial-breast radiotherapy after breast conservation surgery for patients with early breast cancer (UK IMPORT LOW trial): 5-year results from a multicentre, randomised, controlled, phase 3, non-inferiority trial. Lancet 2017; 390:1048–1060.
13. Whelan TJ, Julian JA, Berrang TS, et al. External beam accelerated partial breast irradiation versus whole breast irradiation after breast conserving surgery in women with ductal carcinoma in situ and node-negative breast cancer (RAPID): a randomised controlled trial. Lancet 2019; 394:2165–2172.
14. Vicini FA, Cecchini RS, White JR, et al. Long-term primary results of accelerated partial breast irradiation after breast-conserving surgery for early-stage breast cancer: a randomised, phase 3, equivalence trial. Lancet 2019; 394:2155–2164.
15. Hickey BE, Lehman M, Francis DP, et al. Partial breast irradiation for early breast cancer. Cochrane Database Syst Rev 2016; 7:CD007077.
16. Marta GN, Macedo CR, Carvalho Hde A, et al. Accelerated partial irradiation for breast cancer: systematic review and meta-analysis of 8,653 women in eight randomized trials. Radiother Oncol 2015; 114:42–49.
17. Livi L, Meattini I, Marrazzo L, et al. Accelerated partial breast irradiation using intensity-modulated radiotherapy versus whole breast irradiation: 5-year survival analysis of a phase 3 randomised controlled trial. Eur J Cancer 2015; 51:451–463.
18. Strnad V, Ott OJ, Hildebrandt G, et al. 5-year results of accelerated partial breast irradiation using sole interstitial multicatheter brachytherapy versus whole-breast irradiation with boost after breast-conserving surgery for low-risk invasive and in-situ carcinoma of the female breast: a randomised, phase 3, non-inferiority trial. Lancet 2016; 387:229–238.
19. Al-Ghazal SK, Fallowfield L, Blamey RW. Does cosmetic outcome from treatment of primary breast cancer influence psychosocial morbidity? Eur J Surg Oncol 1999; 25:571–573.
20. Shah C, Vicini F. Accelerated partial breast irradiation: redefining the treatment target for women with early stage breast cancer. Breast J 2019; 25:408–417.
21. Meattini I, Saieva C, Miccinesi G, et al. Accelerated partial breast irradiation using intensity modulated radiotherapy versus whole breast irradiation: health-related quality of life final analysis from the Florence phase 3 trial. Eur J Cancer 2017; 76:17–26.

22. Schafer R, Strnad V, Polgar C, et al. Quality-of-life results for accelerated partial breast irradiation with interstitial brachytherapy versus whole-breast irradiation in early breast cancer after breast-conserving surgery (GEC-ESTRO): 5-year results of a randomised, phase 3 trial. Lancet Oncol 2018; 19:834–844.
23. Perez M, Schootman M, Hall LE, et al. Accelerated partial breast irradiation compared with whole breast radiation therapy: a breast cancer cohort study measuring change in radiation side-effects severity and quality of life. Breast Cancer Res Treat 2017; 162:329–342.
24. Jacobs DH, Horeweg N, Straver M, et al. Health-related quality of life of breast cancer patients after accelerated partial breast irradiation using intraoperative or external beam radiotherapy technique. Breast 2019; 46:32–39.
25. Lyman GH. Economics of cancer care. J Oncol Pract 2007; 3:113–114.
26. Feinstein AJ, Soulos PR, Long JB, et al. Variation in receipt of radiation therapy after breast-conserving surgery: assessing the impact of physicians and geographic regions. Med Care 2013; 51:330–338.
27. Shah C, Vicini F, Shaitelman SF, et al. The American Brachytherapy Society consensus statement for accelerated partial-breast irradiation. Brachytherapy 2018; 17:154–170.
28. Lazovich DA, White E, Thomas DB, et al. Underutilization of breast-conserving surgery and radiation therapy among women with stage I or II breast cancer. JAMA 1991; 266:3433–3438.
29. Murray Brunt A, Haviland JS, Wheatley DA, et al. Hypofractionated breast radiotherapy for 1 week versus 3 weeks (FAST-Forward): 5-year efficacy and late normal tissue effects results from a multicentre, non-inferiority, randomised, phase 3 trial. Lancet 2020; 395:1613–1626.
30. Shah C, Ward MC, Tendulkar RD, et al. Cost and cost-effectiveness of image guided partial breast irradiation in comparison to hypofractionated whole breast irradiation. Int J Radiat Oncol Biol Phys 2019; 103:397–402.
31. Lanni T, Keisch M, Shah C, et al. A cost comparison analysis of adjuvant radiation therapy techniques after breast-conserving surgery. Breast J 2013; 19:162–167.
32. Sumodhee S, Levy J, Chamorey E, et al. Accelerated partial breast irradiation for elderly women with early breast cancer: a compromise between whole breast irradiation and omission of radiotherapy. Brachytherapy 2017; 16:929–934.
33. Kinj R, Chand ME, Gal J, et al. Five-year oncological outcome after a single fraction of accelerated partial breast irradiation in the elderly. Radiat Oncol 2019; 14:234.
34. Dickler A. Xoft Axxent electronic brachytherapy: a new device for delivering brachytherapy to the breast. Nat Clin Pract Oncol 2009; 6:138–142.
35. Hepel JT, Leonard KL, Sha S, et al. Phase 2 trial of accelerated partial breast irradiation (APBI) using noninvasive image-guided breast brachytherapy (NIBB). Int J Radiat Oncol Biol Phys 2020; 108:1143–1149.
36. Hepel JT, Hiatt JR, Sha S, et al. The rationale, technique, and feasibility of partial breast irradiation using noninvasive image-guided breast brachytherapy. Brachytherapy 2014; 13:493–501.
37. Buwenge M, Cammelli S, Ammendolia I, et al. Intensity modulated radiation therapy for breast cancer: current perspectives. Breast Cancer (Dove Med Press) 2017; 9:121–126.
38. Mondal D, Sharma DN. External beam radiation techniques for breast cancer in the new millennium: new challenging perspectives. J Egypt Natl Canc Inst 2016; 28:211–218.
39. Pignol JP, Olivotto I, Rakovitch E, et al. A multicenter randomized trial of breast intensity-modulated radiation therapy to reduce acute radiation dermatitis. J Clin Oncol 2008; 26:2085–2092.
40. Vaidya JS, Tobias JS, Baum M, et al. Intraoperative radiotherapy for breast cancer. Lancet Oncol 2004; 5:165–173.
41. Vaidya JS, Wenz F, Bulsara M, et al. An international randomised controlled trial to compare TARGeted Intraoperative radioTherapy (TARGIT) with conventional postoperative radiotherapy after breast-conserving surgery for women with early-stage breast cancer (the TARGIT-A trial). Health Technol Assess 2016; 20:1–188.
42. Vaidya JS, Bulsara M, Baum M, et al. Long-term survival and local control outcomes from single dose targeted intraoperative radiotherapy during lumpectomy (TARGIT-IORT) for early breast cancer: TARGIT-A randomised clinical trial. BMJ 2020; 370:m2836.
43. Mirnezami R, Chang GJ, Das P, et al. Intraoperative radiotherapy in colorectal cancer: systematic review and meta-analysis of techniques, long-term outcomes, and complications. Surg Oncol. 2013;22:22–35.
44. Sarria GR, Sperk E, Han X, et al. Intraoperative radiotherapy for glioblastoma: an international pooled analysis. Radiother Oncol 2020; 142:162–167.
45. Sedlmayer F, Reitsamer R, Wenz F, et al. Intraoperative radiotherapy (IORT) as boost in breast cancer. Radiat Oncol 2017; 12:23.
46. Veronesi U, Orecchia R, Maisonneuve P, et al. Intraoperative radiotherapy versus external radiotherapy for early breast cancer (ELIOT): a randomised controlled equivalence trial. Lancet Oncol 2013; 14:1269–1277.

47. Fastner G, Reitsamer R, Urbanski B, et al. Toxicity and cosmetic outcome after hypofractionated whole breast irradiation and boost-IOERT in early stage breast cancer (HIOB): first results of a prospective multicenter trial (NCT01343459). Radiother Oncol 2020; 146:136–142.

48. Maranzano E, Arcidiacono F, Italiani M, et al. Accelerated partial-breast irradiation with high-dose-rate brachytherapy: mature results of a phase II trial. Brachytherapy 2019; 18:627–634.

49. Gaudet M, Pharand-Charbonneau M, Wright D, et al. Long-term results of multicatheter interstitial high-dose-rate brachytherapy for accelerated partial-breast irradiation. Brachytherapy 2019; 18:211–216.

50. Esposito E, Anninga B, Harris S, et al. Intraoperative radiotherapy in early breast cancer. Br J Surg 2015; 102:599–610.

51. Kosaka Y, Mitsumori M, Yamauchi C, et al. Feasibility of accelerated partial breast irradiation using three-dimensional conformal radiation therapy for Japanese women: a theoretical plan using six patients' CT data. Breast Cancer 2008; 15:108–114.

52. Njeh CF, Saunders MW, Langton CM. Accelerated partial breast irradiation (APBI): a review of available techniques. Radiat Oncol 2010; 5:90.

53. Huang J, Barbera L, Brouwers M, et al. Does delay in starting treatment affect the outcomes of radiotherapy? A systematic review. J Clin Oncol 2003; 21:555–563.

54. Pan L, Ye C, Chen L, et al. Oncologic outcomes and radiation safety of nipple-sparing mastectomy with intraoperative radiotherapy for breast cancer. Breast Cancer 2019; 26:618–627.

55. Petit JY, Veronesi U, Orecchia R, et al. Nipple-sparing mastectomy in association with intra-operative radiotherapy (ELIOT): a new type of mastectomy for breast cancer treatment. Breast Cancer Res Treat 2006; 96:47–51.

56. Trifiletti DM, Showalter TN, Libby B, et al. Intraoperative breast radiation therapy with image guidance: findings from CT images obtained in a prospective trial of intraoperative high-dose-rate brachytherapy with CT on rails. Brachytherapy 2015; 14:919–924.

Chapter 11

Evolving trends in localisation techniques in breast surgery

Oshi Abeyakoon, Gloria Petralia, Pankaj Roy

INTRODUCTION

Increased public awareness, breast cancer screening programmes, advances in imaging {tomosynthesis, higher resolution [magnetic resonance imaging (MRI)]} and image-guided biopsy have resulted in a rise in the diagnosis of early-stage breast cancer which is often impalpable. Treatment of impalpable cancer requires image-guided localisation to direct surgery. Smaller lesions can be excised while conserving the remaining healthy breast tissue, thus reducing the disfiguring and long-term morbidity of mastectomy. Wire-guided localisation has been the established method of localisation to facilitate breast-conserving surgery. However, there are several disadvantages which include incomplete surgical excision requiring re-operation, removal of excess normal breast tissue, patient discomfort and decreased efficiency in theatre workflow due to limitations in scheduling.

In node-positive disease undergoing neoadjuvant systemic treatment, surgery to the axilla may similarly be de-escalated with potential benefit to the patient. It is reported that marking biopsied axillary nodes before neoadjuvant treatment can improve the diagnostic performance of sentinel lymph node biopsy (SLNB) [1,2] although there are as yet no data from randomised controlled trials supporting this approach.

New techniques such as radioactive seed localisation (RSL), magnetic seed/trace localisation, non-radioactive radar localisation and radiofrequency identification tags (RFIT) are promising new alternatives. In this chapter, we explore advantages and disadvantages of using these techniques and currently available outcome data on localisation systems approved for clinical use.

BACKGROUND

Breast cancer is a heterogeneous disease, which requires accurate stratification and treatment planning to achieve the best outcome. Timing and choice of treatment depend on disease profile and patient characteristics and are aimed at improving survival and quality of life. Treatment options for breast cancer include surgery, radiotherapy, chemotherapy, endocrine therapy and immunotherapy; risks, indications and benefits of which need to be balanced to facilitate an informed choice for the patient. Initial treatment paradigms of breast cancer were based on Halsted's radical mastectomy. As surgical and imaging techniques evolved, there was a shift from radical to minimally disfiguring surgery. The benefits of breast-conserving surgery for non-palpable breast cancer have been validated in several randomised controlled trials [3–5].

Successful breast-conserving surgery of non-palpable early-stage breast cancer is dependent on achieving clear margins; thus re-operation (re-excision) rate is used as a quality indicator in breast cancer treatment [6]. To achieve the best oncological and cosmetic outcome, breast cancer must be accurately staged (size and location) and excised with an adequate clear margin whilst limiting the resection of normal breast tissue [7]. Worldwide re-operation rates after breast-conserving surgery range from 14% to 70% [8], in some regional reports the average is as high 30–40% [9]. The reasons for the variability and high re-operation rates are multifactorial; however, inaccurate localisation is an important factor.

Although dyes have been used in the past as means of marking impalpable areas [10,11], the most commonly used method to localise non-palpable breast cancer is wire-guided localisation (**Figure 11.1a to c**). It is a relatively inexpensive method and can be performed

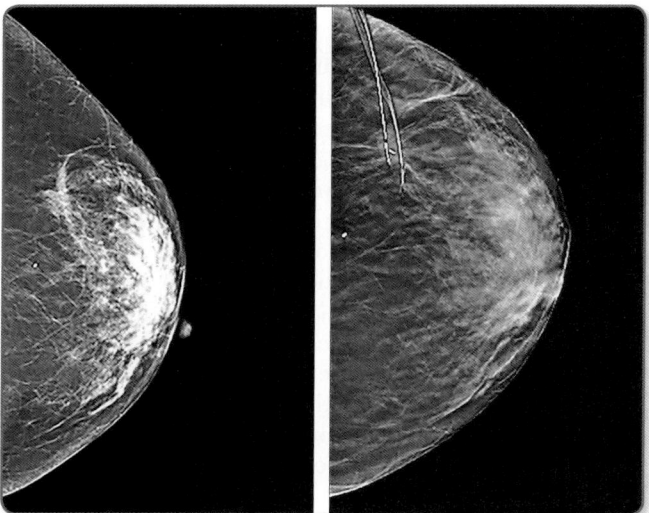

Figure 11.1a Mammograms showing location of tumours before and after bracket localisation with flexible hook wires craniocaudal (CC) views.

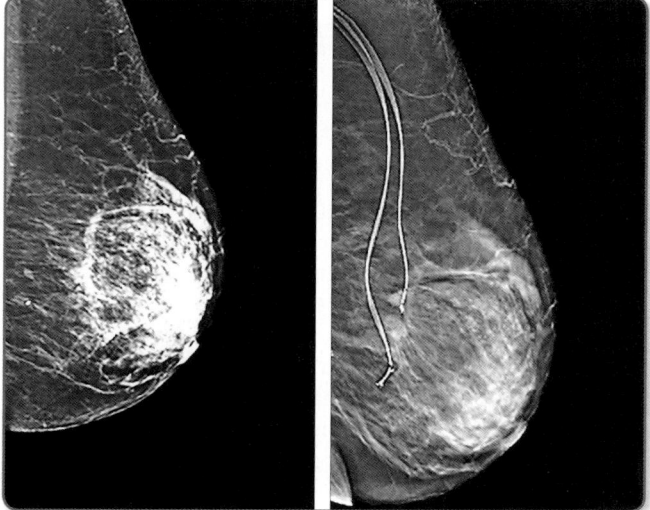

Figure 11.1b Mammograms showing location of tumours before and after bracket localisation with flexible hook wires mediolateral oblique (MLO) views.

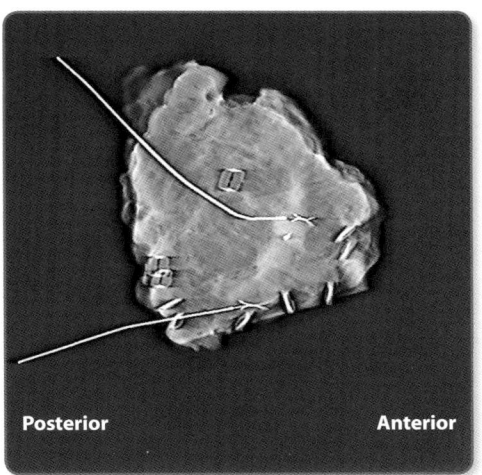

Figure 11.1c Specimen radiograph imaged using tomosynthesis showing the tumours, with wires to the marker clips (shaped like an X). The specimen is oriented with clips (done during surgery after removing the specimen). The specimen radiograph helps the surgeon to take extra shaves during surgery, if needed.

Posterior   Anterior

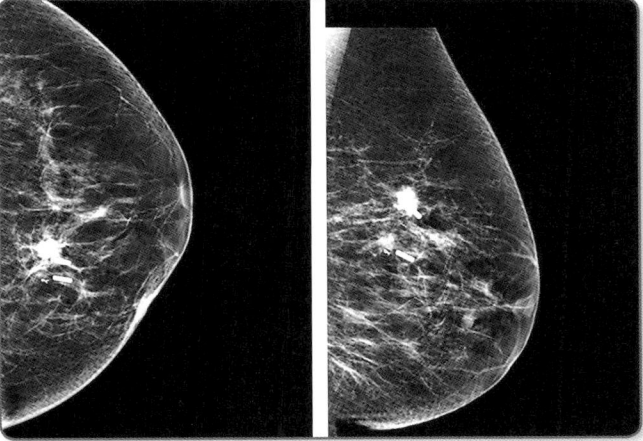

Figure 11.2a Mammograms showing location of tumours along with marker clips (inserted during biopsy) and bracket localisation with radiofrequency (RF) seeds (inserted couple of days before surgery) craniocaudal (CC) and mediolateral oblique (MLO) views.

under ultrasound, mammographic and MR guidance. The skill of placing a wire to localise a small breast cancer can be learned easily, however wires can displace, transect or fracture resulting in an inaccurate target for surgery thus increasing a risk of incomplete surgical resection and re-operation. Clear margin rates with wire-guided localisation are reported in 70.8–87.4% of cases [7]. There are significant limitations: (a) workflow efficiency as wires often need to be inserted on the same day of surgery creating logistical challenges and inefficiency in the use of operating room time; (b) patient experience as the external component of the wire needs to be taped to the skin and post-procedure mammograms need to be performed to document position, resulting in increased discomfort and pain for the patient.

To overcome these challenges, alternative approaches such as RSL [12] (**Figure 11.2a and b**), non-radioactive radar location (SAVI Scout) [13], magnetic seed localisation (Magseed) (**Figure 11.3a to c**) and RFID have been developed and are entering clinical practice having received the Food and Drug Administration (FDA) approval and

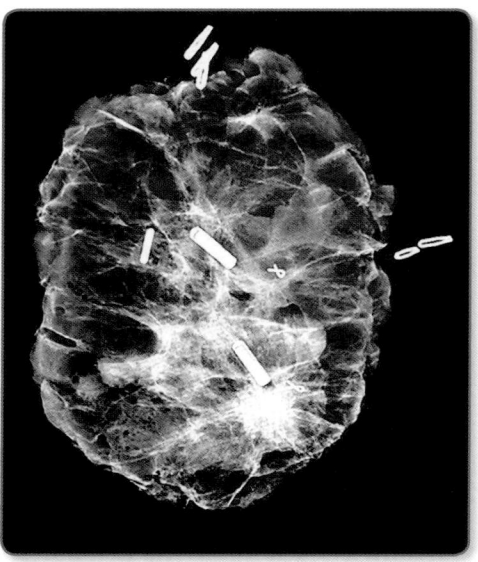

Figure 11.2b Specimen radiograph showing the tumours, marker clips (shaped like the pink ribbon symbol adopted by several breast cancer charities) and radiofrequency (RF) seeds. The specimen is oriented with clips (done during surgery after removing the specimen) with 1 clip (anterior), 2 clips (medial) and 3 clips (inferior). The orientation clips on the specimen radiograph helps the surgeon to take extra shaves during surgery, if needed.

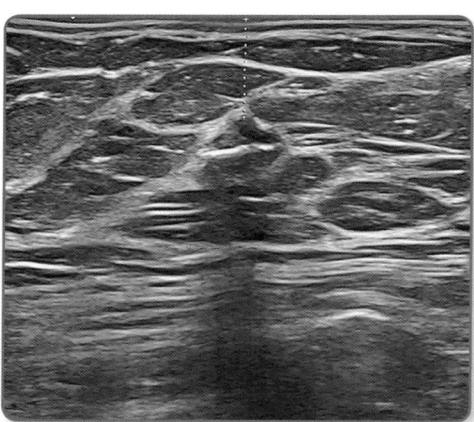

Figure 11.3a Ultrasound picture showing tumour with Magseed.

Conformitè Europëenne (CE) marking for clinical use. A summary of advantages and disadvantages of localisation techniques is summarised in **Table 11.1**.

COSMESIS AND PATIENT SATISFACTION

Similar outcomes have been published in terms of cosmesis when comparing wire localisation (WL) versus seed localisation (SL) techniques.

The cosmetic outcome of procedures is related to the amount of tissue removed in relation to the size of the breast. As demonstrated in Cheang's review [7] multiple

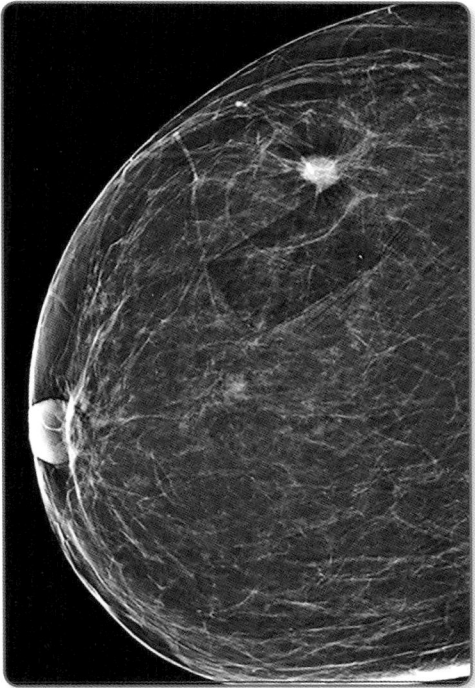 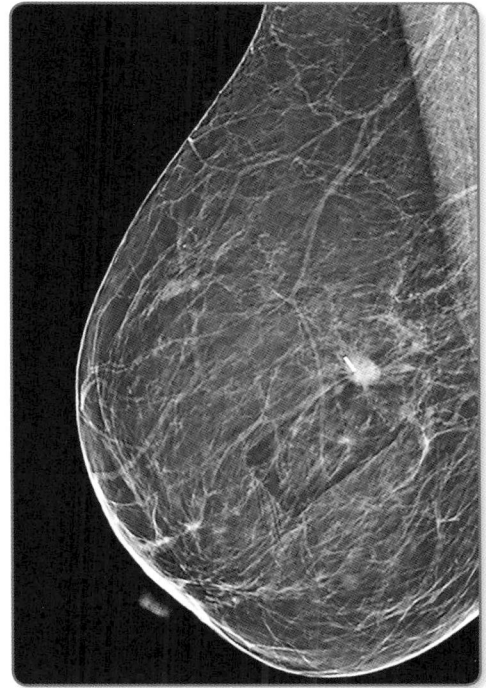

Figure 11.3b Mammogram showing location of tumour along with localisation with Magseed (inserted couple of days before surgery) in craniocaudal (CC) view.

Figure 11.3c Mammogram showing location of tumour along with localisation with Magseed (inserted couple of days before surgery) in mediolateral oblique (MLO) view.

randomised studies showed no statistically significant difference in the weight/volume of tissue excised when using WL versus SL.

Surgical scars are known to contract over time. A one-year follow-up study [14] found no difference in the clinical cosmetic score between patients receiving WL versus SL (97.1% vs. 98.6%; p = 0.5). Parvez et al [15]. conducted a randomised trial comparing cosmetic outcome in patients treated with RS versus WL at 1- and 3-year post-surgery. Frontal photographs were taken 1- and 3-year post-surgery. The European Organisation for Research and Treatment of Cancer Cosmetic Rating System was used to evaluate cosmesis outcomes by the patient and a panel of 5 raters. The study enrolled 73 patients (WL, n = 38; RSL, n = 35). Most patients rated their overall cosmesis as 'excellent' or 'good' (76% WL, 80% RSL). Patient and panel ratings on all cosmetic outcomes were similar between groups. Multivariable regression for overall cosmesis found larger specimen volume and re-operation to be predictors of worse ratings.

When considering patient satisfaction, several papers [16–18] demonstrated procedure convenience was greater with SL than WL. Pain perception with respect to RSL versus WL has a more varied outcome. Lovrics et al [19]. and *Bloomquist EV et al [18]* demonstrated higher pain ratings with WL. (p = 0.038 and 0.058 respectively). *Langhans et al [8]* did not show any difference between the RSL and WL groups.

Table 11.1 Summary of localisation methods

Localisation technique Year first reported	System components/targets	Advantages	Disadvantages
Dye: low-cost (cheaper than wire)			
Pigmented dyes (i.e.: methylthioninium chloride, Patent V) *Radioactive dyes* (Technetium-99m)	• Can target breast • Can target axilla	Routinely used for sentinel lymph node biopsy. Historically used to mark lesions in the breast/axilla	Difficult to identify breast lesions if not palpable, no longer routinely used in clinical practice outside SLNB
Charcoal tattooing Circa 1987	Injected via needle, under ultrasound guidance • Can target breast • Can target axilla	Can tattoo breast and cytology-proven metastatic axillary nodes A needle-point injection track can be made to the skin of the axilla to guide the surgeon	Charcoal granuloma mimicking cancer
Magtrace Endomag	Injected via a needle into the breast. • Axillary nodes	Avoids exposure to radiation Ease of scheduling patients avoiding a need for radionuclide injection on the morning of the surgery	Bruise-like discoloration which fades over time
External component: risk of migration, fracture or transection.			
Wire-guided localisation 1966	Wire Needle/trocar delivery system • Can target breast	Safe and established as routine clinical practice, inexpensive Can be placed under mammogram, US or MRI guidance	Wire migration, fracture or transection leading to incomplete resection/re-operation/poor cosmesis due to inaccurate tumour localisation Workflow scheduling and operating room inefficiencies as placed on day of surgery *Patient discomfort:* external component of the wire needs to be taped to the skin and post-procedure mammograms performed to document the position
Seeds: scheduling flexibility. No external component risks. Better cosmesis due to greater flexibility in choice of surgical approach. Increased cost per unit in comparison to wire localisation			
Radioactive seed localisation (RSL) 1999	Iodine 125 (half-life approximately 60 days) labelled titanium seed implant Needle delivery system *Detector:* Gamma probe/ion chamber • Can target breast	Increased flexibility in scheduling Uses same detector routinely used for sentinel node biopsy	Radiation safety precautions must be adhered to (only 7 days prior to surgery in some countries) Radiation exposure of staff No repositioning once deployed Cannot be placed under MRI guidance

Continues opposite

Table 11.1 *Continued*

Localisation technique Year first reported	System components/targets	Advantages	Disadvantages
Non-radioactive radar localisation (SAVI Scout) 2016	Implantable non-radioactive reflector Needle delivery system Detector Console • Can target breast • Can target axilla	Scheduling flexibility (FDA long-term implant clearance) No radiation exposure/safety precautions needed	Limitations in depth (6 cm) No repositioning once deployed Cannot be placed under MRI guidance Interference with halogen lights in theatre Contains nickel (could provoke reaction in patients with a nickel allergy)
Magnetic seed (Magseed) 2017	Stainless steel seed implant Needle delivery system Detector probe magnetises the seed and temporarily converts it to a magnet • Can target breast • Can target axilla	Scheduling flexibility (placed up to 30 days in advance) No radiation exposure/safety precautions needed Stainless steel seed (no issue with nickel allergy) Count indicates distance to seed	Depth limitation (probe to seed maximum distance 4 cm) No repositioning once deployed MRI bloom up to 4 cm (depending on sequence used) Should not be used in the left breast if pacemaker in situ Cannot be used in conjunction with a wire. Interference from metal operating instruments
Radiofrequency identification tags 2015	RFID localisation tag Needle delivery system Pencil probe system for intra-operative detection of RFID system • Can target breast • No axillary licence/used in research studies	Scheduling flexibility (long-term implantability over 30 days) No radiation exposure/safety precautions needed No issue with nickel allergy Tags are uniquely distinguishable from one another allowing a more complex mark-up of multifocal disease or bracketing the margins of the lesion, and accurate identification of a misplaced tag system Pencil probe detector provides a tag to probe precise distance Can be used in conjunction with a wire. Can be placed under MRI guidance The tag can be identified 6 cm from the skin surface	No repositioning once deployed MRI bloom up to 2–3 cm (depending on sequence used) Has not been used in patients with pacemakers Size of the clip Difficult to place in axilla due to its size

(FDA: Food and Drug Administration; MRI: magnetic resonance imaging)

OUTCOMES AND SAFETY

Fung et al [20]. compared local recurrence rates in 146 patients who received RSL and 152 patients who received WL at 5 years follow-up. There was no statistically different rate of recurrence between the two groups. (2/146 in RSL vs. 6/152 in WL; p = 0.28). The small sample size and low event rate were major limitations with the study.

Overall outcomes data for SL have been summarised in **Table 11.2**.

DISCUSSION

There is an expected learning curve with every new technique. It is possible that the data we see with SAVI Scout, Magseed and RFID do not reflect the true potential of the techniques as currently they are in the early phase of introduction into clinical practice. Increase in experience may demonstrate better outcomes when the technique itself is mastered.

A second important consideration is that the localisation system alone is one component of communicating information to the surgeons in the operating room. High-quality preoperative work-up using multimodality imaging, attention to detail in proving multifocality and multicentricity will refine the selection of cases, which are most suitable for breast-conserving surgery. The information from preoperative imaging will further enhance the surgeon's ability to resect the tumour facilitating negative margins and good cosmetic outcomes. Where neoadjuvant chemotherapy is used to downgrade the tumour prior to resection attention to detail between the original footprint of the tumour, fragmentation pattern and end of treatment appearances play a critical role in the planning and localisation of residual abnormality prior to surgery.

Future research must pay attention to matching the comparative groups for tumour size, histological subtype, grade, molecular profile, breast density, nodal status, preoperative imaging protocols and surgical preferences in removing healthy tissue surrounding the tumour to achieve a negative margin. These are important co-founders in the interpretation of data and best addressed within randomised controlled trials.

We can conclude that the introduction of new methods of localisation such as RSL, SAVI Scout, Magseed and RFID hold the promise of improved workflow, cosmesis and patient satisfaction.

Key points for clinical practice

- The most commonly used technique to localise non-palpable breast cancer is wire-guided localisation
- Alternative techniques include pigmented dyes or charcoal tattooing, RSL, non-radioactive radar location (e.g.,: SAVI Scout), magnetic SL and RFID
- Available data on alternative techniques are mainly based on cohort studies demonstrating high rates of successful localisation and variable rates of re-excision
- There is a need for randomised controlled trials in order to enable comparison between techniques and determine the optimal techniques for specific indications

Table 11.2 Summary of available outcome data for each localisation system. Modified from Cheang et al [7]

Reference Year of publication	Study design	Method	Malignant lesions	Mean/range time to operation (days)	Placement failure (%)	Re-operation rate (%)	Seed/reflector migration (%)
Cox et al 2003 [21]	Prospective	RSL	64/134	0–5	4/124 (3.0)	17/64 (26.5%)	0/134 (0)
Van Riet et al 2010 [22]	Prospective	RSL	325/325	4	3/325 (0.9%)	15/325 (4.6%)	0/325 (0)
Alderliesten et al 2011 [23]	Prospective	RSL	46/48	59.5 (3–136)	0/100 (0)	2/46 (4.3)	0/35 (1)
McGhan et al 2011 [24]	Retrospective	RSL	767/978	0–5	3/978 (0.3%)	118/767 (15.4%)	1/978 (0.1%)
Harvey et al 2018 [25]	Prospective	Magseed	29/29	5 (1–15)	0/29 (0)		
Price et al 2018 [26]	Prospective	Magseed	58/73	3 (0–40)	0/73 (0)	9/58 (12%)	0/73 (0)
Lamb et al 2018 [27]	Prospective	Magseed	142/213	211 placed on day of surgery	7/213 (3.2%) Placed by tomo	30/137 (21.9%)	0
Hersi et al 2019 [28]	Prospective	Magseed and Magtrace	32/32	3(0–25)	0	0	0
Zacharioudakis 2019 [29]	Prospective	Magseed	104/104	-	4/104 (3.8%)	16/104 (16%)	2/104
Thekkinkattil 2019 [30]	Prospective	Magseed	126	7 (0–30)	0/1	18/126 (14%)	0
Cox et al 2016 [31]	Prospective	SAVI Scout	101/153	1/154 (0.6)	1.8 (0–7)	17/101 (16.8)	1
Mango et al 2017 [32]	Retrospective	SAVI Scout	54/110	0–8	0/123 (0)	4/54 (7.4)	5/110

Continues overleaf

Table 11.2 Continued

Reference Year of publication	Study design	Method	Malignant lesions	Mean/range time to operation (days)	Placement failure (%)	Re-operation rate (%)	Seed/reflector migration (%)
Dauphine C et al 2015 [33]	Prospective	Radiofrequency identification technology	15/20	0	0/12 (0)	4/15 (27%)	
McGugin et al 2019 [34]	Retrospective	Radiofrequency identification technology	94/147	1–22 (in a cohort of 19)	0/147	18/95 (19.1%)	
DiNome et al 2019 [35]	Prospective	Radiofrequency identification technology	33/50	1.4 average (earliest 14 days)	0/50	2/33 (6%)	
Wazir et al 2020 [36]	Prospective	Radiofrequency identification technology	7/11	0	0	0/7	
Lowes et al 2020 [37]	Prospective	Radiofrequency identification technology	177/177	0–71 Average 7.8 days	174/177	(8.7%)	

(RSL: radioactive seed localisation)

REFERENCES

1. Caudle AS, Yang WT, Krishnamurthy S, et al. Improved axillary evaluation following neoadjuvant therapy for patients with node-positive breast cancer using selective evaluation of clipped nodes: implementation of targeted axillary dissection. J Clin Oncol 2016; 34:1072–1078.
2. Choy N, Lipson J, Porter C, et al. Initial results with preoperative tattooing of biopsied axillary lymph nodes and correlation to sentinel lymph nodes in breast cancer patients. Ann Surg Oncol 2015; 22:377–382.
3. Fisher B, Anderson S, Bryant J, et al. Twenty-year follow-up of a randomized trial comparing total mastectomy, lumpectomy, and lumpectomy plus irradiation for the treatment of invasive breast cancer. N Engl J Med 2002; 347:1233–1241.
4. Veronesi U, Cascinelli N, Mariani L, et al. Twenty-year follow-up of a randomised study breast-conserving surgery with radical mastectomy for early breast cancer. N Engl J Med 2002; 347:1227–1232.
5. Houssami N, Macaskill P, Marinovich ML, et al. Meta-analysis of the impact of the surgical margins on local recurrence in women with early-stage invasive breast cancer treated with breast-conserving therapy. Eur J Cancer 2010; 46:3219–3232.
6. Tamburelli F, Maggiorotto F, Marchiò C, et al. Reoperation rate after breast-conserving surgery as quality indicator in breast cancer treatment: a reappraisal. Breast 2020; 53:181–188.
7. Cheang E, Ha R, Thornton CM, et al. Innovations in image guided preoperative breast lesion localization. Br J Radiol 2018; 91:20170740.
8. Langhans L, Jensen MB, Talman MM, et al. Reoperation Rates in Ductal Carcinoma In Situ vs Invasive Breast Cancer After Wire-Guided Breast-Conserving Surgery. JAMA Surg 2017; 152:378–384.
9. Landercasper J. Why do re-operation rates vary so much after lumpectomy for breast cancer? Examining the re-operation puzzle and Massachusetts general hospital. Ann Sug Oncol 2018; 25:2506–2508.
10. Dufrane P, Mazy G, Vanhaudenaerde C. Prebiopsy localization of non-palpable breast cancer. J Belge Radiol 1990; 73:401–404.
11. Mok CW, Tan SM, Zheng Q, et al. Network meta-analysis of novel and conventional sentinel lymph node biopsy techniques in breast cancer. BJS Open 2019; 3:445–452.
12. Gray RJ, Salud C, Nguyen K, et al. Randomized prospective evaluation of a novel technique for biopsy or lumpectomy of non-palpable breast lesions: radioactive seed versus wire localization Ann Surg Oncol 2001; 8:711–715.
13. Patel SN, Mango VL, Jadeja P, et al. Reflector guided breast tumor localization versus wire localization for lumpectomies: a comparison of surgical outcomes. Clin Imaging 2018: 47:14–17.
14. Sharek D, Zuley ML, Zhang JY, et al. Radioactive seed localization versus wire localization for lumpectomies: a comparison of outcomes AJR Am J Roentgenol 2015; 204:872–877.
15. Parvex E, Cornacchi SD, Hodgson N, et al. A cosmesis outcome substudy in a prospective randomized trial comparing radio-guided seed localization with standard wire localization for non-palpable, invasive and in situ breast carcinomas. Am J Surg 2014; 208:711–718.
16. Gray RJ, Pockaj BA, Karstaedt PJ, et al. Radioactive seed localization of non-palpable breast lesions is better than wire localization. AM J Surg 2004; 188:377–380.
17. Rao R, Moldrem A, Sarode V, et al. Experience with seed localization for nonpalpable breast lesions in a public health care system. Ann Surg Oncol 2010; 17:3241–3246.
18. Bloomquist EV, Ajkay N, Patil S, et al. A randomized prospective comparison of patient-assessed satisfaction and clinical outcomes with radioactive seed localization versus wire localization. Breast J 2016; 22:151–157.
19. Lovrics PJ, Goldsmith CH, Hodgson N, et al. A multicentred, randomized, controlled trial comparing radioguided seed localization for non-palpable, invasive and site breast carcinomas. Ann Surg Oncol 2011; 18:3407–3414.
20. Fung F, Cornacchi SD, Reedijk M, et al. Breast cancer recurrence following radioguided seed localization and standard wire localization of non-palpable invasive and in situ cancers: 5-Year follow-up from a randomized controlled trial. Am J Surg 2017; 213:798–804.
21. Cox CE, Furman B, Stowell N, et al. Radioactive seed localization breast biopsy and lumpectomy: can specimen radiographs be eliminated? Ann Surg Oncol 2003; 10:1039–1047.
22. Van Riet YE, Maaskant AJ, Creemers GJ, et al. Identification of residual breast tumour localization after neo-adjuvant chemotherapy using a radioactive 125 Iodine seed. Eur J Surg Oncol 2010; 36:164–169.
23. Alderlstien T, Loo CE, Pengel KE, et al. Radioactive seed localization of breast lesions: an adequate localization method without seed migration. Breast J 2011; 17:594–601.
24. McGhan LJ, McKeever SC, Pockaj BA, et al. Radioactive seed localization for non-palpable breast lesions: review of 1,000 consecutive procedures at a single institution. Ann Surg Oncol 2011; 18:3096–3101.

25. Harvey JR, Lim Y, Murphy J, et al. Safety and feasibility of breast lesion localization using magnetic seeds (Mag seeds): a multi-centre, open label-cohort study. Breast Cancer Res Treat 2018; 169:531–536.
26. Price ER, Khoury AL, Esserman LJ, et al. Initial Clinical experience with an inducible magnetic seed system for preoperative breast lesions localization. AJR Am J Roentgenol 2018; 210:913–917.
27. Lamb LR, Bahl M, Specht MC, et al. Evaluation of a Nonradioactive Magnetic Marker Wireless Localization Program. AJR Am J Roentgenol 2018; 211:940–945.
28. Hersi AF, Eriksson S, Ramos J, et al. A combined, totally magnetic technique with a magnetic marker for non-palpable tumour localization and superparamagnetic iron oxide nanoparticles for sentinel lymph node detection in breast cancer surgery. Eur J Surg Oncol 2019; 45:544–549.
29. Zacharioudakis K, Down S, Bholah Z, et al. Is the future magnetic? Magseed localisation for non palpable breast cancer. A multi-centre non randomised control study. Surg Oncol 2019; 45:2016–2021.
30. Thekkinkattil D, Kaushik M, Hoosein MM, et al. A prospective, single-arm, multicentre clinical evaluation of a new localisation technique using non-radioactive Magseeds for surgery of clinically occult breast lesions. Clin Radiol 2019; 74:974.e7–974.e11.
31. Cox CE, Garcia-Henriquez N, Glancy MJ, et al. Pilot study of a new non-radioactive surgical guidance technology for locating non palpable breast lesions. Ann Surg Oncol 2016; 23:1824–1830.
32. Mango VL, Wynn RT, Feldman S, et al. Beyond wires and seeds: reflector-guided breast lesion localization and excision. Radiology 2017; 284:365–371.
33. Dauphine C, Reicher JJ, Reicher MA, et al. A prospective clinical study to evaluate the safety and performance of wireless localization of non-palpable breast lesion using radiofrequency identification technology. AJR Am J Roentgenol 2015; 204:W720–W723.
34. McGugin C, Spivey T, Coopey S, et al. Radiofrequency identification tag localization is comparable to wire localization for non-palpable breast lesions. Breast Cancer Res Treat 2019; 177:735–739.
35. DiNome ML, Kusske AM, Attai DJ, et al. Microchipping the breast: an effective new technology for localizing non-palpable breast lesions for surgery. Breast Cancer Res Treat 2019; 175:165–170.
36. Wazir U, Tayeh S, Perry N, et al. Wireless Breast Localization Using Radio-frequency Identification Tags: The First Reported European Experience in Breast Cancer. In Vivo 2020; 34:233–238.
37. Lowes S, Bell A, Milligan R, et al. Use of Hologic LOCalizer radiofrequency identification (RFID) tags to localise impalpable breast lesions and axillary nodes: experience of the first 150 cases in a UK breast unit. Clin Radiol 2020; 75:942–949.

Chapter 12

Advances in genetic risk of breast cancer

Ava Kwong, Stephanie Wing Yin Yu

INTRODUCTION

Genetic screening for hereditary breast and ovarian cancer (HBOC) has become one of the gold standards for risk management of breast cancer over the past decades. The initial discovery of germline pathogenic variants in *BRCA1* and *BRCA2* genes, which are the strongest risk factors for the development of breast and ovarian cancers, have led to a clinical practice change to include intensive surveillance and preventative measures to individuals and family members at risk. With the development of advanced sequencing technology, pathogenic variants in other high- to moderate-risk genes have also been described; however, management guidelines for individuals who are carriers of such pathogenic variants are more variable, as much intervention still lacks support from concrete evidence [1–5].

As such, for individuals who undergo genetic testing, it is important to have the expertise to order the appropriate testing with adequate interpretation. Increasingly so, due to the complexity of available multi-gene panel testing methods, interpretations from molecular tumour boards and genetic testing have been incorporated into the multi-disciplinary management of breast cancers. The identification of individuals with varying risk levels arising from different gene mutations, along with variable evidence and guidelines, have resulted in the need for more personalised decisions on the appropriate choice of management. Preventative measures, including chemoprevention and preventative surgery (such as risk-reducing mastectomy, risk-reducing salpingo-oophorectomy, and the choice of breast conservation surgery versus mastectomy), are available for genetic mutation carriers diagnosed with breast cancer, and the appropriate management choices require personalised counselling and multi-disciplinary input.

GENETIC PREDISPOSITION AND GENETIC TESTING

Although most breast and ovarian cancers are sporadic, approximately 6–10% of breast cancer and 15–20% of ovarian cancer cases are caused by pathogenic variants in the *BRCA1* and *BRCA2* genes, and an additional 5–7% are associated with other high- to moderate-risk gene mutations such as *PALB2*, *TP53* (associated with Li-Fraumeni syndrome), *PTEN* (associated with Cowden syndrome), *CDH1* (associated with diffuse gastric and lobular breasts cancer syndrome) and *STK11* (associated with Peutz–Jeghers syndrome), to name a few [1–4]. (**Figure 12.1**). These genes not only result in an increased risk of breast cancer, but may also have phenotypic presentations of other cancer types as well (**Table 12.1**).

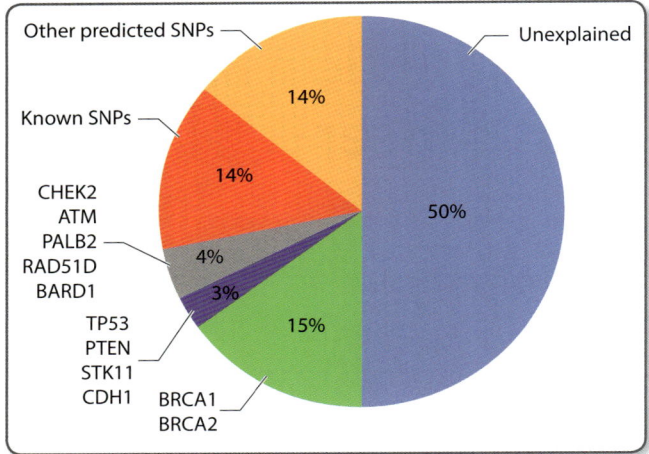

Figure 12.1 Genes with highest increased risk of breast cancer development.
SNP, single nucleotide plymorphism

Table 12.1 Commonly mutated genes in breast cancer: frequency and accounted risk					
Gene	Other susceptible tumour	Population frequency	Proportion of all breast cancers	Proportion of hereditary breast cancers	Lifetime risk of breast cancer (in women)
BRCA 1	ovary, prostate, colorectal	0.1%	1.5%	40%	60–85%
BRCA 2	Ovary, prostate, pancreas, Fanconi	0.1%	1.5%	40%	50–85%
TP53 LFS	Sarcoma, glioma Adrenal	0.0005%	0.02%	2%	80–90%
PTEN Cowden	Thyroid colorectal	0.5%	0.004%	0.3%	25–50%
CHEK2	Prostate, colorectal	0.5%	0.5%	0%	18–20%
ATM	Lymphoma, leukaemia	0.001%	0.5%	0%	20%
STK11	Colorectal	0.1%	0.001%	0.6%	50%
BRIP1	Fanconi	0.1%	0.1%	0%	20%
PALB2			0.1%	0%	20%
RAD51C	Fanconi	0.1%	0.1%	0%	14–20%
RAD51D	Fanconi	0.1%	0.1%	0%	14–20%
CDH1	Stomach	0.005%	0.05%	0%	39–52%
Total		**80% for any**	**5%**	**83%**	

Genetic testing and genetic counselling

The assessment of an individual's risk for breast cancer is complex. The traditional key criteria for hereditary risk evaluation and possible testing include a personal history of cancer such as breast and ovarian cancers, young onset of cancer with multiple cancers in the family spanning over two generations, which later expanded to include more cancer types as we understood more about *BRCA* and other gene pathogenic variants. There are also specific cancer biology characteristics which are more likely to be associated with the presence of pathogenic variants, such as triple negative breast cancer and high grade serous adenocarcinomas of the ovaries, in the setting of *BRCA* mutation carriers. Over the past decade, international guidelines such as National Comprehensive Cancer Network (NCCN) guidelines and ESMO Advanced Breast Cancer (ABC 4) guidelines have broadened their recommendations regarding genetic screening criteria, particularly for *BRCA* mutations. Whereas traditionally, family history and age of onset of cancer were regarded to be the most important criteria for selection of an individual for genetic testing, recent guidelines have also recommended that 'regardless of family history, some individuals with a *BRCA*-related cancer may benefit from genetic testing'. Testing maybe important to determine eligibility for targeted treatment such as poly (ADP-ribose) polymerase 1 (PARP) inhibitors for metastatic human epidermal growth factor receptor 2 (HER2)-positive breast cancers, and some have emphasised the future potential utility of identifying somatic or germline *BRCA* mutations in informing the optimal management of breast cancer [6,7]. In general, however, most countries' guidelines include similar criteria for genetic testing (**Tables 12.2** and **12.3**) [8,9].

In addition, there are a number of risk assessment models developed to ascertain the risk that an individual harbours a pathogenic variant in the breast cancer susceptibility

---

Table 12.2 Referral criteria for BRCA1, BRCA2 or TP53 mutation screening (NICE Clinical Guideline, 2019) [10]

Personal history of breast cancer

- Triple negative breast cancer diagnosed at <40 year old
- Of Jewish ancestry
- With personal history of glioma, childhood adrenal cortical carcinoma, or multiple cancers at a young age
- With family history of sarcoma diagnosed at <45 year old
- With paternal family history of breast cancer in 4 relatives diagnosed at <60 years old

Formal risk assessment with risk estimates of

- ≥10% chance of familial gene mutation
- >8% risk of developing breast cancer in next 10 years, or >30% lifetime risk of developing breast cancer

Significant family history of breast cancer

- 2 close relatives* diagnosed at an average age of <50 year old
- 3 close relatives* diagnosed at an average age of <60 year old
- 4 relatives[†] diagnosed at any age

Family hostory of ovarian cancer, and on the same side

- Breast cancer in 1 close relative* diagnosed at <50 year old
- Breast cancer in 2 close relatives* diagnosed at an average age of <60 year old
- Another ovarian cancer at any age

Significant family history of bilateral breast cancer

- 1 close relative[‡] diagnosed at <50 year old
- 1 close relative* diagnosed at any age, and 1 close relative diagnosed with breast cancer at <60 years old

Family history of male breast cancer, and on the same side

- Breast cancer in 1 close relative* diagnosed at <50 year old
- Breast cancer in 2 close relative* diagnosed at an average age of <60 year old

* First- or second-degree relative
[†] At least one a first-degree relative
[‡] First-degree relative

Table 12.3 Candidates for genetic counselling and possible testing (2015 practice guideline from the American College of Medical Genetics and Genomics and the National Society of Genetic Counsellors) [9]

Personal characteristics

- Ashkenazi Jewish adults

Personal history of cancers

- Triple-negative breast cancer, diagnosed at ≤60 years old
- ≤2 primary breast cancers, first diagnosed at <50 years old
- Breast cancer in males
- Invasive ovarian or fallopian tube cancer, or primary peritoneal cancer
- Exocrine pancreatic cancer
- Metastatic prostate cancer
- High-grade (Gleason score >7) prostate cancer with Ashkenazi Jewish ancestry

Family history of cancers

- Relative with breast cancer diagnosed at ≤50 years old or any cancers listed above, with personal history of breast cancer diagnosed at any age
- A first- or second-degree relative meeting the criteria for genetic testing

Genetic analyses

- *BRCA1/2* or other specific pathogenic variants identified from tumour genomic analysis
- Pathogenic variant in an actionable gene (such as *BRCA1/2*) identified in a relative

Risk assessment models

>5% model-based probability of carrying a *BRCA1/2* pathogenic variant

genes *BRCA1* and *BRCA2*, and to estimate the risk of developing breast cancer in women. Each of these models were developed based on different cohort studies with varying inclusion criteria, such that different weighting used in each models results in a slightly different probability prediction. Largely used to assess risk in individuals who have a positive family history, common risk-prediction models include BRCAPRO, BOADICEA (or CanRisk) and Claus and Tyrer-Cuzick, where the latter two are used only in women without a history of breast cancer. No models are perfect and some models, such as the BOADICEA, have incorporated pathology information and also additional genetic information, to improve their prediction accuracy [11–15]. More often than not, however, clinically qualitative criteria are used to identify appropriate individuals for genetic testing.

It is not uncommon for an unaffected individual with strong family history, to request genetic testing due to the concerns about hereditary cancer risk. Whenever possible, it is ideal for a physician to initiate genetic testing in a family member who is most likely to test positive for a pathogenic variant, who usually is the cancer patient with the youngest age at diagnosis. The inheritance of pathogenic variants related to cancer is often that of an autosomal dominant inheritance (**Figure 12.2**); hence if an unaffected individual is found not to carry a mutation, it can be one of two reasons: either he/she did not inherit a pathogenic variant which exists within the family, or there is no such pathogenic variant in the family. The cancer risk estimation would therefore be difficult to interpret unless the most likely person to carry a pathogenic variant has been tested.

Traditional genetic counselling consists of two components: pretesting counselling and post-testing counselling. Pretesting counselling usually include a detailed medical history, family history and pedigree evaluation, which would usually include all details from

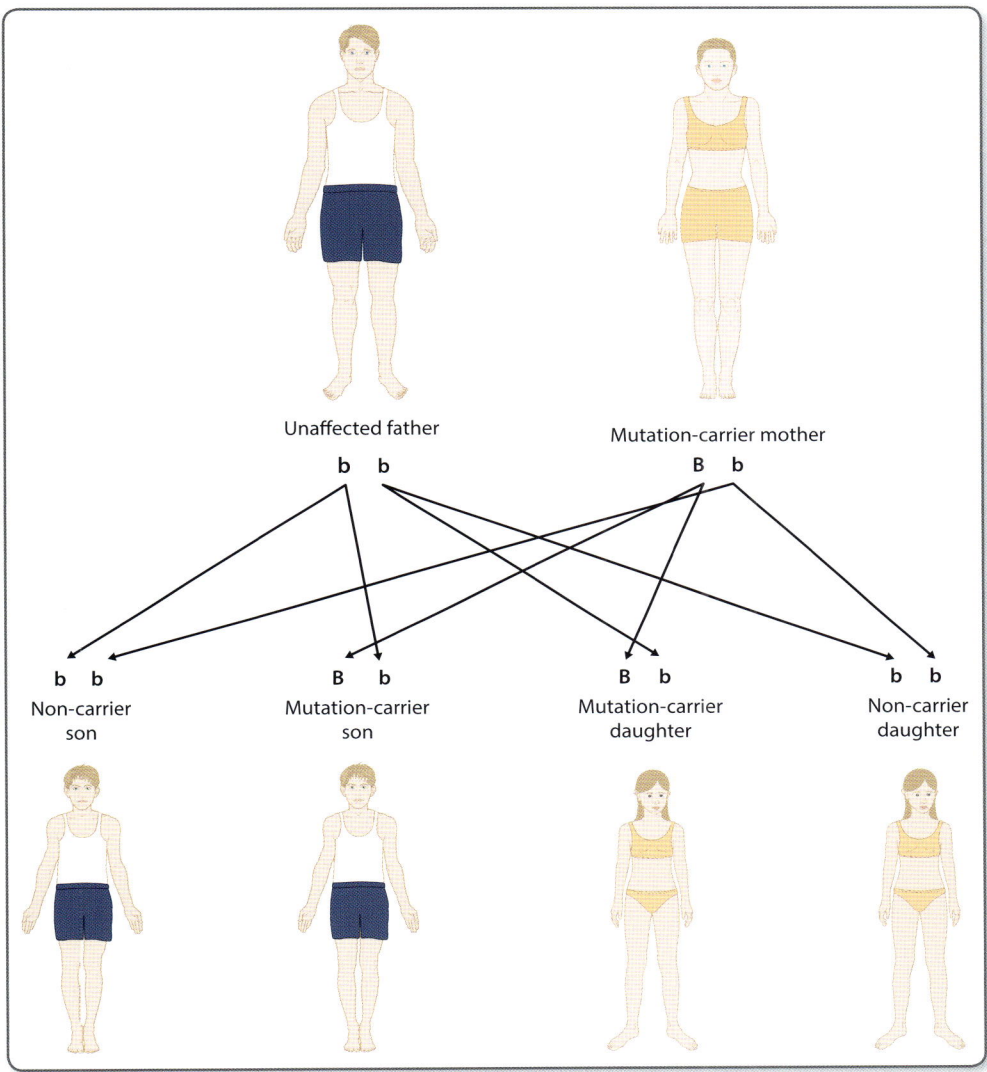

Figure 12.2 Inheritance pattern of autosomal dominant mutations.

multiple generations including the type of cancers, age of onset and biological type of the cancer, and history of any family members receiving genetic testing results. Risk assessment is then made including with the use of mathematical models. A recommendation for genetic testing, including the choice of multi-gene panel testing versus testing for *BRCA1* and *BRCA2* pathogenic variant alone, is then made after explanation of the implications of genetic testing, including the potential benefits, limitations and the risks. In additional, clinical management for various outcomes would be discussed. The discussion of financial and legal implications, including that of genetic discrimination, varies in different countries.

Post-testing counselling allows for the disclosing of genetic testing results, and also for providing more information to patients and their family members where appropriate. Sharing of information to other family members is encouraged, such that those who should be tested can get tested.

The practice of genetic counselling has traditionally been one-on-one, face-to-face counselling sessions done by genetic counsellors or trained physicians including oncologists, surgeons, and geneticists. However, the recent increase in uptake of cancer genetic testing has created the need for alternative genetic counselling techniques to cater for the increase needs.

There are various reasons accounting for an increase in the uptake of genetic testing, including:

- The availability of advanced technologies, including next generation sequencing, has allowed for the investigation of multiple genes at a lower cost and shorter time. These are now available both in academic centres and on a direct-to-consumer basis [16]
- The increased therapeutic indications, such as targeted therapies including PARP inhibitors, which are of relevance to HBOC syndrome
- The increased use of somatic tumour gene panels to identify pathogenic variants or microsatellite instabilities to guide therapy in cancer patients, resulting in more pathogenic variants being identified and requiring confirmatory germline testing [17,18]

With such increase in demand, the traditional one-on-one technique has been replaced in some centres by other techniques particularly pretest counselling. These include telephone counselling, group counsellor, electronic-based education, decision-making tools and also oncologist-led genetic counselling. These cater for somatic testing and therapeutic implications in the first instance, while deferring genetic counselling for germline pathogenic variants, if any were to be found, to a later stage (**Figure 12.3**). Although these newer techniques are increasingly practiced, it has been reported an individual's anxiety may not be well addressed using these alternative techniques [19–21].

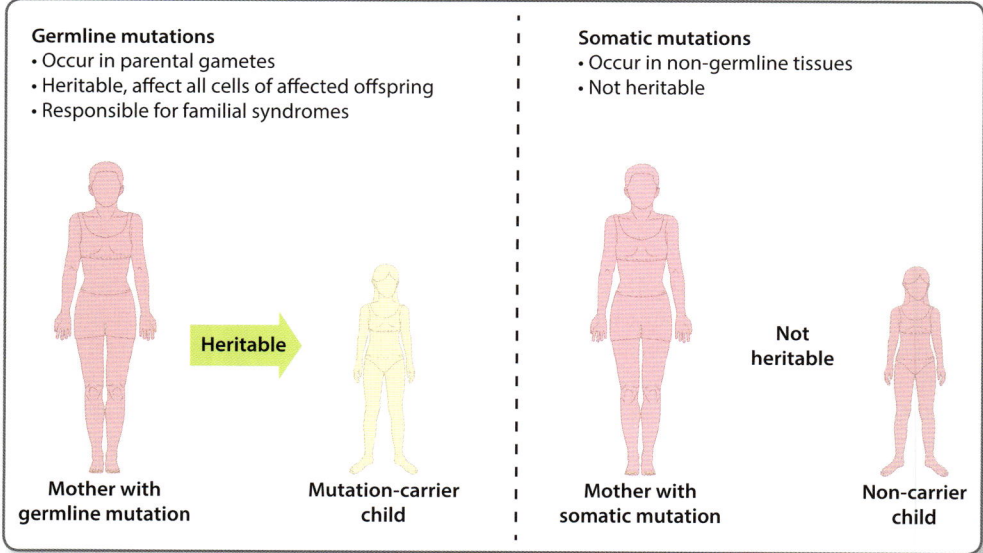

Figure 12.3 Germline versus somatic mutations.

Multi-gene panel testing

Although the use of multi-gene panel testing is an attractive option allowing for the investigation of multiple genes at a much lower cost, there are still a lot of unknowns about the genes that are being testing, and it is not uncommon to identify a large number of variants of uncertain significance (VUS). Next-generation sequencing (NGS) can produce simultaneous information on several genetic variants with different functions and consequences. Accordingly, determining the status of the patient or consultant and interpreting sequencing results from many genes can largely increase the complexity of genetic counselling. With unknown definitive positive or negative results, VUS and also some negative results can be uninformative and poise interpretation difficulties, and hence decisions for clinical management may not be simple and could lead to misinterpretation by patients and healthcare professionals. Studies have found inconsistencies in the interpretation of results which can lead to inappropriate management [22]. In larger multi-gene panels, many of the genes which are included are rare and some of them relatively new and less well characterised, with no guidelines for medical management. In individuals with VUS, the role of predictive testing for family members is even less certain. Multi-gene panels should therefore be used with caution, and to date are not recommended as the gold standard in many countries. Multi-gene sequencing could have a role for some specific individuals and families, for example in cases where there are multiple different types of cancer, or for individuals who have a strong family history of cancer but have previously been tested negative for *BRCA1* and *BRCA2* mutations [23–25].

MANAGEMENT STRATEGIES

When a pathogenic variant has been identified, four management principles can be applied:
1. Surveillance
    a. Commencing at an earlier age
    b. Increased frequency
    c. Using additional imaging modalities
2. Prevention
    a. Risk-reducing surgery
    b. Chemoprevention
3. Therapeutic implications
    a. Targeted therapies
    b. Therapeutic surgical options
4. Testing of family members

For individuals with moderate-penetrance pathogenic gene variants for breast and ovarian cancer

To date, definitive guidelines exist more for high penetrant pathogenic variants such as *BRCA1* and *BRCA2* genes, and less for moderate-penetrant pathogenic variants which are much less understood due to their rarity. The appropriate management of individuals harbouring such moderate-penetrance genetic variants is unclear, and most guidelines are only suggestive guidelines. Decisions are based on a multi-disciplinary approach, through the experience of genetic counsellors and specialists along with discussions with the patient for more personalised management decisions. It is important to note that extrapolation of guidelines for the management of individuals with high-penetrance variants gene mutations to the clinical care of moderate-penetrance gene mutations, could result in substantial harm [26].

High-penetrance pathogenic gene variants for breast cancer

To date, the most solid guidelines for risk management are still for *BRCA1* and *BRCA2* mutation carriers. This group of patients can be divided into two groups: those who do not have a personal history of breast cancer, and those who do.

Overview of recommendations of breast cancer surveillance

Mammography (MMG) has been the gold standard for breast cancer screening in the general population, but recent prospective studies have shown that for women at high risk of breast cancer, MMG carries a lower sensitivity, with the rate of developing interval cancers ranging from 29 to 50%, and an overall nodal involvement rate 20–56% [27–29]. This poorer performance could be attributed to many factors, such as earlier cancer onset, higher breast density in a relatively younger population requiring high risk surveillance, and more aggressive tumour associated with *BRCA* mutations [30]. On the other hand, contrast-enhanced magnetic resonance imaging (CE-MRI), unlike MMG, mainly relies on abnormal density and distortion, which provides additional information regarding neovascularity and functional assessment of breast tissues [31]. A systematic review found that MMG sensitivity ranges from 25 to 59% with a pooled sensitivity of 39%, while MRI sensitivity ranges from 68 to 100% with a pooled sensitivity of 77% [32]. The two modalities were found to be complementary with a combined sensitivity of 94%. When MRI was added to high risk screening, the majority of cancers detected were either in-situ or very early invasive cancers with a node-positive rate of 12–26%. Many guidelines recommend a multi-modal screening approach for individuals who carry a familial risk including that of *BRCA* pathogenic variants, with some variations between countries. For pathogenic variants in moderate-risk or other high-penetrance genes, there are even less consistent guidelines available due to the lack of evidence support. In general, annual MRI has now been incorporated into breast screening guidelines for *BRCA* mutation carriers starting from age 25 to 30 years old, at 6-month intervals to MMG screening, including the National Comprehensive Cancer Network (NCCN) [33], National Institute for Health and Care (NICE) [10], European Society for Medical Oncology (ESMO) [34] and Cancer Care Ontario (CCO) [35] (**Table 12.4**). Of note however, despite data supporting the early stage of diagnosis of breast cancer when MRI is used, there is no survival benefit attributed by such intensive surveillance compared to standard screening programmes, although survival was seen to be higher with the combined use of breast MRI and MMG as compared to no intensive screening group (95.3% vs. 73.7 %, p = 0.002). Therefore, it is important to balance the benefits of surveillance with its harms, including over diagnosis, false positive results and radiation exposure [36–40].

SURGICAL STRATEGIES

For individuals who carry the *BRCA1* and *BRCA2* pathogenic variants, and who do not have cancer, the major goal of surgical intervention would be for reduction of breast cancer

Table 12.4 Screening recommendations for women with no personal history of breast cancer (NICE Clinical Guideline, 2019) [10]			
Imaging modality	Recommendations according to risk		
	Moderate risk, or high risk of non-*BRCA/TP53*-related breast cancers	Known *BRCA1* or *BRCA2* mutation	Known *TP53* mutation
Mammography	• Annually between 40 and 59 years old • As part of screening programme at age 60 years old or above	• Annually between 30 and 69 years old • As part of screening programme at age 70 years old or above	Do not offer
MRI breasts	Do not offer	Annually between 30 and 49 years old	Annually between 20 and 49 years old
(MRI: magnetic resonance imaging)			

risk, which can be achieved by risk-reducing bilateral mastectomy with or without bilateral salpingo-oophorectomy.

Bilateral risk-reducing mastectomy, reduces the risk of breast cancer by up to 90% in moderate to high risk individuals, but to date there are no randomised trials showing any survival benefits. It would also be highly unlikely that such a trial design would be ethically acceptable. A Cochrane review has looked at 61 studies to determine the degree of risk reduction and the incidence of breast cancer and disease-specific mortality of women who underwent risk-reducing mastectomy (RRM) with contralateral risk-reducing mastectomy (CRRM). In particular, for women who carry the *BRCA1* or *BRCA2* pathogenic variants, 26 studies found that CRRM consistently reduces the incidence of breast cancer, but improvements in disease-specific survival are inconsistent. Seven studies found no difference in overall survival in women who received CRRM. One study found a significant improvement in survival following CRRM, but after adjusting for risk-reducing bilateral salpingo-oophorectomy (RRBSO), the CRRM effect on all-cause mortality was no longer significant [41].

Another study investigated the expected benefit of RRM on breast cancer incidence and mortality in *BRCA* mutation carriers by age, using a simulated hypothetical cohort of women, and found that the actuarial risk of developing breast cancer before the age of 80 years old, is at an estimated 70.8% with an actual risk was 64%. The probability of an individual being alive at age 80 years, having had a mastectomy at the age of 25 years, was increased by 8.7%. However, if RRM was performed at a later age, the improvement of survival was much less, suggesting that the benefits of RRM declines rapidly with age [42]. Another study developed a Monte Carlo Model for breast screening, RRM and RRBSO to study the most effective intervention for risk reduction in *BRCA* mutation carriers. The study found that RRM at age 25 years with RRBSO at age 40 years, maximises the survival probability. However, substituting MMG and MRI screening for RRM, seems to offer a comparable survival, indicating that *BRCA1* and *BRCA2* mutation carriers should be given the choice between risk-reducing surgery and intensive breast surveillance, particularly if RRBSO were to be performed [43]. **Table 12.5** shows the 2019 NICE recommendations regarding RRM and RRBSO.

A common choice for RRM is the nipple areolar sparing mastectomy (NSM). In *BRCA* mutation carriers, when NSM is performed, RRM-related incidental cancers are reported in

Table 12.5 ScreeningRisk-reducing surgeries for mutation carriers (NICE Clinical Guideline, 2019) [10]
Risk-reducing mastectomy
• Consider in carriers of: *BRCA1, BRCA2, TP53, PTEN, PALB2, CDH1, ATM CHEK2* • Full genetic counselling prior to surgery • Discussion on risk factors, family history, psychosocial and sexual consequences, reconstruction options
Risk-reducing bilateral salpingo-oophorectomy
• Consider in carriers of: *BRCA1, BRCA2, PTEN, BRIP1, RAD51C, RAD51D* • Full genetic counselling if family completed • Discussion on risk factors, family history, effects of early menopause, psychosocial and sexual consequences

1–2.7% of the mastectomy specimens but with no nipple areolar complex (NAC) involvement. There is also a 2% chance of cancer events at 31.6 months follow-up. In contrast, the incidental cancer rate in therapeutic NSMs is estimated to be 3.9%, with a NAC involvement rate of 5.8–10% and a comparable 2% rate of cancer events. Hence, NSM in RRM has been regarded as oncologically safe. Another report has found that in both the therapeutic or risk-reducing settings, even in cases of recurrence, the recurrence did not occur in the NAC [44,45]. However, it has to be emphasised that even RRM is not without risks, including those of surgical complications such as bleeding, skin flap necrosis, loss of the NAC, infection, implant loss and myocutaneous flap failure. Mutation carriers who do not have cancer, need to also understand and accept that RRM is irreversible and may not result in the expected body image, as newly re-constructed breasts appear different to the natural breasts even if they are aesthetically re-constructed. There may be some loss of sensation with negative impact on psychosexual function and adverse psychological effect, but studies have shown that the majority of the women are satisfied with the postoperative result [46].

Breast conservation surgery

Breast conservation surgery (BCS) has comparable survival outcomes compared with mastectomy in sporadic breast cancers, and has the additional advantage of carrying a favourable cosmetic outcome. Similar to RRM and CRRM, there are no randomised controlled studies, and it is unlikely we will see such trials, to compare the oncological and survival outcomes of breast conservation surgery with mastectomy in carriers of high-penetrance breast susceptibility. Although there is good data to support the increased risk of contralateral breast cancer in *BRCA* mutation carriers and hence the consideration of CRRM, the oncological outcomes in this group of patients have been less consistent. A 2020 systemic review of 18 studies found that although ipsilateral breast cancer recurrence rate at 5, 10, and 15 years were higher in the BCS group compared with the mastectomy group (8.2%, 15.5%, and 23% vs. 3.4%, 4.9%, and 6.4% respectively), the overall 5-, 10- and 15-year survival rates were comparable to that of mastectomy (89.7%, 89.2%, and 83.6% vs. 82.9%, 86.0%, and 83.2% respectively). Hence, breast conservation surgery should still be offered to mutation carriers as an option, but the decision should take into account tumour size, stage at presentation and tumour biology [47] (**Table 12.6**).

Study (authors, year	Design	Stage	Overall survival					
			5-year		10-year		15-year	
			BSC	M	BCS	M	BCS	M
Robson et al. 2005	Case series	T1-2	85/87 (97.8%)	N/A	78/87 (89.7%)	N/A	N/A	N/A
Garcia-Etienne et al. 2009	Retrospective cohort	T1-3	N/A	N/A	278/302 (92.1%)	324/353 (91.8%)	264/302 (87.3%)	317/353 (89.8%)
Martin et al. 2014	Prospective cohort	Stage I-III	36/45 (80.0%)	97/117 (82.9%)	31/45 (68.9%)	80/117 (68.4%)	26/45 (57.9%)	74/117 (63.2%)
Pierce et al. 2000	Retrospective cohort	N/A	61/71 (85.9%)	N/A	N/A	N/A	N/A	N/A
Overall pooled			182/203 (89.7%)	97/117 (82.9%)	387/434 (89.2%)	404/470 (86.0%)	290/347 (83.6%)	391/470 (83.2%)

Table 12.6 Overall survival of breast conserving surgery and mastectomy in BRCA mutation carriers [47]

BCS, breast-conservation surgery; M, mastectomy; N/A data not available

OTHER CONSIDERATIONS FOR RISK-REDUCTION MEASURES

Risk-reducing bilateral salpingo-oophorectomy is one option for women who carry the *BRCA1* or *BRCA2* pathogenic variant, but may not be relevant to other high- to moderate-penetrance genes mutations. The risk of ovarian, peritoneal and fallopian tube cancer is much increased in *BRCA* mutation carriers to around 45%. RRBSO has been shown to reduce the risk of not only ovarian and fallopian tube cancers but also of breast cancer, and has been shown to reduce the all-cause mortality in *BRCA* mutation carriers by 46–56%. Although RRBSO does result in early surgical menopause, other options of preventive and surveillance measures are much limited. In general, RRBSO can be offered after completion of child bearing and as early as age 35 years old, as the benefit of the procedure decreases with age [48].

Other means of breast cancer prevention include the use of selective oestrogen-receptor modulators, namely tamoxifen and raloxifene. A subgroup analysis of the National Surgical Adjuvant Breast and Bowel Project (NSABP) trial evaluated the effect of tamoxifen on *BRCA* breast cancer risk. Among the 288 incident cases, there were 8 *BRCA1* and 11 *BRCA2* mutation carriers. Although the sample size was small, the study concluded that a potential reduction in *BRCA2* (risk ratio 0.38; 95% CI 0.06–1.56) but not *BRCA1*-associated breast cancer (risk ratio 1.67; 95% CI 0.32–10.7) with tamoxifen use. There have not been any primary prevention trials of tamoxifen or raloxifene conducted specifically among women with a *BRCA1* or *BRCA2* mutation, but increasing number of studies are looking at the use of other chemoprevention drugs to reduce the breast cancer risk [49].

CONCLUSION

Genetic testing can now be considered as a gold standard in management of breast cancer. With the complexity of multi-gene panel testing, decisions for individuals found to carry a pathogenic variant will require a multi-disciplinary approach. Patients and clinicians should work together to make an informed decision so that the most appropriate management options can be implemented.

Key points for clinical practice

- A number of high risk and moderate – penetrance genes have been identified which confers an increased risk of breast cancer.
- Genetic testing can be considered standard of care. Management of such individuals with increased risk of cancer requires a multi-disciplinary approach.
- The traditional one-on-one and face-to-face genetic counselling can no longer cater for the increased demands for genetic counselling.
- Management of individuals who carry a risk due to a pathogenic variant in high-penetrance genes involves intensive surveillance and preventative measures.

REFERENCES

1. Couch FJ, Shimelis H, Hu C, et al. Associations Between Cancer Predisposition Testing Panel Genes and Breast Cancer. JAMA Oncol 2017; 3:1190–1196.
2. LaDuca H, Stuenkel AJ, Dolinsky JS, et al. Utilization of multigene panels in hereditary cancer predisposition testing: analysis of more than 2,000 patients. Genet Med 2014; 16:830–837.
3. Kurian AW, Ward KC, Howlader N, et al. Genetic Testing and Results in a Population-Based Cohort of Breast Cancer Patients and Ovarian Cancer Patients. J Clin Oncol 2019; 37:1305–1315.
4. Kwong A, Shin VY, Chen J, et al. Germline Mutation in 1338 BRCA-Negative Chinese Hereditary Breast and/or Ovarian Cancer Patients: Clinical Testing with a Multigene Test Panel. J Mol Diagn 2020; 22:544–554.
5. Jatoi I. Risk-Reducing Options for Women with a Hereditary Breast Cancer Predisposition. Eur J Breast Health 2018; 14:189–193.
6. Robson ME, Bradbury AR, Arun B, et al. American Society of Clinical Oncology Policy Statement Update: Genetic and Genomic Testing for Cancer Susceptibility. J Clin Oncol 2015; 33:3660–3667.
7. Forbes C, Fayter D, de Kock S, et al. A systemic review of international guidelines and recommendations for the genetic screening, diagnosis, genetic counseling, and treatment of BRCA-mutated breast cancer. Cancer Manag Res 2019; 11:2321–2337.
8. NCCN. (2020). National Comprehensive Cancer Network. "Genetic/Familial High-Risk Assessment: Breast and Ovarian." NCCN Clinical Practice Guidelines in Oncology. [online] Available from https://www.genomeweb.com/sites/default/files/nccn_genetic_cancer_risk_assessment.pdf [Last accessed January, 2021].
9. Hampel H, Bennett RL, Buchanan A, et al. A practice guideline from the American College of Medical Genetics and Genomics and the National Society of Genetic Counselors: referral indications for cancer predisposition assessment. Genet Med 2015; 17:70–87.
10. NICE. (2019). National Institute for Health and Care Excellence (NICE). "Familial breast cancer: classification, care and managing breast cancer and related risks in people with a family history of breast cancer", NICE Clinical Guideline 164. [online] Available from https://www.nice.org.uk/guidance/cg164/evidence [Last accessed January, 2021].
11. Lee AJ, Cunningham AP, Tischkowitz M, et al. Incorporating truncating variants in PALB2, CHEK2 and ATM into the BOADICEA breast cancer risk model. Genet Med 2016; 18:1190–1198.
12. Mazzola E, Blackford A, Parmigiani G, et al. Recent Enhancements to the Genetic Risk Prediction Model BRCAPRO. Cancer Inform 2015; 14:147–157.

13. (2004). U.T. Southwestern Medical Center at Dallas and The BayesMendel Group. "CancerGene with BRCAPRO, MMRpro, PancPRO, and MelaPRO." [online] Available from www4.utsouthwestern.edu/breasthealth/cagene/ [Last accessed January, 2021].

14. Lee AJ, Cunningham AP, Kuchenbaecker KB, et al. BOADICEA breast cancer risk prediction model: updates to cancer incidences, tumour pathology and web interface. Br J Cancer 2014; 110:535–545.

15. University of Cambridge. CanRisk Web Tool. Version 1.1.2. 2020. [online] Available from https://www.canrisk.org. [Last accessed January, 2021].

16. Stadler, ZK, Scahrader KA, Vijai J, et al. Cancer Genomics and inherited risk. J Clin Oncol 2014; 32:687–698.

17. Jain R, Savage MJ, Forman AD, et al. The Relevance of Hereditary Cancer Risks to Precision Oncology: What Should Providers Consider When Conducting Tumor Genomic Profiling? J Natl Compr Canc Netw 2016; 14:795–806.

18. Mandelker D, Zhang L, Kemel Y, et al. Mutation Detection in Patients With Advanced Cancer by Universal Sequencing of Cancer-Related Genes in Tumor and Normal DNA vs Guideline-Based Germline Testing. JAMA 2017; 318:825–835.

19. Platten U, Rantala J, Lindblom A, et al. The use of telephone in genetic counseling versus in-person counseling: a randomized study on counselees' outcome. Fam Cancer 2012; 11:371–379.

20. Schwartz MD, Valdimarsdottir HB, Peshkin BN, et al. Randomized noninferiority trial of telephone versus in-person genetic counseling for hereditary breast and ovarian cancer. J Clin Oncol 2014; 32:618–626.

21. Kinney AY, Butler KM, Schwartz MD, et al. Expanding access to BRCA1/2 genetic counseling with telephone delivery: a cluster randomized trial. J Natl Cancer Inst 2014; 106:dju328.

22. Cheon JY, Mozersky J, Cook-Deegan R. Variants of uncertain significance in BRCA: a harbinger of ethical and policy issues to come? Genome Med 2014; 6:121.

23. Yang M, Kim JW. Principles of Genetic Counseling in the Era of Next- Generation Sequencing. Ann Lab Med 2018. 38:291–295.

24. Eggington JM, Bowles KR, Moyes K, et al. A comprehensive laboratory-based program for classification of variants of uncertain significance in hereditary cancer genes. Clin Genet 2014; 86:229–237.

25. Turner SA, Rao SK, Morgan RH, et al. The impact of variant classification on the clinical management of hereditary cancer syndromes. Genet Med 2019; 21:426–430.

26. Tung N, Domchek SM, Stadler Z, et al. Counselling framework for moderate-penetrance cancer-susceptibility mutations. Nat Rev Clin Oncol 2016; 13(9):581–588.

27. Vasen HF, Tesfay E, Boonstra H, et al. Early detection of breast and ovarian cancer in families with BRCA mutations. Eur J Cancer 2005; 41:549–554.

28. Brekelmans CT, Seynaeve C, Bartels CC, et al. Effectiveness of breast cancer surveillance in BRCA1/2 gene mutation carriers and women with high familial risk. J Clin Oncol 2001; 19:924–930.

29. Rosenberg RD, Hunt WC, Williamson MR, et al. Effects of age, breast density, ethnicity, and estrogen replacement therapy on screening mammographic sensitivity and cancer stage at diagnosis: review of 183,134 screening mammograms in Albuquerque, New Mexico. Radiology 1998; 209:511–518.

30. Sardanelli F, Podo F, Santoro F, et al. Multicenter surveillance of women at high genetic breast cancer risk using mammography, ultrasonography, and contrast-enhanced magnetic resonance imaging (the high breast cancer risk italian 1 study): final results. Invest Radiol 2011; 46:94–105.

31. Morris EA. Diagnostic breast MR imaging: current status and future directions. Magn Reson Imaging Clin N Am 2010; 18:57–74.

32. Warner E, Messersmith H, Causer P, et al. Systematic review: using magnetic resonance imaging to screen women at high risk for breast cancer. Ann Intern Med 2008; 148:671–679.

33. Daly MB, Axilbund JE, Buys S, et al. Genetic/familial high risk assessment: Breast and ovarian. Natl Compr Canc Netw 2010; 8:562–594.

34. Paluch-Shimon S, Cardoso F, Sessa C, et al. Prevention and screening in BRCA mutation carriers and other breast/ovarian hereditary cancer syndromes: ESMO Clinical Practice Guidelines for cancer prevention and screening. Ann Oncol 2016; 27:v103–v110.

35. Warne E, Messersmith H, Causer P, et al. Magnetic Resonance Imaging Screening of Women at High Risk for Breast Cancer: A Clinical Practice Guideline. A Quality Initiative of the Program in Evidence-based Care (PEBC), Can Care Ontario. 2007.

36. Saslow D, Boetes C, Burke W, et al. American Cancer Society guidelines for breast screening with MRI as an adjunct to mammography. CA Cancer J Clin 2007; 57:75–89.

37. Bernstein-Molho R, Kaufman B, David MAB, et al. Breast cancer surveillance for BRCA1/2 mutation carriers – is "early detection" early enough. Breast 2020; 49:81–86.

38. Santoro F, Podo F, Sarrdanelli F. MRI screening of women with hereditary predisposition to breast cancer" diagnostic performance and survival analysis. Breast Cancer Res Treat 2014; 147:685–687.
39. Evans DG, Kesavan N, Lim Y, et al. MRI breast screening in high-risk women: cancer detection and surgical analysis. Breast Cancer Res Treat 2014; 145:663–672.
40. Passaperuma K, Warner E, Causer PA, et al. Long-term results of screening with magnetic resonance imaging in women with BRCA mutations. BR J Cancer 2012; 107:24–30.
41. Carbine NE, Lostumbo L, Wallace J, et al. Risk-reducing mastectomy for the prevention of primary breast cancer. Cochrane Database Syst Rev 2018; 4:CD002748.
42. Giannakeas V, Narod SA. The expected benefit of preventive mastectomy on breast cancer incidence and mortality in BRCA mutation carriers, by age at mastectomy. Breast Cancer Res Treat 2018; 167:263–267.
43. Kurian AW, Sigal BM, Plevritis SK. Survival Analysis of Cancer Risk Reduction Strategies for BRCA1/2 Mutation Carriers. J Clin Oncol 2010; 28:222–231.
44. Peled AW, Irwin CS, Hwang ES, et al. Total skin-sparing mastectomy in BRCA mutation carriers. Ann Surg Oncol 2014; 21:37–41.
45. Yao K, Liederbach E, Tang R, et al. Nipple-sparing mastectomy in BRCA1/2 carriers: An interim analysis and review of the literature. Ann Surg Oncol 2015; 22:370–376.
46. Razdan SN, Tael V, Jewell S, et al. Quality of life among patients after bilateral prophylactic mastectomy: a systemic review of patient-reported outcomes. Qual Life Res 2016; 25:1409–1421.
47. Co M, Liu T, Leung J, et al. Breast Conserving Surgery for BRCA Mutation Carriers- a Systematic Review. Clin Breast Cancer 2020; 20:e244–e250.
48. Eisen A, Rebbeck TR, Wood WC, et al. Prophylactic surgery in women with a hereditary predisposition to breast and ovarian cancer. J Clin Oncol 2000; 18:1980–1995.
49. Kotsopoulos J. BRCA mutations and breast cancer prevention. Cancers (Basel) 2018; 10:524.

Section 7

Abdominal surgery

Chapter 13

Para-oesophageal hernias

Damon Bizos

INTRODUCTION

Para-oesophageal hernias (POHs) are uncommon but important hernias that present mainly in the elderly. Also known as rolling hernias, POHs are a form of hiatus hernia (HH) that have become more relevant to surgical practice as populations age. They need to be differentiated from the more common sliding HH as their presentation and indication for surgical repair differ.

Sliding HHs predispose patients to gastro-oesophageal reflux, which may be asymptomatic or symptomatic. POHs may be truly asymptomatic or may cause dysphagia, obstruction, respiratory symptoms and may present as an emergency with gastric volvulus and strangulation.

Para-oesophageal hernias usually requires surgical repair, unless the patient is very frail. Laparoscopic surgery is now the approach of choice. The indications for, and technical aspects of, surgery will be covered in this chapter.

ANATOMY OF THE DIAPHRAGMATIC HIATUS AND DIFFERENTIAL DIAGNOSIS

The oesophageal hiatus is situated level with T10 and forms part of the muscular diaphragm. Surgeons often refer to the left and right crurae when repairing a HH. The hiatus is actually formed entirely by sling formed by the right crus, which splits to form an ellipse or inverted teardrop shape. The correct terminology is the right and left hiatal pillars or bundles of the right crus [1]. The left crus lies posterolaterally. The thoracic aorta lies just below the arcuate ligament, a fact that should be appreciated when a posterior crural repair is done. There may be an inferior crural artery on the left, which can cause troublesome bleeding when dissecting the left pillar. The anterior and posterior vagal nerves accompany the oesophagus as it traverses the hiatus. The endoabdominal fascia which covers the undersurface of the diaphragm, fuses with tranversalis fascia to form the phreno-oesophageal ligament anteriorly which then attaches the adventitia of the oesophagus at the gastro-oesophageal junction (GOJ) to the diaphragm [1]. This allows for shortening of the oesophagus during swallowing. The abdominal oesophagus is mainly retroperitoneal. (**Figure 13.1**).

A sliding HH results in the stomach sliding up retroperitoneally into the thorax without a sac. A rolling hernia occurs when a sac develops and the stomach fundus rolls up next to the oesophagus (**Table 13.1**). This is termed as POH. On plain chest radiographs, an air

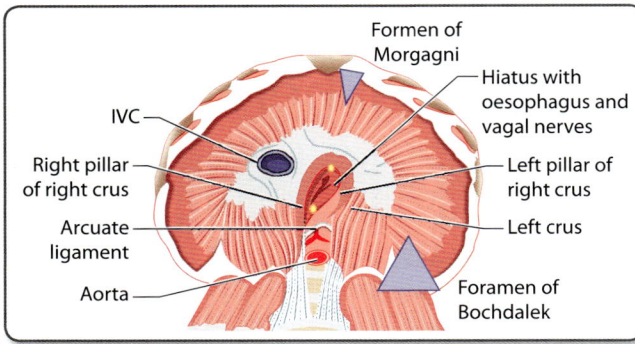

Figure 13.1 Anatomy of the diaphragm. (IVC, inferior vena cava)

Table 13.1 Classification of hiatus hernia (HH)			
Type I	**Type II**	**Type III**	**Type IV**
Sliding HH	Rolling HH = True POH	Mixed sliding and rolling HH	Type II or III - containing stomach and other viscera
95% of HH	4% of POH	76% of POH	20% of POH
No sac	Sac present	Sac present	Sac present
Oesophageal shortening possible	No shortening of oesophagus	Oesophageal shortening possible	Oesophageal shortening possible
GOJ above diaphragm	GOJ at diaphragm	GOJ above diaphragm	GOJ variable
Mainly reflux symptoms	Mainly obstructive symptoms	Obstructive and reflux symptoms	Obstructive and reflux symptoms
Volvulus not possible	Volvulus most likely	Volvulus possible	Volvulus possible

(POH, para-oesophageal hernias; GOJ, gastro-oesophageal junction)

bubble may be seen on the anteroposterior and lateral views (**Figure 13.2**). Conditions that may mimic a POH are a large sliding HH, traumatic diaphragmatic hernia (blunt or penetrating), congenital defects with herniation such as Bochdalek (posterolateral) and Morgagni (anterior), eventration of the diaphragm due to phrenic palsy, hydropneumothorax, pulmonary abscess [2] and parahiatal hernias. Parahiatal hernias are rare and may be primary, or secondary to previous hiatal hernia repairs. They most commonly form in the left pillar of the right crus [3].

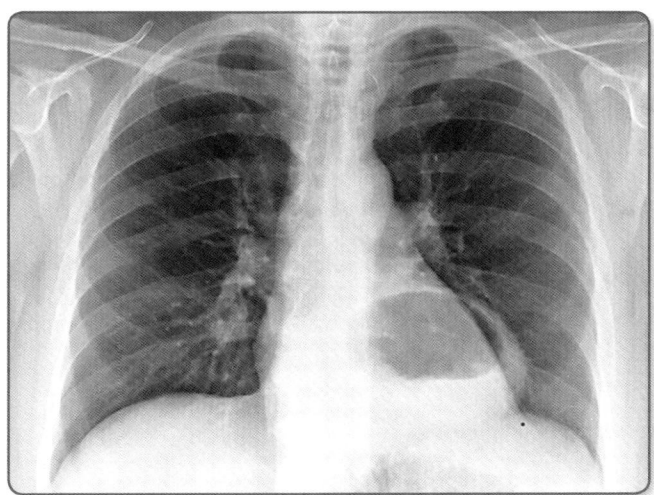

Figure 13.2 Erect chest radiograph with air bubble behind heart due to POH (Rolling HH).
(POH, para-oesophageal hernias; HH, hiatus hernia)

PHYSIOLOGY OF THE OESOPHAGUS/MOTILITY

Video-swallows, manometry and, more recently, high-resolution manometry (HRM) have given insight into the normal motility of the oesophagus and the function of the lower oesophageal sphincter (LOS), as well as the contribution of the diaphragm to the LOS pressure. Patients with HH and reflux often have altered motility. This may be due to or may result in reflux disease. Manometry is recommended before anti-reflux surgery, although oesophageal dysmotility has not been conclusively shown to be a factor in the choice of anti-reflux procedure. Prior to POH repair, anatomical factors may make preoperative motility testing difficult and is often omitted.

CLASSIFICATION

Hiatus hernias are divided into four types (**Table 13.1**).

Type I, sliding hernia comprises 95% of HH. There is no sac formed and the stomach slides up retroperitoneally with the GOJ above the crurae [1]. Most sliding HH are treated conservatively.

Types II–IV are para-oesophageal hernias.

Type II are true POH and are uncommon. The GOJ remains in its normal position (**Figure 13.3**) and the stomach starts to roll up through an enlarging hiatus. With time, most of the stomach herniates into the chest and there is usually some degree of organoaxial and mesenteroaxial (mesoaxial) volvulus of the stomach. The pylorus then rides higher than the GOJ. A sac is present. The stomach then assumes an upside down appearance (**Figure 13.4**) and the greater curvature of the stomach is often to the right of the oesophagus within the chest. If there is a wide diastasis of the crural pillars, the herniation may be mostly posterior. This allows large retroperitoneal fat pads to slide into the mediastinum behind the sac and these mediastinal lipomas need to be excised or pulled back into the abdomen before any attempt at posterior closure is attempted [1].

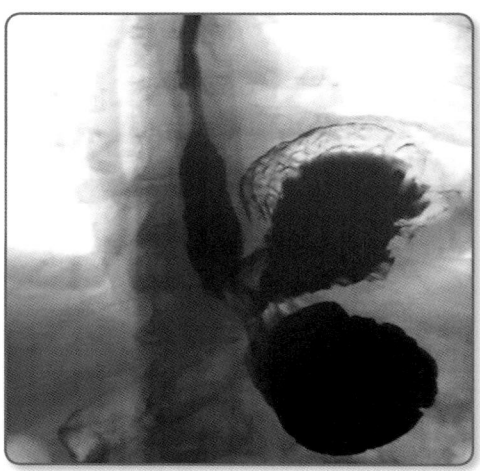

Figure 13.3 Type II hiatus hernia with GOJ at hiatus. (GOJ, gastro-oesophageal junction)

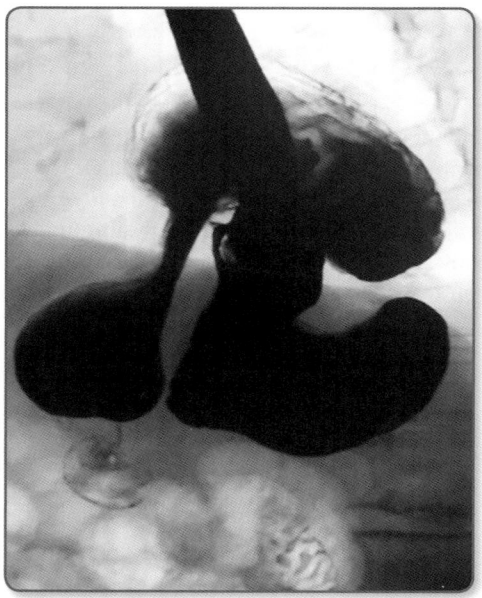

Figure 13.4 Type II hernia with upside down stomach.

Type III or mixed POH is more common. Here, there is a combination of a sliding and a rolling hernia (**Figure 13.5**). These patients may present with reflux as well as mechanical symptoms. From an operative point of view, there is a possibility of a shortened oesophagus, which adds complexity to decision-making and operative techniques.

Type IV hernias have organs other than the stomach within the intra-thoracic sac. This can be difficult to diagnose unless a computed tomography (CT) scan is performed. Other organs such as the colon, omentum, spleen, small bowel, liver, and pancreas may become incarcerated and strangulate.

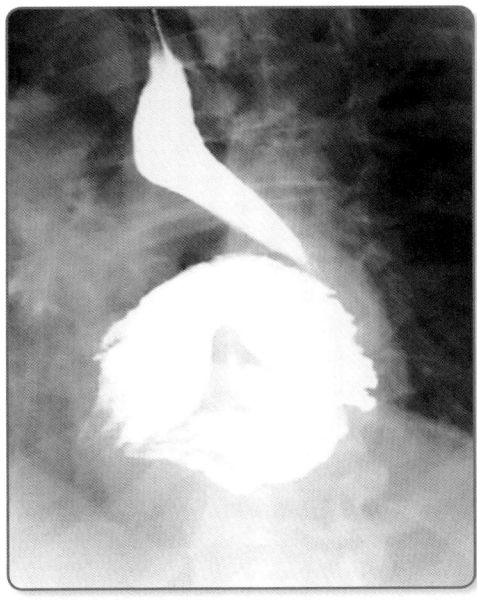

Figure 13.5 Type III hernia with GOJ above the diaphragm and upside-down stomach. (GOJ, gastro-oesophageal junction)

In a study of 270 patients with POH, 4% were type II, 76% type III, and 20% type IV. The percentage of stomach within the chest was estimated to be less than 50% in 12%, 50–74% in 32% and 75–100% in 56% [4].

Aetiology, incidence, and natural history

The underlying cause of hiatal herniation is often unclear. Predisposing factors include gastro-oesophageal reflux causing damage to the oesophagus and oesophageal shortening which pulls up the stomach. Increased abdominal pressure due to chronic cough, pregnancy, heavy labour, heavy weight training and chronic constipation may be associated [2]. There is some evidence that defective collagen formation may play a role as there is an association with other abdominal hernias [5].

Kyphosis predisposes to development of a POH. A historical overview, which includes a review of 4 studies from the 21st century, concluded that there is an association between the two conditions and that postoperative respiratory complication were more common if kyphosis was present [6].

Para-oesophageal hernias represent approximately 5–15% of all HHs. The incidence of HH varies widely with higher rates in the USA and lower rates in China and Japan. Analysis of the US National Inpatient Sample documented 63,812 POH repairs between 2001 and 2013 [7].

The natural history of POH has not been evaluated in prospective trials. However, these herniae are unlikely to get smaller, but there is no study describing increase in size over time. The risk of presenting with a life-threatening complication is probably low, but there are quality of life (QOL) issues which need to be taken into account There is good evidence that QOL after POH repair in the elderly is substantially and sustainably improved over baseline [8].

CLINICAL PRESENTATION

Para-oesophageal hernia may be picked up incidentally. The diagnosis is often suspected on a chest radiograph taken for another reason, which shows a retrocardiac air containing viscus (**Figure 13.2**). A careful and comprehensive history and examination is required to ensure that patients do not have gradually worsening symptoms such as early satiety, dyspnoea and symptoms of anaemia which have been attributed to ageing [4]. The onset of dysphagia and breathlessness is often insidious and careful history taking and respiratory function testing is required [9].

Others present with symptoms of reflux (especially in type III hernias), dysphagia, post-prandial fullness, postprandial chest pain, postprandial breathlessness, regurgitation, and aspiration. The symptoms of reflux may be oesophageal in nature or extra-oesophageal symptoms (pulmonary and laryngeal). If the stomach is obstructed, nausea, vomiting epigastric and chest pain may predominate. Occasionally, patients have haematemesis or anaemia from venous engorgement and Cameron's ulcers [5,9,10]. If anaemia is present, colonic lesions should be excluded.

A retrospective review of 270 patients, operated on for POH found that typical symptoms of reflux were present in 65% which is higher than previous reports. The other symptoms were chest pain (48%), dyspnoea (48%), regurgitation (47%) and anaemia (41%). Practically all had at least one symptom and the median number of symptoms was four. Types II and III hernias were more likely to have heartburn and type IV was associated with dyspnoea [4].

Symptoms of incarceration and strangulation with a gastric volvulus include complete dysphagia, severe chest and upper abdominal pain, excessive salivation and retching, and haemodynamic instability. Borchardt described the clinical triad of chest pain, retching without the ability to vomit and the inability to pass a nasogastric tube (NGT) beyond the intra-thoracic stomach that retains his name. The mortality associated with strangulation with necrosis of an organ has been reported to be as high as 90% in some early studies but this has decreased considerably in recent years [2].

Organoaxial volvulus may cause problems, but mesoaxial volvulus has been reported to be more dangerous. The antrum is high up in the chest. A sub-diaphragmatic closed loop obstruction of the fundus and the rest of the stomach above the diaphragm gives the appearance of a double air fluid level on plain radiograph [2].

Investigations

Elective cases require extensive investigations. A full cardiopulmonary assessment is required. Close collaboration between the patient, surgeon, anaesthetist and pulmonary physician is required.

A contrast meal and swallow is usually diagnostic. In order to diagnose a POH the stomach should be higher that the GOJ with a rolling component. An intra-thoracic stomach (ITS) of greater that 30% [10] or greater than 50% [2] is defined as a giant POH. A contrast swallow delineates the anatomy better than a CT. The hernia normally sits in the left chest and behind the heart but with increasing size can encroach the right chest [2]. These hernias may be reducible in the upright position.

Upper endoscopy is recommended to check for other pathology such as Barrett's metaplasia, tumour or a Cameron's ulcer. The position of the GOJ can be determined which will help to differentiate type II from the more common type III POH. Occasionally, endoscopy is incomplete especially in types III and IV hernias with an upside down stomach.

A CT scan of the chest and abdomen may confirm a type IV hernia, diagnose complications such as perforation, help exclude other diaphragmatic hernias and eventration, and may be used to measure the size and morphology of the hiatal defect [11].

Twenty four hour pH monitoring is not recommended as the patient often requires the operation for reasons other than reflux [5]. Manometry is recommended by some who prefer to tailor the type of fundoplication if there is oesophageal hypomotility. Placement of the manometry catheter may be technically challenging due to obstruction [9].

Indications for operation

Over time, the propensity of surgeons to operate on POHs has varied. Initial reports suggested that all POHs should be repaired as the risk of mortality for emergency repairs was so high [12,13]. This was followed by a period when it was recommended that only symptomatic patients should undergo repair [14]. This change was partly due to new evidence that the probability of requiring an emergency operation was low, and that the morbidity and mortality of emergency surgery had decreased with improved surgical techniques and perioperative care.

Sliding HH predisposes patients to gastro-oesophageal reflux which may be asymptomatic or symptomatic. Symptoms may be typical or extra-oesophageal. The ICARUS (International Consensus regarding preoperative examinations and clinical characteristics assessment to select adult patients for AntiReflUx Surgery) consensus document on workup and indications for surgery has recently been agreed using a Delphi process. There is only one statement on the indication for operation for POH which states that symptomatic cases should undergo repair, although evidence quality was Grade C [15].

Patients presenting with obstructive symptoms or features of strangulation need a period of resuscitation and conservative measures such as decompression with a NGT. If placement of the NGT fails, an attempt with radiological guidance may succeed. Fluoroscopic guidance is recommended due to a high perforation with blind NGT placement [16]. An endoscopic detorsion may be attempted. This should be done with endotracheal intubation to prevent aspiration. If there is no gastric necrosis, a NGT should be inserted under endoscopic guidance and left in place. Further resuscitation and optimisation for surgery may then be employed. This approach is successful in 67–75% of cases with acute symptoms [16,17]. Less than 10% of cases presenting as an emergency require immediate operation but repair on the same admission is strongly recommended. If patients are unfit for surgery, a percutaneous endoscopic gastrostomy (PEG) in the gastric body may be performed if there is no gastric necrosis. This acts as a gastropexy. A second PEG in the antrum is also recommended if definitive repair is not possible [9,18].

If decompression fails, urgent surgery is required. If there is necrosis of part of the stomach, this needs to be resected. Any resection at, or near the GOJ, should be performed with a large diameter oesophageal bougie in place to prevent narrowing of the GOJ. If the patient is unstable on the operating table and there is no necrosis, reduction of as much stomach as possible followed by a gastropexy and gastrostomy has been recommended as a bailout option [19].

If the POH is discovered incidentally and the patient is truly asymptomatic, then patient age, cognitive function, comorbidities, operative risk, availability of expert team at a high volume centre and patient wishes will determine whether watchful waiting or operative repair is employed. Initial reports by Belsey and Hill suggested that all POH should be repaired due to the risk of strangulation requiring emergency surgery which was associated with a high mortality [12,13]. The risk of mortality with emergency surgery has decreased from prior estimations of 17% to 5.4% in 1997 [14] and further to 2.5% between 2011 and 2016 [20]. This may be used to reassure the asymptomatic patient. The need for emergency surgery was estimated to be less than 2% per annum [17]. However, the mortality of emergency repairs remains higher than for elective repairs, whether done open or laparoscopically [20]. The cost of watchful waiting is estimated to be less, but QOL post-repair in minimally symptomatic patients was improved in a cost benefit analysis [21]. Respiratory function reliably improves after POH repair [22]. The morbidity and mortality of elective repairs has decreased substantially due to improved laparoscopic techniques and surgeon expertise, sophisticated endoscopic and ancillary equipment and regionalisation of care [23]. Chronic iron deficiency anaemia often improves with successful repair.

Younger patients (< 50 years old) should be offered an operative repair even if asymptomatic [5]. Others suggest surgery for those younger than 65 years old providing they are fit for operation [9].

Operative techniques

The steps of a laparoscopic repair of a giant POH are well described by Auyang and Pellegrini [24] as well as Antonoff [25]. There are areas of debate as to whether all steps are necessary. The main steps are:

- Reduction of the contents of the sac
- Systematic resection of the hernia sac
- Oesophageal mobilisation or lengthening
- Crural repair with or without mesh reinforcement
- Fundoplication

Reduction of sac contents

This should be attempted with care. Careful inspection of the contents is necessary to ensure that any non-viable necrotic tissue is identified and appropriate resection undertaken.

Sac excision

Complete sac excision is generally recommended. This allows for identification of structures and for oesophageal mobilisation. Care should be taken not to injure the pleura and the posterior vagus nerve. The sac is usually quite thin and the plane of dissection can easily be lost. If the pleura is inadvertently entered, there is usually no major issue providing there is no lung injury but some surgeons prefer to place an intercostal underwater drain. Failure to resect the sac has been associated with unacceptable rates of recurrence [9]. During excision of the sac it is important to preserve the peritoneal lining of the crura [24,26].

Both crural pillars need to be well visualised with dissection proceeding posteriorly until the posteroinferior 'V' is seen. This ensures that the subsequent crural repair does not leave a posterior gap. A few of the uppermost short gastric vessels may need division to free up the posterior aspect of the left crural pillar and to loosen the fundus for the fundoplication. Thick fibrous attachments are often encountered in this area and must be divided.

Mobilisation of the oesophagus

At least 3–4 cm of oesophagus should be below the crural repair [26–28]. Failure to ensure adequate oesophageal length, the size of the hiatus and age are the main determinants of recurrence [28]. Extensive mobilisation of the oesophagus, up to the carina if necessary, is required before diagnosing a short oesophagus.

Oesophageal lengthening procedure, in the form of a Collis gastroplasty is performed often by some experts [25,27,29] and rarely by others [24,28]. The overall rate of a shortened oesophagus is estimated to be 10% and the need for oesophageal lengthening with a Collis gastroplasty is 3%. It is suggested that high dissection of the oesophagus up to the carina will obviate the need for Collis lengthening procedures with decreased chance of leaks, necrosis, and abnormal acid secretion [28]. The open Collis technique has been serially modified for laparoscopic procedures and if done, a wedge Collis gastroplasty is usually now performed [24]. Advocates of Collis gastroplasty often do minimal oesophageal dissection. Routine use of Collis gastroplasty in redo POH repair has been recommended [28].

Crural repair

Closure of the crural pillars posteriorly is performed using non-absorbable sutures. The crural pillars are usually approximated posteriorly, due to the inverted teardrop shape of the hiatal defect. Anterior closure is tempting but the tension on the suture closure is greater. If too many sutures are needed posteriorly, the oesophagus may have to loop over the posterior closure which causes a step and occasionally some sutures are required anteriorly. Preservation of the glistening peritoneal layer and endoabdominal fascia is highly recommended. In order to ensure that the repair starts at the 'V' posteriorly, any mediastinal lipomas must be removed or displaced back into the abdomen. Care should be taken not to injure the aorta with the first stitch or two. The hiatal size and surface area should be calculated or estimated to guide the likelihood of needing to augment the repair [30,31]. Recently, the shape of the hiatus which can be described as 'slit', 'D', 'teardrop' or 'oval' has been shown to influence the tension of the repair [32].

If there is excessive tension on the pillars on attempted closure, a left lateral (occasionally right) crural relaxing incision may be performed. The inferior vena cava must be identified and avoided and the incision must not extend anterior to the phrenic vein. This relaxing incision is patched with mesh which is then not in contact with the oesophagus and hopefully prevents mesh erosion [29,33]. Another option is to use a bridging mesh to cover the posterior defect but this has fallen out of favour. Deflating the pneumoperitoneum to the minimum required for technical completion may be attempted. Closure may be with simple or figure of 8 non-absorbable sutures, with or without pledgets. Some authors omit the pledget on the final posterior suture to prevent erosion into the oesophagus [19]. Judging the tightness of the closure requires experience. Some authors recommend a 56F Bougie to be placed in the oesophagus. In experienced hands, snug closure onto a non-distended oesophagus suffices. A single suture placed anteriorly though the diaphragmatic fascia is recommended by some to decrease anterior recurrence. If a mesh is to be used it may be placed before or after the fundoplication.

Fundoplication

This has become a standard component of POH repair. Even if reflux was not a major symptom preoperatively, omission of a fundoplication results in unacceptably high rates of postoperative reflux. Fundoplication may also help to prevent recurrence of the HH by acting as a buttress [9]. There is no consensus on whether a complete or partial fundoplication should be performed. In one study, a Dor fundoplication was associated with less dysphagia than a 360° wrap but these were short term outcomes [34]. The use of a 56F Bougie for calibration of a complete wrap is advocated by some authors [25].

Other procedures and adjuncts

The Hill operation, where anchoring the phreno-oesophageal membrane to the median arcuate ligament reconstructs a competent anti-reflux mechanism, is advocated by authors from Seattle [16].

Magnetic sphincter augmentation (MSA) with the LINX™ device (Johnson and Johnson, New Brunswick, NJ) has been used with fundal gastropexy [26].

Bariatric or metabolic operations – morbidly obese patients are predisposed to HH and obesity predicts hernia recurrence. Performance of a Roux-en-Y gastric bypass may be indicated in the morbidly obese and should be discussed with the patient. A sleeve gastrectomy is advocated by some but it is associated with reflux disease and probably should be avoided as an adjunct [5,9]. Bariatric procedures may be used for recurrent hernias in the morbidly obese.

Concomitant PEG placement during elective laparoscopic repair is advocated for older and frailer patients and was performed in 2% of cases in a retrospective USA analysis. This may allow earlier feeding [35,36].

ISSUES REGARDING THE USAGE OF MESH IN PARA-OESOPHAGEAL HERNIA REPAIR

Late recurrence of POH after repair has been decreasing but remains a major challenge. Recurrence rates of 5–59% have been reported. Many recurrences are radiological and the patients are minimally symptomatic. The need for reoperation is less than 5% [28].

Meshes have been used with great success in other forms of abdominal hernioplasty and therefore there has been some interest in using meshes to reduce recurrence rates for primary POH repair, or for redo procedures. An array of mesh designs and types, some preformed, have been described for POH repair, including bridging and reinforcing meshes.

Initial promising results with non-absorbable meshes at the hiatus, for all types of HH, were tempered by reports of serious complications with erosion of the mesh into the oesophagus and stomach. Although uncommon, these reported cases result in severe morbidity [37]. This prompted the use of absorbable biologic meshes, with fewer complications reported and promising early results. However, disappointing long-term recurrence rates have dampened enthusiasm. Despite conflicting evidence, approximately 40% of surgeons in the USA use mesh [37]. In a retrospective review of 795 patients in 2017, Tam showed that dysphagia was more common with a mesh (placed in 13% of patients) but recurrence rates were similar with or without a mesh. A systematic review in 2016 concluded that mesh placement decreased long-term recurrence by 49% but did not statistically decrease the need for re-operation. The quality of data was reported to be poor and the infrequent but serious complication of mesh erosions was mentioned [38]. A systematic review and meta-analysis by Campos in 2020 concluded that there was no difference in recurrence rate or other outcomes when a mesh was used [39]. Trials of slowly absorbable synthetic meshes are ongoing [27,40,41].

Mesh may be unavoidable if releasing incisions are performed, or if there is an inability to get secure approximation by sutured crural closure alone. The use of mesh should be considered when there are predictors of recurrence (large hiatal surface area, age and obesity, and redo surgery) [7].

The shape and position of the mesh is not standardised. U-shaped meshes are commonly used. Due to contraction of the mesh and possible stenosis, circular or keyhole meshes are generally avoided. Recurrences have been noted to occur anterior and to the left of the oesophagus with U-shaped meshes and the keyhole pattern has recently been shown to have good results [42].

Fixation of the mesh may be effected by suture, glue or tacks. Tacking runs the risk of vascular, cardiac and pulmonary complications [43]. A non-absorbable mesh may be covered by the mobilised hernia sac to help prevent erosion [44].

SURGICAL ACCESS METHODS

Prior to the introduction of minimal access surgery (MAS) in the mid-1990s, the operative approach was either by laparotomy or thoracotomy. The purported advantage of a left thoracotomy was the ease of resection of the sac and easier mobilisation of the oesophagus. A transthoracic anti-reflux procedure such as a Belsey Mark IV was often added. The disadvantage of this approach was the morbidity of a thoracotomy and the difficulty of the fundoplication [17]. Some units continued with the open approach well after laparoscopic procedures became established because of initial reports of high conversion and recurrence rates.

A review of 97,393 patients operated in the USA from 2002 to 2012 showed that the use of MAS increased from 9.8% in 2012 to almost 80% in 2012. This was associated with decreased morbidity, mortality and length of hospital stay [45]. Most cases are now done laparoscopically and this should be the standard of care [46]. A MAS approach is also recommended for emergency procedures unless perforation is suspected [20].

Robotic POH repair has been reported as feasible in a retrospective study and was performed more often for recurrent cases. This resulted in fewer conversions and lengthening procedures than the laparoscopic group due to improved oesophageal mobilisation, as well as a decreased length of stay [47].

There are no prospective randomised trials comparing different approaches. The type and route of repair should be tailored to the patient's general condition, size, and nature of the hernia as well as the surgical expertise and equipment available [30].

OUTCOMES AND COMPLICATIONS OF SURGERY

Immediate perioperative complications have reduced considerably due to the adoption of laparoscopic surgery [45]. Conversion to open surgery is now uncommon. Splenectomy is very uncommon with the laparoscopic approach. Possible inadvertent luminal perforations should be excluded with a postoperative contrast swallow. Early gas-bloat needs decompression and take down of the repair while acute re-herniation into the chest requires emergency decompression and re-operation.

Early dysphagia may be an issue if a complete wrap is fashioned. Dietary modifications and the inability to burp or vomit needs to be discussed with the patients. Dysmotility, fundoplication and a mesh may result in dysphagia but this often responds to endoscopic dilation. Vagal injury may result in gastroparesis.

The high reported recurrence rate remains an issue despite numerous proposed solutions such as oesophageal mobilisation and lengthening procedures, and mesh cruraplasties. Radiographic recurrence does not correlate with symptoms [29], and patients are often unaware of their recurrence [48]. Postoperative reflux may become an issue and can usually be treated with anti-secretory medication. Occasionally, if the stomach herniates through the wrap (slipped fundoplication), reflux may be difficult to manage and redo operation may be indicated. Recurrent massive HH usually requires re-operation with a Collis gastroplasty.

Mesh erosion is a feared complication. The mesh may erode into the oesophagus or stomach, and rarely may involve the bronchi, pericardium, ventricles, and aorta. Occasionally, the entire mesh extrudes into the lumen of the stomach or oesophagus and may be removed endoscopically without further issues. Synthetic meshes are more likely to erode, whereas biodegradable meshes tend to cause obstruction requiring dilation. Partial mesh extrusion often requires re-operation which is usually complex and may need organ resection [37].

Quality of life postoperatively needs to be carefully considered in the elderly. There is good evidence that the QOL postoperatively in selected aged patients can be good, even if their life expectancy is short. Respiratory function almost always improves as does reflux and other symptoms [4].

Surgical volume and perioperative outcomes

There is now good evidence that high volume centres, doing more than 20 POH repairs a year, have better outcomes than those performing fewer cases. Emergency decompression and stabilisation of the patient and referral to a specialist centre is recommended [7,17]. Analysis of the US National Inpatient Sample documented 63,812 repairs of POHs between 2001 and 2013. The rate of POH repair increased in high-volume centres (> 20 cases per year) from 65.8 to 94.4%, with 67% being performed laparoscopically in high volume centres. The majority were females (64%). The mean age was 65 in low volume centres and 54 in high volume centres. Low volume centres (< 6 cases per year) were less likely to treat elective cases (57%) versus high volume centres (78%). Mortality was 0.8% in high volume centres versus 2.9% in low volume centres [7].

CONCLUSION

Para-oesophageal hernias present important challenges for the surgeon. A detailed knowledge of the anatomy and physiology of the oesophagus, stomach diaphragm and their embryological origin is essential. Sliding and rolling types of POH can be distinguished by clinical and radiological methods. Clinical presentation may vary from incidental findings with minimal symptoms through to acute surgical emergency presentation with gastric volvulus or strangulation producing severe constitutional upset and sepsis. The balance of risk between elective prophylactic surgery and the risk of emergency presentation should be carefully considered taking into account patient factors such as comorbidity. Multiple operations and technical modifications have been reported for POH repair. This reflects the complexity and variable outcomes of this type of surgery. Meticulous dissection are to avoid iatrogenic damage to the distal oesophagus and surrounding structures is essential. The role of surgical adjuncts such as fundoplication, sphincter augmentation or combined bariatric procedures remains controversial and provide scope for ongoing research.

Key points for clinical practice

- Para-oesophageal hernias are distinct from sliding hernias and the indications for operative repair are different
- Very few patients who have POH are truly symptomatic. Gradual onset of postprandial breathlessness, early satiety and difficulty in swallowing are often attributed to ageing
- Centralisation of care in high volume centres has been shown to improve results
- Almost all patients presenting with acute symptoms need surgery, but temporising measures with decompression usually allows transfer to a specialist centre
- Symptomatic cases should be offered an elective repair providing their operative risk is not prohibitive
- Truly asymptomatic patients may be offered "watchful waiting" but those aged < 65 years should be considered for repair
- Laparoscopic repair with excision of the sac, extensive mobilisation of the oesophagus, occasional lengthening procedures, posterior crural closure with judicious use of mesh cruroplasty and a fundoplication is advised

REFERENCES

1. Petrov RV, Su S, Bakhos CT, et al. Surgical Anatomy of Paraesophageal Hernias. Thorac Surg Clin 2019; 29:359–368.
2. Duranceau A. Massive hiatal hernia: a review. Dis Esophagus 2016; 29:350–366.
3. Li J, Guo C, Shao X, et al. Another type of diaphragmatic hernia to remember: parahiatal hernia. ANZ J Surg 2020; 90:2180–2186.
4. Carrott PW, Hong J, Kuppusamy M, et al. Clinical ramifications of giant paraesophageal hernias are underappreciated: making the case for routine surgical repair. Ann Thorac Surg 2012; 94:421–426.
5. Andolfi C, Jalilvand A, Plana A, et al. Surgical treatment of paraesophageal hernias: a review. J Laparoendosc Adv Surg Tech 2016; 26:778–773.
6. Polomsky M, Peters JH, Schwartz SI. Hiatal hernia and disorders of the spine : a historical perspective. Dis Esophagus 2012; 25:367–372.
7. Schlottmann F, Strassle PD, Allaix ME, et al. Paraesophageal Hernia Repair in the USA : trends of utilization stratified by surgical volume and consequent impact on perioperative outcomes. J Gastrointest Surg 2017; 21:1199–1205.
8. Merzlikin OV, Louie BE, Farivar AS, et al. Repair of symptomatic paraesophageal hernias in elderly (> 70 years) patients results in sustained quality of life at 5 years and beyond. Surg Endosc. 2017;31:3979–3984.
9. Lebenthal A, Waterford SD, Fisichella PM. Treatment and controversies in paraesophageal hernia repair. Front Surg 2015; 2:13.
10. Tam V, Luketich JD, Levy RM, et al. Mesh cruroplasty in laparoscopic repair of paraesophageal hernias is not associated with better long-term outcomes compared to primary repair. Am J Surg 2017; 214:651–656.
11. Kumar D, Zifan A, Ghahremani G, et al. Morphology of the esophageal hiatus: is it different in 3 types of hiatus hernias? J Neurogastroenterol Motil 2020; 26:51–60.
12. Skinner DB, Belsey RH. Surgical management of esophageal reflux and hiatus hernia. Long-term results with 1,030 patients. J Thorac Cardiovasc Surg 1967; 53:33–54.
13. Hill LD. Incarcerated paraesophageal hernia. A surgical emergency. Am J Surg 1973; 126:286–291.

14. Stylopoulos N, Gazelle GS, Rattner DW. Paraesophageal Hernias : operation or observation ?Ann Surg 2002; 236:492–500.
15. Pauwels A, Boecxstaens V, Andrews CN, et al. How to select patients for antireflux surgery? The ICARUS guidelines (international consensus regarding preoperative examinations and clinical characteristics assessment to select adult patients for antireflux surgery). Gut 2019; 68:1928–1941.
16. Wirsching A, El Lakis MA, Mohiuddin K, et al. Acute Vs. Elective Paraesophageal Hernia Repair: endoscopic gastric decompression allows semi-elective surgery in a majority of acute patients. J Gastrointest Surg 2018; 22:194–202.
17. Dreifuss NH, Schlottmann F, Molena D. Management of paraesophageal hernia review of clinical studies: timing to surgery, mesh use, fundoplication, gastropexy and other controversies. Dis Esophagus 2020; 33.
18. Coleman C, Musgrove K, Bardes J, et al. Incarcerated paraesophageal hernia and gastric volvulus: Management options for the acute care surgeon, an Eastern Association for the Surgery of Trauma master class video presentation. J Trauma Acute Care Surg 2020; 88:E146–E148.
19. Siegal SR, Dolan JP, Hunter JG. Modern diagnosis and treatment of hiatal hernias. Langenbeck's Arch Surg 2017; 402:1145–1151.
20. Sherrill W, Rossi I, Genz M, et al. Non-elective paraesophageal hernia repair: surgical approaches and short-term outcomes. Surg Endosc 2020.
21. Morrow EH, Chen J, Patel R, et al. Watchful waiting versus elective repair for asymptomatic and minimally symptomatic paraesophageal hernias: a cost-effectiveness analysis. Am J Surg 2018; 216:760–763.
22. Wirsching A, Klevebro F, Boshier PR, et al. The other explanation for dyspnea: Giant paraesophageal hiatal hernia repair routinely improves pulmonary function. Dis Esophagus 2019;32.
23. Sorial RK, Ali M, Kaneva P, et al. Modern era surgical outcomes of elective and emergency giant paraesophageal hernia repair at a high-volume referral center. Surg Endosc 2020; 34:284–289.
24. Auyang ED, Pellegrini CA. How I Do It: laparoscopic paraesophageal hernia repair. J Gastrointest Surg 2012; 16:1406–1411.
25. Antonoff MB, D'Cunha J, Andrade RS, et al. Giant paraesophageal hernia repair: technical pearls. J Thorac Cardiovasc Surg 2012; 144:S67–S70.
26. Allman R, Speicher J, Rogers A, et al. Fundic gastropexy for high risk of recurrence laparoscopic hiatal hernia repair and esophageal sphincter augmentation (LINX) improves outcomes without altering perioperative course. Surg Endosc 2020;1–5.
27. Abdelmoaty WF, Dunst CM, Filicori F, et al. Combination of Surgical Technique and Bioresorbable Mesh Reinforcement of the Crural Repair Leads to Low Early Hernia Recurrence Rates with Laparoscopic Paraesophageal Hernia Repair. J Gastrointest Surg 2020; 24:1477–1481.
28. Flores LE, Armijo PR, Xu T, et al. How high is too high? Extensive mediastinal dissection in patients with hiatal hernia repair. Surg Endosc. 2020.
29. Luketich JD, Nason KS, Christie NA, et al. Outcomes after a decade of laparoscopic giant paraesophageal hernia repair. J Thorac Cardiovasc Surg 2010; 139:395–404.
30. Grubnik VV, Malynovskyy AV. Laparoscopic repair of hiatal hernias: new classification supported by long-term results. Surg Endosc 2013; 27:4337–4346.
31. Moten AS, Ouyang W, Hava S, et al. In vivo measurement of esophageal hiatus surface area using MDCT: description of the methodology and clinical validation. Abdom Radiol(NY) 2020; 45:2656–2662.
32. Bradley DD, Louie BE, Farivar AS, et al. Assessment and reduction of diaphragmatic tension during hiatal hernia repair. Surg Endosc 2015; 29:796–804.
33. Greene CL, DeMeester SR, Zehetner J, et al. Diaphragmatic relaxing incisions during laparoscopic paraesophageal hernia repair. Surg Endosc 2013; 27:4532–4538.
34. Trepanier M, Dumitra T, Sorial R, et al. Comparison of Dor and Nissen fundoplication after laparoscopic paraesophageal hernia repair. Surgery 2019; 166:540–546.
35. Roberts I, Shakur-Still H, Afolabi A, et al. (2020). Effects of a high-dose 24-h infusion of tranexamic acid on death and thromboembolic events in patients with acute gastrointestinal bleeding (HALT-IT): an international randomised, double-blind, placebo-controlled trial. Lancet 2020; 395:1927–1936.
36. Yheulon CG, Balla FM, Lin E, et al. Who gets a PEG? An analysis of simultaneous PEG placement during elective laparoscopic paraesophageal hernia repair. Surg Endosc 2020; 34:686–695.
37. Spiro C, Quarmby N, Gananadha S. Mesh-related complications in paraoesophageal repair: a systematic review. Surg Endosc 2020; 34:4257–4280.
38. Tam V, Winger DG, Nason KS. A systematic review and meta-analysis of mesh vs suture cruroplasty in laparoscopic large hiatal hernia repair. Am J Surg 2016; 211:226–238.

39. Campos V, Palacio DS, Glina F, et al. Laparoscopic treatment of giant hiatal hernia with or without mesh reinforcement: a systematic review and meta-analysis. Int J Surg 2020; 77:97–104.
40. Panici Tonucci T, Asti E, Sironi A, et al. Safety and Efficacy of Crura Augmentation with Phasix ST Mesh for Large Hiatal Hernia: 3-year single-center experience. J Laparoendosc Adv Surg Tech A 2020; 30:369–372.
41. Iossa A, Silecchia G. Mid-term safety profile evaluation of Bio-A absorbable synthetic mesh as cruroplasty reinforcement. Surg. Endosc 2019; 33:3783–3789.
42. Keville S, Rabach L, Saad AR, et al. Evolution From the U-shaped to Keyhole-shaped Mesh Configuration in the Repair of Paraesophageal and Recurrent Hiatal Hernia. Surg Laparosc Endosc Percutan Tech 2020; 30:339–344.
43. Vidrio Duarte R, Vidrio Duarte E, Gutierrez Ochoa J, et al. Cardiac Tamponade by Tack Fixation of a Hiatal Mesh. Should Tacks Still Be Used in the Diaphragm? Cureus 2020; 12:e8416.
44. Braghetto I, Korn O, Rojas J, et al. Hiatal hernia repair: prevention of mesh erosion and migration into the esophagogastric junction. Arq Bras Cir Dig 2020; 33:e1489.
45. McLaren PJ, Hart KD, Hunter JG, et al. Paraesophageal Hernia Repair Outcomes Using Minimally Invasive Approaches. JAMA Surg 2017; 152:1176–1178.
46. Schlottmann F, Strassle PD, Farrell T, et al. Minimally Invasive Surgery Should Be the Standard of Care for Paraesophageal Hernia Repair. J Gastrointest Surg 2017; 21:778–784.
47. Gerull WD, Cho D, Arefanian S, et al. Favorable peri-operative outcomes observed in paraesophageal hernia repair with robotic approach. Surg Endosc. 2020.
48. Dallemagne B, Kohnen L, Perretta S, et al. Laparoscopic repair of paraesophageal hernia: long-term follow-up reveals good clinical outcome despite high radiological recurrence rate. Ann Surg 2011; 253:291–296.

Chapter 14

Idiopathic non-cirrhotic portal hypertension

Arunima Verma, Sunil Kumar

INTRODUCTION

Idiopathic non-cirrhotic portal hypertension (INCPH) is a rare vascular liver disease resulting in portal hypertension (PHT) with near normal hepatic venous pressure gradient (HVPG). There is no universally accepted definition, and the nomenclature is also confusing, with several terms in current use including:
- Non-cirrhotic portal fibrosis (NCPF) used in the Indian subcontinent
- Idiopathic portal hypertension (IPH) used in Japan and other Asian countries
- Idiopathic non-cirrhotic portal hypertension used in the West [1,2]

Various terms such as nodular regenerative hyperplasia (NRH), partial nodular transformation, incomplete septal cirrhosis, obliterative portal venopathy, hepatoportal sclerosis, besides NCPF and IPH, have also been used to describe one disease with heterogeneous morphological aspects, and the term INCPH has been introduced to avoid confusion. INCPH has both clinical and histopathological features of the disease [3]. Any disorder known to cause PHT in the absence of cirrhosis and any other cause of chronic liver disease, excluding those with splanchnic venous thrombosis, allows the diagnosis of INCPH [4,5].

EPIDEMIOLOGY

Idiopathic non-cirrhotic portal hypertension has a worldwide distribution but is more prevalent in Asia. Approximately 23% of cases of PHT from India [1,6]and 14–27% of cases in the Western world [7–9] are due to INCPH. It is more prevalent in lower socioeconomic groups that is reflected in the geographical distribution which is higher in Asia, decreasing in Japan and low in the Western countries. There are also indications of a decrease in NCPF in India since 1990, due to improvements in sanitation and hygiene, reflected also in a decreased incidence of hepatitis A infection, and reduction in umbilical sepsis [1,10,11]. Gender and age disparity are seen across geographical regions, with median age at diagnosis being 40 with male preponderance in the Western world, and younger age at diagnosis with males more affected in the Indian population, whereas, females in their fifth decade are those most affected in the Japanese population [2,3,5,12,13].

AETIOLOGY

A variety of rare disorders are implicated in the causation of INCPH as classified in **Table 14.1**. Multifactorial aetiology can also be encountered.

All these disorders involve the pre-hepatic, intrahepatic or posthepatic sites. Of those that are intrahepatic, the site of involvement may be pre-sinusoidal, sinusoidal or post-sinusoidal. Some disorders may also affect multiple sites (**Table 14.2**).

PATHOPHYSIOLOGY

The pathophysiological mechanism resulting in INCPH remains largely unknown and is an area of ongoing research. Several theories have been proposed to explain the aetiopathogenesis. Sarin and Kumar proposed the *Unifying common hypothesis* for both

	Table 14.1 Aetiological classification of INCPH	
	Aetiology	**Examples**
1.	Immunological disorders	• Common variable immunodeficiency syndrome. • Crohn's disease. • Systemic sclerosis and systemic lupus erythematosus (SLE). • Coeliac disease. • Ulcerative colitis. • Hypogammaglobulinemia. • Rheumatoid arthritis. • Autoimmune thyroid disease. • Solid organ transplant. • Primary antibody-deficiency syndrome.
2.	Exposure to medications or toxins	• Azathioprine. • 6-thioguanine. • Arsenic. • Vinyl chloride. • Didanosine. • Oxaliplatin. • Vitamin A. • Fowler's solution. • Busulfan. • Arabinoside. • Bleomycin
3.	Chronic infections	• Infant umbilical sepsis. • Bacterial intestinal infections. • HIV infection.
4.	Genetic predisposition	• Familial aggregation. • Adams-Oliver syndrome. • Turner syndrome. • Phosphomannose isomerase deficiency. • Cystic fibrosis.
5.	Prothrombotic conditions	• Inherited and acquired thrombophilias. • Myeloproliferative disorders. • Anti-phospholipid syndrome. • ADAMTS13 deficiency
(INCPH, idiopathic non-cirrhotic portal hypertension; HIV, human immunodeficiency virus)		

Table 14.2 Anatomical site of involvement in idiopathic non-cirrhotic portal hypertension (INCPH)		
Pre-hepatic: Disruption of vascular system proximal to liver		
• Extrahepatic portal vein obstruction (EPHVO)		
• Portal vein thrombosis		
• Splenic vein thrombosis		
• Splanchnic arteriovenous fistulas		
• Massive splenomegaly – infiltrative and storage diseases		
Intrahepatic: The hepatic parenchyma may be involved at three levels – pre-sinusoidal, sinusoidal or post-sinusoidal		
Pre-sinusoidal	Sinusoidal	Post-sinusoidal
• Developmental anomalies – adult polycystic liver disease, congenital hepatic fibrosis, and arteriovenous fistula	• Fibrosis of space of Disse – metabolic, inflammatory, drugs/ toxins	• Sinusoidal obstruction syndrome (previously called veno-occlusive disease) – hepatic irradiation, toxins, and drugs
• Biliary diseases – biliary cholangitis, primary sclerosing cholangitis, autoimmune cholangiopathy, toxic biliary injury from vinyl chloride	• Amyloid or light-chain deposition in the space of Disse
• Sinusoidal defenestration – early alcoholic liver disease	• Budd-Chiari syndrome
• Phlebosclerosis of hepatic veins – alcoholic liver disease, chronic radiation injury, and hypervitaminosis A
• Neoplastic occlusion of the intrahepatic portal vein – lymphoma, epithelial malignancies, chronic lymphocytic leukaemia, and epithelioid hemangioendothelioma	• Sinusoidal destruction or collapse in the setting of acute hepatic injury
• Sinusoidal infiltration – mastocytosis, Gaucher disease, agnogenic myeloid metaplasia	• Primary vascular malignancies – epithelioid hemangioendothelioma, angiosarcoma
• Granulomatous liver lesions – schistosomiasis, mineral oil granuloma, and sarcoidosis	• Sinusoidal compression by markedly hypertrophied hepatocytes, as seen with microvesicular steatosis	• Granulomatous phlebitis – *Mycobacterium avium* or *Mycobacterium* intra-cellulare infection, sarcoidosis
• Hepatoportal sclerosis
• Non-cirrhotic portal fibrosis
• Idiopathic portal hypertension		• Lipogranulomas – mineral oil granuloma
Posthepatic: Disruption of vascular system distal to liver.		
• Obstruction of hepatic veins or inferior vena cava – Budd–Chiari syndrome.		
• Cardiac diseases – constrictive pericarditis and restrictive cardiomyopathy.		

NCPF/IPH and extrahepatic portal vein obstruction (EHPVO), according to which EHPVO occurs due to a major thrombotic event in the main portal vein (PV) at a young age, while repeated microthrombotic events in the smaller and medium-sized branches lead to NCPF [14].

Schouten et al. presented the *dual theory* implicating both intrahepatic vascular obstruction (obliterative venopathy) and increased splanchnic blood flow due to high levels of inducible nitric oxide synthase (iNOS), as well as endothelial nitric oxide synthase (eNOS) in splenic endothelial cells which causes dilatation of splenic sinuses and increased splenic venous inflow [3]. Nakanuma pointed out the similarity, in small portal veins and skin findings, between patients with INCPH and those with scleroderma and found this to be a result of an increase in transforming growth factor-β (TGF-β), connective tissue growth factor, and vascular endothelial growth factor, in serum, skin, and portal veins, which led to portal vein occlusion in INCPH.

Further to this, Sato and Nakanuma described a third concept of *endothelial mesenchymal transition* for IPH, whereby the vascular endothelial cells of portal venules acquire myofibroblastic features, as evidenced by reduced expression of the vascular endothelial cell marker CD34, and increased expression of mesenchymal cell markers. Following cell transformation, they synthesise type I collagen, which causes obliterative portal venopathy and pre-sinusoidal PHT [15–17].

Immunological conditions: The preponderance of INCPH in females, especially in the Western world, has been found to be associated with immunological disorders such as systemic sclerosis and systemic lupus erythematosus (SLE). Various autoantibodies have been found in the serum of affected patients which cause obliteration of small vessels. There is increased fibrogenesis in systemic sclerosis and immunoglobulin interference in prostacyclin formation leading to microthrombosis in SLE [18,19].

Chronic infections: Repeated intestinal infection with *Escherichia coli (E. coli)* in early childhood leads to septic embolisation and subsequent intrahepatic portal vein occlusion with subsequent development of INCPH in early adulthood. This concept has been supported by animal studies in rabbits by injecting *E. coli* into the portal system which resulted in development of non-cirrhotic portal fibrosis [20,21]. INCPH has been increasingly reported in human immunodeficiency virus (HIV) – infected patients in the Western countries. Multiple factors have been implicated. Independent risk factors include prolonged monotherapy or short-term combination treatment with didanosine and stavudine, with potential mitochondrial toxicity leading to INCPH; genetic predisposition to develop INCPH in HIV patients when exposed to didanosine. Vascular obstruction due to a high prevalence of pre-existing hypercoagulability, mainly due to protein S deficiency, has also been reported in patients with HIV-related INCPH [12,13,22–27].

Exposure to medications and toxins: Several drugs such as azathioprine, 6-thioguanine, arsenic and Fowler's solution lead to INCPH by causing fibrosis in the space of Disse. However, only a small proportion of patients exposed to these medications develop INCPH, which indicates the role of an additional pathogenetic mechanism in affected patients [3].

Genetic disorders: Potential genetic pathogenesis is suggested by reports of familial aggregation of INCPH, high frequency of human leucocyte antigen (HLA)-DR3 and presence of its key histologic features in congenital disorders (e.g., Adams–Oliver syndrome, Turner disease). A shared mutation in the deoxyguanosine kinase (*DGUOK*) gene, required for mitochondrial deoxyribonucleic acid (DNA) replication, was identified in a study of eight patients with I NCPH [28,29].

Prothrombotic conditions: Thrombophilia plays a dominant role as suggested by certain pathological features in liver specimens of INCPH patients. Evidence of prothrombotic disorders in 30–50% of INCPH patients with development of portal vein and extrahepatic portal vein thrombosis (PVT) has been reported [30,31].

CLINICAL PRESENTATION

Clinical presentation may range from asymptomatic patients to those with florid presentation of PHT. Typically, patients present with moderate to massive splenomegaly (average size 11 cm below costal margin), features of hypersplenism or anaemia, with episodes of upper gastrointestinal (UGI) bleeding following development of oesophageal varices as a complication of PHT [4,2]. In 15% of patients, dilated superficial abdominal veins can be seen, and in 50 percent of patients, mild hepatomegaly (< 4 cm below the right subcostal margin) can be found [6]. Hepatic function is usually well preserved and patent hepatic and portal veins are usually found. Presentation varies across geographical regions. In a large Indian study 72% of patients with INCPH presented with gastrointestinal

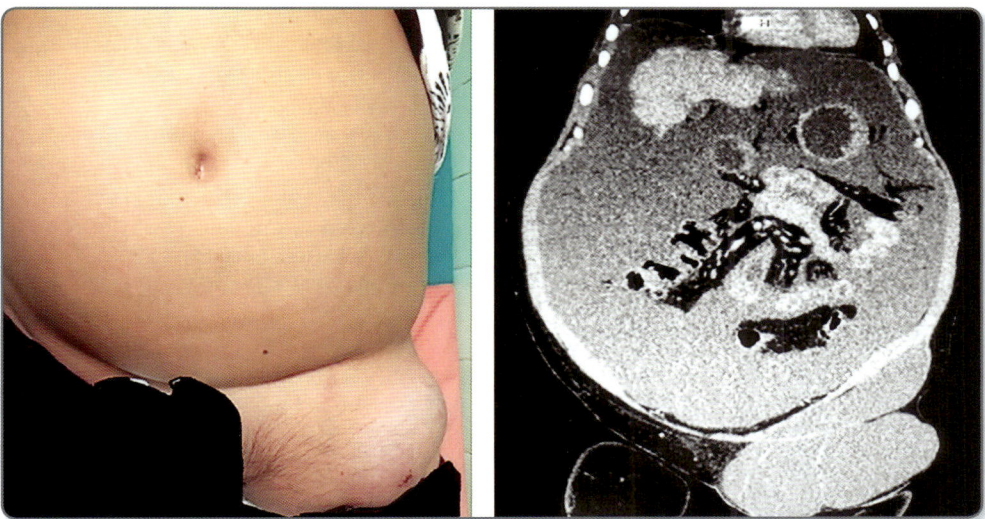

Figure 14.1: Ascites with left inguinal hernia in a case of idiopathic non-cirrhotic portal hypertension (INCPH) in a case of Budd–Chiari syndrome.

haemorrhage, while only 14% presented with splenomegaly [1,32]. Conversely, initial presentation with splenomegaly and liver function disturbances, in contrast to UGI bleed, has been found in Japanese and Western patients [30,33]. Ascites (**Figure 14.1**) is present in 50% of the patients, usually secondary to a precipitating factor such as variceal bleeding or infection, and is also related to hypoalbuminemia, prolonged duration of PHT and progressive deterioration of liver function [3,34,35]. PVT is reported in 13–46% [32,37,38]. Liver-related complications such as hepatic encephalopathy and liver failure may occur in INCPH, but the incidence is low compared to cirrhotics. Hepatopulmonary syndrome, which was considered to be a rare complication of INCPH, has been found to be present in 10% of INCPH patients reported by various authors [36,37].

DIAGNOSIS

The diagnosis of INCPH is one of exclusions, made clinically with support from imaging modalities. The diagnostic criteria are discussed in **Table 14.3**. Diagnostic work-up for these patients should include:

- Detailed medical history
- Imaging
- Laboratory tests
- Liver biopsy

Medical history

A detailed family history along with past history of infection and other known medical conditions, drug/medication intake or exposure to toxins should be elicited. The aetiological conditions listed in **Table 14.1** should be kept in mind during history taking.

Table 14.3 Diagnostic criteria for INCPH

APASL criteria for INCPH [1]	Japanese criteria for IPH [2]	EASL criteria for INCPH [47]
• Presence of moderate to massive splenomegaly • Evidence of portal hypertension, varices, and/or collaterals • Patent spleno-portal axis and hepatic veins on ultrasound Doppler • Test results indicating normal or near-normal liver functions • Normal or near-normal HVPG • Liver histology – no evidence of cirrhosis or parenchymal injury	• Clinical disorder of unknown aetiology with • Splenomegaly, anaemia and portal hypertension with • Absence of cirrhosis, blood disease, parasites in the hepatobiliary system, and occlusion of the hepatic and portal veins	All five criteria must be fulfilled: 1. More than one clinical sign of portal hypertension* (anyone of the following) a. Splenomegaly/hypersplenism b. Oesophageal varices c. Ascites (non-malignant) d. Increased hepatic venous pressure gradient e. Portovenous collaterals 2. Exclusion of cirrhosis on liver biopsy 3. Exclusion of chronic liver disease** causing cirrhosis or non-cirrhotic portal hypertension including: a. Chronic viral hepatitis B and/or C b. Non-alcoholic steatohepatitis/alcoholic steatohepatitis c. Autoimmune hepatitis d. Hereditary haemochromatosis e. Wilson's disease f. Primary biliary cirrhosis 4. Exclusion of conditions causing non-cirrhotic portal hypertension: a. Congenital liver fibrosis b. Sarcoidosis c. Schistosomiasis 5. Patent portal and hepatic veins (on Doppler ultrasound or computed tomography)
Other features • Absence of signs of chronic liver disease • No decompensation after variceal bleed except occasional transient ascites • Absence of serum markers of hepatitis B or C virus infection • No known aetiology of liver disease • Imaging with ultrasound or other imaging techniques showing dilated and thickened portal vein with peripheral pruning and periportal hyperechoic areas	**Additional points***** • Normal to near-normal liver function tests • Varices demonstrable by endoscopy or radiography • Decrease of one or more of the formed blood elements • Liver scan not typical of cirrhosis • Patent hepatic veins with a normal to slightly elevated WHVP • Grossly non-cirrhotic liver surface • Hepatic histology not indicative of cirrhosis • Patent extrahepatic portal vein with frequent collateral vessels • Elevated portal pressure	

* Splenomegaly must be accompanied by additional signs of portal hypertension to fulfil this criterion.
** Chronic liver disease must be excluded because severe fibrosis may be under-staged on liver biopsy.
*** Not all these investigations are required for diagnosis
(APASL, Asian pacific association for the study of liver; EASL, European association for the study of the liver; INCPH, idiopathic non-cirrhotic portal hypertension; IPH, idiopathic portal hypertension; HVPG, hepatic venous pressure gradient; WHVP, wedged hepatic venous gradient)

Imaging

There is a role for standard as well as emerging imaging modalities in assisting the diagnosis and management of INCPH. The goal of liver imaging is to determine the radiological signs of PHT such as splenomegaly, collateral vessels or ascites, and the patency of the hepatic veins and the portosplenomesenteric venous axis need to be evaluated for diagnosis of INCPH. First-line imaging is ultrasonography which assesses liver size, echotexture, and evidence of PHT including splenomegaly, ascites and an initial assessment of the portal venous system. Doppler studies can identify PVT and portal cavernous transformation. However, this is operator-dependent, hence further evaluation with computed tomography (CT) and magnetic resonance (MR) angiography is required. Contrast-enhanced ultrasonography is a promising technique which may help in differentiating NCPF from cirrhosis.

For differentiating PVT due to cirrhosis from PVT in the setting of INCPH, there is a role for transient elastography, which measures liver stiffness. Patients with INCPH have liver stiffness values lower than those in cirrhosis which is < 13 kPa [38]. Magnetic resonance elastography (MRE) can also be used for assessing liver stiffness as it has advantages over transient elastography in that the entire liver may be easily imaged without acoustical window limitations [39]. However, further studies are needed to establish its role in INCPH.

Laboratory tests

Liver function tests usually remain within normal parameters in INCPH but need to be done to rule out other causes of liver disease. Blood tests performed are shown in **Table 14.4** and include liver function tests, haematologic and coagulation profile tests for immunological derangements and autoimmunity and a few special tests, although their exact role still needs to be confirmed by larger studies.

Liver biopsy

Idiopathic non-cirrhotic portal hypertension resembles cirrhosis and there is no gold standard test to distinguish them. The pathological picture is not straightforward as there is no pathognomonic lesion. Rather, a variety of subtle vascular changes with a wide spectrum of non-specific features, unevenly distributed, are present in needle biopsy of the liver specimen. The approach to liver biopsy may be percutaneous or trans-jugular biopsy, but this may not be sufficient because of the sampling variability. Therefore, patients suspected of having INCPH, who have an equivocal picture on core needle biopsy, may require an open or laparoscopic biopsy. INCPH has histologic changes secondary to obliterative portal venopathy including shunt vessels, phlebosclerosis, increased number of portal vessels, arterialisation of portal veins in the portal tracts and periportal area, incomplete septa, sinusoidal dilatation, aberrant hepatic vessels and also portal fibrosis and NRH seen in the liver parenchyma, in the absence of cirrhosis or fibrosis [1,5,40–45]. Several patterns of injury, involving portal/periportal areas and parenchymal structures need to be recognised, and all of these may not be evident in a single specimen. The variability in the histologic findings may be because of the heterogeneity of the disease and its severity and also due to sampling variability of liver biopsy specimens. Essential for INCPH diagnosis in an adequate-sized liver biopsy is the absence of regenerative nodules with features of possible or definite cirrhosis [1]. Few uncommon histological features such as pseudonodules, piecemeal necrosis and

Table 14.4 Laboratory tests		
Tests		**INCPH**
Liver function tests	• Bilirubin • Liver enzymes • Hepatitis screen	• Jaundice rarely seen • Transient impairment in LFT seen in context of variceal bleed or infection • Hepatitis B and C comparable to non-transfused general population
Haematologic tests	• Hb • TLC • Platelets	• Pancytopenia due to hypersplenism
Coagulation profile	• Prothrombin time • Fibrinogen • Platelet aggregation	• Increased INR • Decreased fibrinogen • Decreased platelet aggregation with low-grade disseminated intravascular coagulation (DIC) may be seen
Immunological tests	• Anti-nuclear • Anti-mitochondrial • Anti-Scl-70 • Anti-SS-A • Anti-centromere • Anti-double-stranded DNA	• Antibody tests done in suspected autoimmune disorders
Special tests	• Vitamin B12	• Serum vitamin B12 levels are significantly lower in patients with INCPH compared to patients with cirrhosis and may be useful in distinguishing between the two entities [44]

(INCPH, idiopathic non-cirrhotic portal hypertension; Hb, haemoglobin; TLC, total leucocyte count; INR, international normalised ratio; LFT, liver function test)

regenerative activity may be seen [46]. In some patients, electron microscopy shows widening of the space of Disse with fibrogenesis in the perisinusoidal space leading to capillarisation of the sinusoids [21].

OTHER INVESTIGATIONS

Haemodynamics may aid in diagnosis. In INCPH, HVPG is usually normal (≤ mmHg), or slightly increased (5–10 mmHg) but below the cut-off for clinically significant PHT in cirrhosis (CSPH; HVPG > 10 mmHg).

Endoscopic features

About 85–90% patients are reported to have oesophagogastric varices in NCPF. In comparison with cirrhosis, gastric varices in NCPH are more common and 44% of patients have both gastric and oesophageal varices associated at the time of diagnosis [20,46]. Antral varices and portal hypertensive gastropathy is less common compared to cirrhosis.

MANAGEMENT

Due to limited available information on the natural clinical history, pathophysiology and clinical outcome of patients with INCPH, the management guidelines for these patients

are the same as the guidelines for PHT in cirrhotic patients. The aims of management strategies are:
- Management of PHT
- Management of PVT
- Elimination and control of etiological factors, e.g. withdrawing toxins or medication
- Treatment of any associated medical conditions

Management of Portal Hypertension

The primary focus is the management of acute variceal bleed followed by secondary prophylaxis to prevent re-bleeding. Management of acute variceal bleed starts with standard UGI bleed care – admission to a critical care unit; airway protection; haemodynamic stability (intravenous fluids and blood transfusion), use of vasoactive drugs such as terlipressin, somatostatin, or octreotide followed by endotherapy. In contrast to cirrhotics, where the role of prophylactic antibiotics in variceal bleed is associated with reduced re-bleed and better survival, no study has been done to establish their role in INCPH [1].

Endoscopic therapy: Endoscopic sclerotherapy (EST) and endoscopic variceal ligation (EVL) have equal efficacy for the eradication of varices and are 80–90% effective in control of acute bleeding from oesophageal varices and prevention of re-bleeding [1]. EVL is generally the preferred method because of its lower complication rate and also faster eradication of varices. However, recurrence of varices is higher with EVL. Glue injection with N-butyl-cyanoacrylate can be given to control bleeding from gastric varices which are more common in INCPH. Endotherapy needs to be repeated every 2–3 weeks until variceal eradication is achieved [1,48]. For prevention of re-bleeding, equivalent efficacy of propranolol and EVL has been reported [49]. However, combined therapy with drugs and endoscopic treatment has been shown to have better control of acute bleeds and lower re-bleed rates, but no difference in mortality. In 8–12% patients, these therapies fail to control the bleed or prevent re-bleed. An endoscopic failure is defined as further variceal bleeding after two endoscopic treatments during a single hospital admission for acute bleeding [50,51]. This group of patients may require other modes of management such as image-guided interventions, trans jugular intrahepatic portosystemic shunt (TIPS), partial splenic embolisation, balloon-occluded retrograde transvenous obliteration (BRTO), percutaneous trans-hepatic obliteration (PTO) or surgery.

Image-guided interventions: The concept behind this modality is to occlude the varices. Options include TIPS, partial splenic embolisation, BRTO and PTO. TIPS is a good option for complications of INCPH, but should be avoided in patients with poor renal function, ascites, and significant extrahepatic comorbidities such as prothrombotic conditions, haematologic malignancy and solid organ transplantation. TIPS is a multistage procedure requiring close surveillance and repeated interventions to maintain shunt patency. Polytetrafluoroethylene (PTFE)-covered stents (stent-grafts) in place of fenestrated stents can be used to prevent TIPS stenosis and occlusions. However, the high cost of stent-grafts in the countries where PHT is common, would still be a challenge. Nevertheless, TIPS can be used in patients with good hepatic function with lower risks of death, overt hepatic encephalopathy and hepatic insufficiency. The other image-guided procedures mentioned above, such as BRTO are less invasive and can be used in patients with poor hepatic reserve and those with large gastric varices [52,1,53].

Surgical management: Surgical management is indicated when endoscopic treatment has failed and includes splenectomy, shunt surgeries, ablative procedures and finally liver transplantation. Splenectomy is indicated in patients with symptomatic hypersplenism (spontaneous bleeding episodes, severe transfusion-dependent anaemia, or repeated splenic infarcts). Shunt procedures such as total or partial and physiological shunts are selected depending upon the shuntable veins. Selective shunts, such as distal splenorenal shunt (DSRS), selectively decompress the gastrosplenic zone and are superior to non-selective shunts such as central (CSRS) or proximal splenorenal shunts (PSRS) in terms of patency, lower re-bleeding and encephalopathy rates. Physiological shunts, such as mesenterico-left PV bypass (MLPVB) or mesoportal (Rex) shunt, maintain the hepatic portal blood flow, while bypassing the level of obstruction and not only control symptoms but also cure the disease reflected by improvement in coagulation status, reduction in spleen size, and hypersplenism and reversal of hepatic encephalopathy [2]. Ablative surgery includes oesophagogastric devascularisation alone or in combination with splenectomy, in cases where there has been shunt failure, or absence of a shuntable vein or as an emergency operation for refractory variceal bleeding. These procedures have high re-bleed and mortality rates and hence are obsolete [54]. Although, many INCPH patients have well-preserved hepatic function, some cases are associated with unmanageable PHT, chronic hepatic encephalopathy, progressive liver failure, hepatopulmonary syndrome, and hepatocellular carcinoma and therefore liver transplant may be indicated. Survival in these patients is usually good and INCPH recurrence is rare [55].

Management of Portal Vein Thrombosis

There is no consensus on the role of anticoagulation therapy in INCPH, but it should be considered in patients with prothrombotic conditions and those with PVT. Anti-coagulation may be an option for patients with a hypercoagulable disorder but is not used for preventing PVT [56,57].

PROGNOSIS

As liver function is well preserved in patients of INCPH, the prognosis is much better compared to cirrhotics with similar degrees of PHT. However, a small group of INCPH patients do develop liver failure, and this subgroup usually have nodular transformation of the liver with extensive hepatic and portal fibrosis and then need liver transplant. A minority of patients have been reported to develop hepatocellular carcinoma but it is not clear if they had other risk factors to account for this, hence screening for carcinoma in INCPH is not recommended. There are very few studies on long-term prognosis of INCPH, and in two of these, development of ascites was reported as a poor prognostic factor [34,35]. Furthermore, the presence of a severe associated disorder (immunological disease or malignancy) is also considered as a poor prognostic factor in INCPH [35].

CONCLUSION

Idiopathic non-cirrhotic portal hypertension (INCPH) is one of the terms used to describe a rare vascular disorder of the liver. Although there are many causes, predisposing factors and clinicopathological features, the resulting portal hypertension is a cause of significant morbidity and mortality. It is important to ensure that cirrhosis has been excluded prior to diagnosing INCPH and to ensure that any underlying causes have been identified and treated if possible. Multiple radiological and biochemical tests of liver structure and function are performed since the differential diagnosis is wide, and there are many important and treatable conditions with similar features which must be excluded. Most patients can be managed with conservative medical, pharmacological, and endoscopic therapies. Surgery is rarely indicated in the absence of complications. Portal hypertension and portal venin thrombosis are serious long-term consequences of INCPH and may portend a poor prognosis and indication for liver transplantation.

Key points for clinical practice

- There is no universally accepted definition of INCPH
- Idiopathic non-cirrhotic portal hypertension is a rare vascular liver disease resulting in PHT with near-normal HVPG
- Idiopathic non-cirrhotic portal hypertension is more common in Asia, but can occur worldwide
- Although the aetiology is unknown, potential causes of INCPH include immunological disorders, chronic infections, exposure to medications or toxins, genetic disorders and prothrombotic conditions
- Clinical presentation may range from asymptomatic patients to those with florid presentation of PHT and complications such as PVT
- The diagnosis of INCPH is one of exclusion, and is based on clinical history, imaging, laboratory tests and liver biopsy
- The management aims at control of PHT and the management of PVT
- As liver function is well preserved in INCPH patients, the prognosis is better than that for cirrhotics with similar degrees of PHT

REFERENCES

1. Sarin SK, Kumar A, Chawla YK, et al. Noncirrhotic portal fibrosis/idiopathic portal hypertension: APASL recommendations for diagnosis and treatment. Hepatol Int 2007;1:398–413.
2. Khanna R, Sarin SK. Non-cirrhotic portal hypertension–diagnosis and management. J Hepatol 2014;60:421–441.
3. Schouten JN, Garcia-Pagan JC, Valla DC, et al. Idiopathic non-cirrhotic portal hypertension. Hepatology 2011; 54:1071–1081.
4. Guido M, Sarcognato S, Sacchi D, et al. Pathology of idiopathic non-cirrhotic portal hypertension. Virchows Arch 2018; 473:23–31.
5. Schouten JN, Verheij J, Seijo S. Idiopathic non-cirrhotic portal hypertension: a review. Orphanet J Rare Dis 2015; 10:67.
6. Dhiman RK, Chawla Y, Vasishta RK, et al. Non-cirrhotic portal fibrosis (idiopathic portal hypertension): experience with 151 patients and a review of the literature. J Gastroenterol Hepatol 2002; 17:6–16.
7. Mahamid J, Miselevich I, Attias D, et al. Nodular regenerative hyperplasia associated with idiopathic thrombocytopaenic purpura in a young girl: a case report and review of the literature. J Pad atr Gastroenterol Nutr 2005; 41:251–255.
8. Nakanuma Y, Hoso M, Sasaki M, et al. Histopathology of the liver in non-cirrhotic portal hypertension of unknown aetiology. Histopathology 1996; 28:195–204.
9. Naber AH, Van Haelst U, Yap SH. Nodular regenerative hyperplasia of the liver: an important cause of portal hypertension in non-cirrhotic patients. J Hepatol 1991; 12:94–99.

10. Dhawan PS, Shah SS, Alvares JF, et al. Seroprevalence of hepatitis A virus in Mumbai, and immunogenicity and safety of hepatitis A vaccine. Indian J Gastroenterol 1998; 17:16–18.
11. Mall ML, Rai RR, Philip M, et al. Seroepidemiology of hepatitis A infection in India: changing pattern. Ind J Gastroenterol 2001; 20:132–135.
12. Sarin SK, Kapoor D. Non-cirrhotic portal fibrosis: current concepts and management. J Gastroenterol Hepatol 2002; 17:526–534.
13. Okuda K. Non-cirrhotic portal hypertension versus idiopathic portal hypertension. J Gastroenterol Hepatol 2002; 17:S204–S213.
14. Sarin SK, Kumar A. Noncirrhotic portal hypertension. Clin Liver Dis 2006; 10:627–651.
15. Sato Y, Nakanuma Y. Role of endothelial-mesenchymal transition in idiopathic portal hypertension. Histol Histopathol 2013; 28:145–154.
16. Nakanuma Y, Sato Y, Kiktao A. Pathology and pathogenesis of portal venopathy in idiopathic portal hypertension: hints from systemic sclerosis. Hepatol Res 2009; 39:1023–1031.
17. Kitao A, Sato Y, Sawada-Kitamura S, et al. Endothelial to mesenchymal transition via transforming growth factor-beta1/Smad activation is associated with portal venous stenosis in idiopathic portal hypertension. Am J Pathol 2009; 175:616–626.
18. Tsuneyama K, Harada K, Katayanagi K, et al. Overlap of idiopathic portal hypertension and scleroderma: report of two autopsy cases and a review of literature. J Gastroenterol Hepatol 2002; 17:217–223.
19. Carreras LO, Defreyn G, Machin SJ, et al. Arterial thrombosis, intrauterine death and "lupus" antiocoagulant: detection of immunoglobulin interfering with prostacyclin formation. Lancet 1981; 1:244–246.
20. Sarin SK, Aggarwal SR. Idiopathic portal hypertension. Digestion 1998; 59:420–423.
21. Kono K, Ohnishi K, Omata M, et al. Experimental portal fibrosis produced by intraportal injection of killed nonpathogenic Escherichia coli in rabbits. Gastroenterology 1988; 94:787–796.
22. Chang PE, Miquel R, Blanco JL, et al. Idiopathic portal hypertension in patients with HIV infection treated with highly active antiretroviral therapy. Am J Gastroenterol 2009; 104:1707–1714.
23. Schouten JNL, Van der Ende ME, Koëter T, et al. Risk factors and outcome of HIV-associated idiopathic noncirrhotic portal hypertension. Aliment Pharmacol Ther 2012; 36:875–885.
24. Mallet V, Blanchard P, Verkarre V, et al. Nodular regenerative hyperplasia is a new cause of chronic liver disease in HIV-infected patients. AIDS 2007; 21:187–192.
25. Vispo E, Moreno A, Maida I, et al. Noncirrhotic portal hypertension in HIV-infected patients: unique clinical and pathological findings. AIDS 2010; 24:1171–1176.
26. Maida I, Garcia-Gasco P, Sotgiu G, et al. Antiretroviral-associated portal hypertension: a new clinical condition? Prevalence, predictors and outcome. Antivir Ther 2008; 13:103–107.
27. Vispo E, Cevik M, Rockstroh JK, et al. Genetic determinants of idiopathic noncirrhotic portal hypertension in HIV-infected patients. Clin Infect Dis 2013; 56:1117–1122.
28. Sarin SK, Mehra NK, Agarwal A, et al. Familial aggregation in non-cirrhotic portal fibrosis: a report of four families. Am J Gastroenterol 1987; 82:1130–1133.
29. Vilarinho S, Sari S, Yilmaz G, et al. Recurrent recessive mutation in deoxyguanosine kinase causes idiopathic non-cirrhotic portal hypertension. Hepatology 2016; 63:1977–1986.
30. Hillaire S, Bonte E, Denninger MH, et al. Idiopathic non-cirrhotic intrahepatic portal hypertension in the West: a re-evaluation in 28 patients. Gut 2002; 51:275–280.
31. Köksal AS, KöKlü S, Ibis M, et al. Clinical features, serum interleukin-6, and interferon-gamma levels of 34 Turkish patients with hepatoportal sclerosis. Dig Dis Sci 2007; 52:3493–3498.
32. Sarin SK. Non-cirrhotic portal fibrosis. J Gastroenterol Hepatol 2002; 17:S214–S223.
33. Okuda K, Kono K, Ohnishi K, et al. Clinical study of eighty-six cases of idiopathic portal hypertension and comparison with cirrhosis with splenomegaly. Gastroenterology 1984; 86:600–610.
34. Schouten JNL, Nevens F, Hansen B, et al. Idiopathic non-cirrhotic portal hypertension is associated with poor survival: results of a long-term cohort study. Aliment Pharmacol Ther 2012; 35:1424–1433.
35. Siramolpiwat S, Seijo S, Miquel R, et al. Idiopathic portal hypertension: natural history and long-term outcome. Hepatology 2014; 59:2276–2285.
36. Krasinskas AM, Eghtesad B, Kamath PS, et al. Liver transplantation for severe intrahepatic noncirrhotic portal hypertension. Liver Transpl 2005; 11:627–634.
37. De BK, Sen S, Sanyal R. Hepatopulmonary syndrome in non-cirrhotic portal hypertension. Ann Intern Med 2000; 132:924.
38. Friedrich-Rust M, Ong MF, Martens S, et al. Performance of transient elastography for the staging of liver fibrosis: a meta-analysis. Gastroenterology 2008; 134:960–974.
39. Mariappan YK, Glaser KJ, Ehman RL. Magnetic resonance elastography: a review. Clin Anat 2010; 23:497–511.

40. Zuo C, Chumbalkar V, Ells PF, et al. Prevalence of histological features of idiopathic noncirrhotic portal hypertension in general population: a retrospective study of incidental liver biopsies. Hepatol Int 2017; 11:452–460.
41. Verheij J, Schouten JNL, Komuta M, et al. Histological features in Western patients with idiopathic non-cirrhotic portal hypertension. Histopathology 2013; 62:1083–1091.
42. Nakanuma Y, Tsuneyama K, Ohbu M, et al. Pathology and pathogenesis of idiopathic portal hypertension with an emphasis on the liver. Pathol Res Pract 2001; 197:65–76.
43. Bioulac-Sage P, Le Bail B, Bernard PH, et al. Hepatoportal sclerosis. Semin Liver Dis 1995; 15:329–339.
44. Goel A, Ramakrishna B, Muliyil J, et al. Use of serum vitamin B12 level as a marker to differentiate idiopathic noncirrhotic intrahepatic portal hypertension from cryptogenic cirrhosis. Dig Dis Sci 2013; 58:179–187.
45. Okudaira M, Ohbu M, Okuda K. Idiopathic portal hypertension and its pathology. Semin Liver Dis 2002; 22:59–72.
46. Amarapurkar DN, Dhawan PS, Chopra K, et al. Stomach in portal hypertension. J Assoc Physicians India 1993; 41:638–640.
47. European Association for the Study of the Liver. EASL clinical practice guidelines: vascular diseases of the liver. J Hepatol 2016; 64:179–202.
48. De Franchis R, Baveno V Faculty. Revising consensus in portal hypertension: report of the Baveno V consensus workshop on methodology of diagnosis and therapy in portal hypertension. J Hepatol 2010; 53:762–768.
49. Sarin SK, Gupta N, Jha SK, et al. Equal efficacy of endoscopic variceal ligation and propranolol in preventing variceal bleeding in patients with non-cirrhotic portal hypertension. Gastroenterology 2010; 139:1238–1245.
50. Dagher L, Burroughs A. Variceal bleeding and portal hypertensive gastropathy. Eur J Gastroenterol Hepatol 2001; 13:81–88.
51. Sarin SK, Shastri HM, Jain M, et al. The natural history of portal hypertensive gastropathy. Influence of variceal eradication. Am J Gastroenterol 2000; 95:2888–2893.
52. Lv Y, Li K, He C, et al. TIPSS for variceal bleeding in patients with idiopathic noncirrhotic portal hypertension: comparison with patients who have cirrhosis. Aliment Pharmacol Ther 2019; 49:926–939.
53. Bissonnette J, Garcia-Pagán JC, Albillos A, et al. Role of the transjugular intrahepatic portosystemic shunt in the management of severe complications of portal hypertension in idiopathic non-cirrhotic portal hypertension. Hepatology 2016; 64:224–231.
54. Sarin SK, Agarwal SR. Extrahepatic portal vein obstruction. Semin Liver Dis 2002; 22:43–58.
55. Dumortier J, Bizollon T, Scoazec JY, et al. Orthotopic liver transplantation for idiopathic portal hypertension: indications and outcome. Scand J Gastroenterol 2001; 36:417–422.
56. Hernández-Gea V, Baiges A, Turon F, et al. Idiopathic portal hypertension. Hepatology 2018; 68:2413–2423.
57. De Franchis R, Baveno VI Faculty. Expanding consensus in portal hypertension: Report of the Baveno VI Consensus Workshop: Stratifying risk and individualizing care for portal hypertension. J Hepatol 2015; 63:743–752.

Chapter 15

Recent advances in complete mesocolic excision surgery for colon cancer

Marieke Rutgers, Afsana Elanko, Jim Khan

INTRODUCTION

The embryological planes that underpin total mesorectal excision (TME) surgery extend proximally to include the entire colon. A resection of the colon according to these principles is called complete mesocolic excision (CME). CME leaves the visceral mesocolic fascia intact to reduce the chances of tumour cell dissemination and central vascular ligation (CVL), where the supplying artery is ligated at its origin. While results of ongoing randomised controlled trials are still awaited, there is current evidence in Europe suggesting approximately 10% increase in survival and lower rates of 5-year local recurrence for stages I–III colorectal cancer (CRC) when this technique is adopted.

Complete mesocolic excision is a technically challenging surgical procedure with potential high morbidity that requires in depth anatomical knowledge and intensive training. This chapter summarises the concepts of CME, anatomical updates, surgical techniques, and evidence for CME surgery in colon cancer.

BACKGROUND

Colorectal cancer is the fourth most common cause of death from cancer, estimated to be responsible for almost 700,000 cancer deaths a year. CRC survival outcome depends on the stage at presentation. The 5-year survival rate for early CRC is 90% compared with 13% for those diagnosed at a late stage. Globally, it is one of the cancers where the incidence continues to rise and the number of cases of CRC is expected to increase by 60% over the next 15 years, which translates to > 2.2 million new cases per year [1].

Even though CRC is often described as a single entity there are significant differences in treatment and survival between colon and rectal cancer. Traditionally, patients with rectal cancer had a worse prognosis compared to patients with a colonic malignancy. However, after the introduction of TME in rectal cancer treatment, the prognosis for rectal cancer has strongly improved and addressed the imbalance [2].

Currently, in many developed counties, the long-term oncologic results are actually better for rectal cancer than for colon cancer. Some of the factors that have been responsible for the improved outcomes in rectal cancer surgery are better staging using magnetic resonance imaging (MRI) assessment, integrated multidisciplinary management, improvement in neoadjuvant treatment, and surgical techniques. However, the same cannot be said for the colon cancers due to late presentation, tumour biology, variation in surgical practice, and the lack of standardisation of therapy [3].

CURRENT TREATMENT OF COLON CANCER

The standard surgical treatment for colon cancer is hemicolectomy (right or left). The major issue with the conventional hemicolectomy technique is lack of standardisation of the procedure, resulting in variable quality of the resected specimen and the resection planes. Over the last 20 years the main debate has been regarding the mode of surgery – open versus laparoscopic, which has been the subject of several clinical trials [2,4,5]. More recently, the use of robotic methods to perform colectomy has been undertaken in developed countries by enthusiastic surgeons who report excellent outcomes [6,7]. However, whatever the advantages of different modes of access, all these approaches adopt the same resectional operation when removing the colon and the variability related to the mesenteric resection remains.

CONCEPT OF COMPLETE MESOCOLIC EXCISION

The concept that the mesocolon should remain intact is not new. In rectal surgery the concept of TME was popularised by Professor Heald in the 1980s [8], although the importance of resecting the rectal tumour with its surrounding vascular supply and lymphatic draining had been recognised in the early 20th century [9]. The mesorectal fascia is used as a guide for the correct plane for dissection for rectal resection, leading to significant improvements in outcomes over the last 30 years [10,11].

A similar concept can be applied to the colon. Understanding of mesenteric anatomy is not new and was described by Carl Toldt (known for the Toldt's fascia) who, in 1879, stated that:

> *"The human mesentery is a continuous anatomic structure from the duodenal-jejunal*
> *flexure to the mesorectum."*

Total mesorectal excision is based on the concept of the "mesorectum" as the rectal mesentery and the mesocolic fascia extend into the pelvis to envelope the mesorectum [12]. Likewise, the colonic mesentery within the protected planes contains the vascular and lymphatic drainage systems of the colon. The aim of resection is to remove all locally invasive and metastatic disease. This is achieved by dissecting all the lymphatic, vascular, and neural tissue in the drainage area of the tumour in a complete mesorectal or mesocolic envelope respectively, with intact mesentery, peritoneum and encasing fascia, thus maximising the lymph node yield.

SURGICAL ANATOMY OF THE MESOCOLON

The midgut, which runs from the sphincter of Oddi to the junction of the middle and distal thirds of the transverse colon, is supplied by the superior mesenteric artery (SMA). The hindgut runs from the distal thirds of the transverse colon to the dentate line and is supplied predominantly by the inferior mesenteric artery (IMA).

Arterial anatomy

The SMA branches to give off two or three major colonic arteries to the right:
- *Ileocolic artery (ICA)*: Is always present, but it comes from behind (posterior to) the superior mesenteric vein (SMV) in 63–79% of cases and in front of the SMV in the rest

- *Middle colic artery (MCA)*: Is divided into two branches (right and left). Anatomic variations of the MCA include complete absence in up to 25% of cases and the presence of an accessory (up to 10%) or double MCA
- *Right colic artery (RCA)*: Is present in up to 63.3% of cadavers. When present, it may not arise from the SMA, but may be a branch of the ileocolic or the MCA

The topography of the ICA and RCA in relation to the SMA is important for vascular ligation during surgery for right sided colon cancer. The ICA runs anterior to the SMV in 17–83% of specimens. The RCA, if present, crosses anteriorly in 63–100% of specimens.

The IMA originates from the ventral side of the abdominal aorta about 3.0–6.3 cm above the aortic bifurcation. The IMA gives off the following branches:

- *Left colic artery*: Which supplies most of the left colon
- *Sigmoid branches*: Between 2 and 6 in number. Sigmoid branches may also arise from the left colic artery or superior rectal artery
- *Superior rectal (haemorrhoidal) artery*: Which is the terminal branch of IMA

Venous anatomy

Venous drainage of the colon follows the arterial anatomy but is also highly variable. Venous blood from the caecum to the proximal transverse colon is directed to the SMV. Clinically, the venous anatomy of the right colic vein (RCV), superior RCV, gastrocolic trunk of Henle, and the middle colic vein (MCV) are of interest. Understanding of these anatomic variations may prevent inadvertent venous injury during CME, especially for right sided colon cancers.

- *The gastrocolic trunk of Henle*: Refers to the confluence of the right gastroepiploic vein, superior RCV, and anterior superior pancreaticoduodenal vein. A gastrocolic trunk is present in 46–70% of individuals. In order to do a radical venous resection the gastrocolic trunk may usually be spared, even with tumours in the transverse colon including those at the hepatic flexure
- *Right colic vein*: May drain into the SMV (56%) or into the gastrocolic trunk (44%)
- *Middle colic vein*: May enter the SMV directly in 84.5% of cases or may drain into the gastrocolic trunk [13]

On the left side the situation is simpler as the superior rectal vein continues as the inferior mesenteric vein (IMV) and drains into the portal vein (PV) with the sigmoid and left colic branches joining en route. Cancer surgeons need to be familiar with both standard vascular anatomy and its variations in order to perform safe CME surgery. There are frequent anatomic variations of the branching vessels from the SMA, SMV, IMA, and IMV.

Splanchnic nerves and lymphatics

It is generally accepted that lymph node metastases from primary colonic cancers follow the draining lymphatics along the course of the supplying arteries. The splanchnic nerves are paired autonomic nerves which supply the abdominal and pelvic viscera. They are composed of motor nerve fibres (visceral efferent fibres) passing to the internal organs, and the sensory nerve fibres (visceral afferent fibres) which originate from these organs. These nerves can be damaged during radical lymph node dissection leading to erratic bowel function postoperatively.

Surgical and pathological terminology related to complete mesocolic excision

As surgical and pathological techniques have developed in order to harvest and analyse a greater number of lymph nodes, so a number of new terms have entered the oncological lexicon which are important in describing CME techniques and obtaining accurate pathological staging and prognostic information.

- *D1 nodes:* Pericolic nodes (**Figure 15.1**)
- *D2 nodes*: Nodes along the trunks of named vessels (ileocolic, right colic, middle colic, superior mesenteric, left colic, inferior mesenteric, and sigmoidal arteries)
- *D3 nodes*: Central, apical or nodes along SMA, SMV, and aorta
- *Regional lymph nodes*: Pericolic lymph nodes and nodes along the trunks of named vessels (ileocolic, right colic, middle colic, superior mesenteric, left colic, inferior mesenteric, and sigmoidal arteries).
- *High tie*: Central ligation of the feeding vessels immediately at their origins from the SMA and SMV (or IMA and IMV), with the resulting maximal distance of the apical lymph node from the primary tumour
- *Isolated tumour cells*: Isolated tumour cells or clusters too small (<0.2 mm) to be identified as metastatic lymph nodes
- *Micrometastasis*: Tumour deposits (<2 mm) identified within lymph nodes with special staining methods
- *Skip metastases*: Metastasis in the D3 area (central or main nodes) without metastasis close to the tumour (D1 area (pericolic)

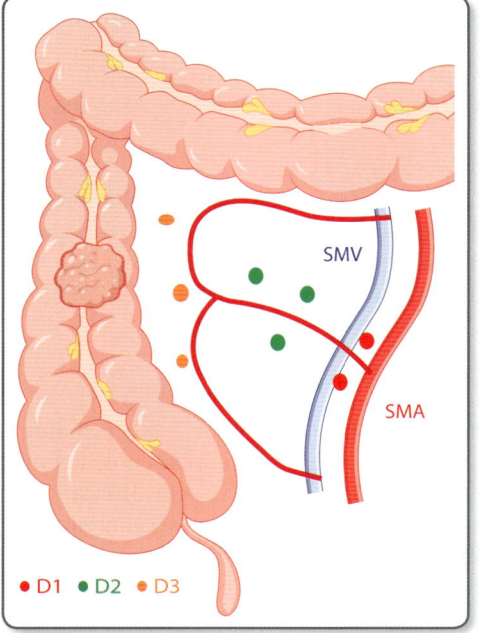

Figure 15.1 Levels of central radicality for right-sided colon cancer.
(SMV, superior mesenteric vein; SMA, superior mesenteric artery)

A good quality CME specimen should have an intact mesocolon on both sides, no defect in the mesentery. The pathologist should be able to measure the distances as shown in **Figure 15.2**.

According to both European CME principles and Japanese guidelines, the lymph nodes around the root of the feeding artery (SMA), the main nodes, should be dissected and removed at the same time as the specimen, but there is a danger of damaging the splanchnic nerves by doing so.

Requirement for complete mesocolic excision

the ultimate goal of attempted curative surgical cancer treatment is to remove the tumour with all potential metastatic spread. For most carcinomas this includes the primary cancer plus the draining lymph nodes and lymphatic vessels. As early as 1908, the famous surgeon Moynihan stated that:

'The surgery of malignant disease is not the surgery of organs.
It is the anatomy of the lymphatic system.'

In order to achieve radical clearance in colon cancer treatment a central zone of nodes should be resected and the resection margins should be oncologically negative. However, the exact magnitude of the margins and lymph node drainage area that is required to be removed in colon cancer is still unclear. Thus, many surgeons divide the mesentery and colon where it is anatomically convenient, usually at the mid-mesenteric or intermediate level. However, up to 25% of patients with stages I and II CRC, who have undergone apparently 'curative surgery' ultimately die as a result of recurrent or metastatic disease. Therefore, it is tempting to assume that a more radical primary resection, with a more extensive lymph node harvest is likely to result in improved oncological outcomes and longer-term survival. It has been hoped that improvements in rectal cancer survival and

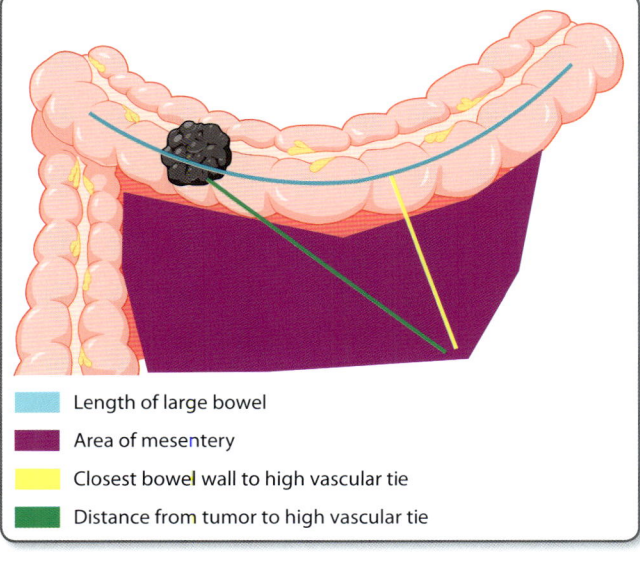

Figure 15.2 Measurements pathologic specimen right-sided complete mesocolic excision (CME).

Length of large bowel

Area of mesentery

Closest bowel wall to high vascular tie

Distance from tumor to high vascular tie

outcome which have occurred since widespread practice of TME [8,10,13–15] could be translated into improvements in outcomes for colonic cancer by performance of CME as the standard of care for colon cancer resection.

PRINCIPLES OF COMPLETE MESOCOLIC EXCISION

In 2009, the Hohenberger group from Germany were among the first, in recent years, to describe CME in order to try to translate the survival advantages of TME to patients with colon cancer [16]. There are three main components to CME:

1. Dissection in the embryological plane (Toldt's space or mesocolic fascia) – which is between the mesenteric plane and parietal fascia, to remove a complete envelope containing the mesenteric fascia and visceral peritoneum together with all draining lymph
2. A CVL – to remove the lymph nodes in the central (vertical) direction. A central division of the feeding arteries at their origins from the SMA is performed for tumours of the right colon and at the origin of the IMA for tumours of the left colon
3. Resection of a sufficient length of bowel to remove the involved pericolic lymph nodes in the longitudinal direction [3,14,15].

This results in a colonic specimen which is larger than that obtained by conventional surgery. The distance from the CVL to the tumour is also longer, integrity of the mesocolon is preserved and the number of retrieved lymph nodes is higher [2,13,17–19].

Over the last decade multiple clinical studies have been done which have looked at the benefits of CME compared to conventional surgery with respect to both patient outcomes and surrogate endpoints such as lymph node harvest. These are summarised in **Table 15.1**.

Preoperative planning

As mentioned above, a comprehensive understanding of the vascular anatomy is essential for successful CME, particularly in the light of the frequency of high anatomical variations. While performing open CME surgery, a surgeon can follow the vasculature alongside SMA and SMV after Kocherizing the duodenum. In minimal invasive surgery this is less easy to achieve. Therefore, a computed tomography (CT) scan with arterial and venous reconstruction is useful for preoperative planning. Arterial and venous phase CT is essential in order to delineate the arterial and venous anatomy respectively. The key questions that these preoperative planning scans can help to clarify are:

- The relation of the ICA to the SMV
- The presence of absence of a RCA
- The length of the MCA
- The presence (or not) of any accessory vessels
- The configuration of Henle's trunk.

The main lymph nodes are located on the ventral side of the SMV and the lymphatic channels run through anteriorly towards the SMA. If the ICA courses behind the SMV, high ligation at the root of the SMA may increase nodal gain. However, as with the arterial and venous anatomy, unusual patterns of lymphatic spread may occur in some cases of colon cancer. Aberrant vessels may connect the hepatic flexure with the sub-pyloric area and there may be lymphatic channels at the posterior of the omentum, which link the greater curvature to the fused colonic mesenteric and omental fascia. Hepatic flexure, sub-pyloric and gastroepiploic locations of lymph node metastases may justify extensive resections in some cases where there are aberrant vessels from the hepatic flexure to the gastroduodenal or gastroepiploic arteries.

Table 15.1 Complete mesocolic excision (CME) studies: Patient populations and outcomes

Lead author	Country	Study type	Number of cases	Right/Left/All	Local recurrence	Overall survival	Disease-free survival	Lymph node harvest (mean)	Follow-up
West [20]	UK	Pathological assessment mesocolic plane	399	All	-	+ 15%, HR 0.57	-	-	5 years
Hohenberger [1]	Germany	Observational	1329	All	3.6%	-	89.1%	32	4 years
Bokey [21]	Australia	Observational	867	All	2.1%	63.7%	76.6%	-	5 years
Storli [22]	Norway	Case control, open versus lap CME	251 (123/128)	All	13%/14.1%	84.5% (80.4%/88.2%)	74.8%/80.0%	12+ (17.5/15.8)	3 years
Olofsson [23]	Sweden	Population	2084	Right	4.0%	79.4%	73.8%	19	3 years
Kotake [24]	Japan	Retrospective, pT3/pT4	3425	All	-	HR 0.814	-	21.8	3 years
Bertelsen [25]	Denmark	Case-control	364	All	11.3	74.9%	85.8%	36.5	4 years
Siani [26]	Finland	Cohort, retrospective	115	Right	-	82.6%	73.8%	31	5years
Kitano [27]	Japan	RCT, cT3/cT4, open versus lap D3	1057	All	-	90.8%/91.8%	80%/79%	22/21	5 years
Karachun [28]	Russia	RCT, D2 versus D3	92	All	-	-	-	27.8	30 days

(RCT: randomised controlled trial)

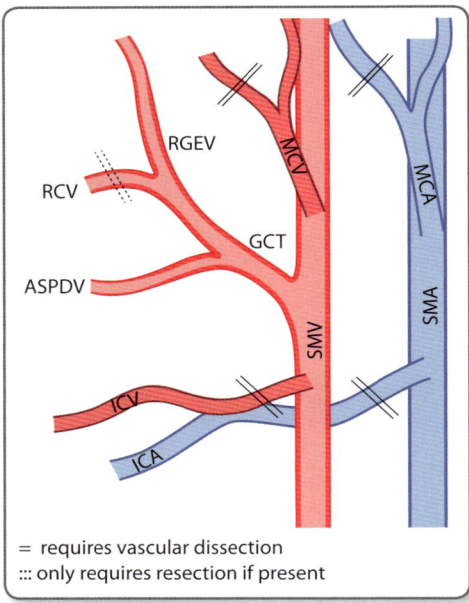

Figure 15.3 Schematic representation of the arterial and venous supply of right colon.
(RCV, right colic vein; RGEV, right gastroepiploic vein; MCV, middle colic vein; ICV, ileocolic vein; SMV, superior mesenteric vein; SMA, superior mesenteric artery; GCT, gastrocolic trunk; ICA, ileocolic artery; MCA, middle colic artery; ASPDV, anterior superior pancreaticoduodenal vein)

= requires vascular dissection
::: only requires resection if present

Standard right hemicolectomy is limited to mesocolic excision for caecal and proximal ascending colon cancers by ligating the right branches of the MCA and MCV and by taking the ileocolic vessels from their origin at the SMV. For hepatic flexure and proximal (15 cm) transverse colon cancers, extended right hemicolectomy is performed and the roots of the MCA and MCV are ligated from the SMV. This extended procedure is performed due to additional channels for lymphatic tumour spread in this region. The gastrocolic truck of Henle, with its inflow from the pancreatic head, is preserved in both standard and extended procedures, unless adjacent lymph nodes are present which can only be removed by sacrificing the trunk for oncological reasons (**Figure 15.3**).

OPERATIVE TECHNIQUE: COMPLETE MESOCOLIC EXCISION WITH CENTRAL VASCULAR LIGATION FOR RIGHT-SIDED COLONIC CANCER

In conventional open surgery, the surgeon Kocherizes the duodenum and performs lateral to medial mobilisation of the right colon and its mesentery, followed by central ligation of feeding vessels. With the uptake of minimal access surgery (MIS) there has been a focus on achieving CME by either laparoscopic or robotic techniques.

Two common approaches for MIS CME are: (1) the SMV approach, and (2) the sub-ileal approach.

Superior mesenteric vein first approach

This approach involves surgical dissection of SMV pedicle as the first stage of the procedure, rather than dissecting the ileocolic pedicle after colonic mobilisation as in a

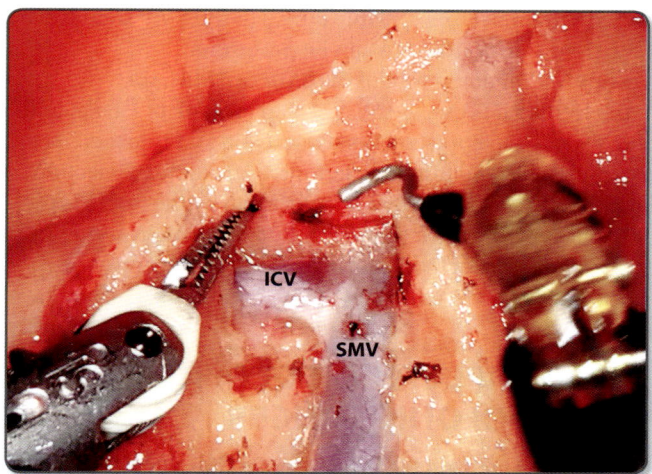

Figure 15.4 Intraoperative view of ileocolic vein (ICV) and superior mesenteric vein (SMV).

standard right colectomy. Early exposure of the SMV is followed by dissection vertically along the superior mesenteric vessels ligating ileocolic, right colic, and middle colic pedicles at their origin (**Figure 15.4**). Dissection continues over the SMV cranially to identify the middle colic trunk and its division into right and left branches as for a standard right colectomy. The right branch of the MCA is divided between clips. The gastrocolic trunk of Henle can be seen over the pancreas, although it may have significant anatomical variations. Careful identification and ligation of the RCV and preservation of pancreaticoduodenal veins, gastroepiploic vein and Henle trunk is required. After the CVL, medial to lateral dissection is then performed to separate the colonic mesentery from Gerota's fascia, duodenum and pancreas. Cranially, this plane is continued to gain entry into the lesser sac. Lateral peritoneal detachment is carried out up to the hepatic flexure. The gastrocolic omentum is divided starting from the level of the falciform ligament and staying outside the gastroepiploic arcade. Colonic and small bowel mesentery is divided up to the intended point of transection. Intra-corporeal division is done with the help of a 60-mm stapler. Side to side isoperistaltic ileocolic anastomosis can be performed with a 60-mm stapler. Two stay stitches are placed, one on either end of the bowel, to facilitate this step. The common enterotomy (stapler ends) is closed by the surgeon's method of choice, for example with two-layer Vicryl 3/0 suture. The specimen is extracted through a suprapubic Pfannenstiel incision, using an appropriate wound protector.

Sub-ileal approach

The terminal ileum and the ascending colon are dissected along the embryological plane. Dissection between the mesocolon and Gerota's fascia continues to the duodenum and head of the pancreas. Once the ileocolic vessels are identified, the mesocolic package containing lymph nodes is cleared along the vessels while exposing the ventral side of the SMV and SMA.

If the ICA runs anterior to the SMV, it is divided close to its origin at the SMA. If the ICA crosses dorsal to the SMV, its division is performed at the level of the right border of the SMV. Using this approach, the SMA often becomes visible dorsal to the SMV so that a complete lymphadenectomy on the right side of the SMA can be performed.

After ligation of the ileocolic vessels (either at the root of the SMV or SMA), the dissection continues cephalad to the right colic vessels, the gastrocolic trunk of Henle, and the middle colic vessels. The right colic vessel, if present, is skeletonised and transected at its root. The gastrocolic trunk has a number of anatomic variations, and careful dissection is necessary to avoid unwanted vascular injury. Unless there is infiltration by the tumour, the anterior superior pancreaticoduodenal vein and right gastroepiploic vein are preserved, and only the RCV and/or superior RCV are transected. Then, the middle colic vessels are identified and skeletonised at the roots of the SMA and SMV.

OPERATIVE TECHNIQUE: COMPLETE MESOCOLIC EXCISION FOR LEFT-SIDED COLONIC CANCER

The left-sided CME procedure is initiated by incising the medial side of the sigmoid mesocolon at the level of the sacral promontory and medial to lateral mobilisation is continued through the avascular plane. With adequate traction, the IMA is lifted up and skeletonised with caution. The goal is not to damage the superior hypogastric plexus around the aortic bifurcation. After complete clearance of lymph nodes around the root of the IMA, the left colic artery or IMA is ligated at their origin depending on the type of procedure planned (left hemicolectomy or anterior resection respectively).

The ureter and gonadal vessels are identified and preserved with further medial to lateral dissection. The IMV is lifted up and dissected cephalad to the ligament of Treitz and ligated at the lower border of the pancreas. The retroperitoneal space is developed between the mesocolon and Gerota's fascia. The root of the transverse mesocolon is freed from the lower border of the pancreas and the lesser sac is entered by dissection along the ventral side of the pancreas. After completing medial colonic mobilisation, the left lateral paracolic attachments are divided.

Dissection continues to the lower pole of the spleen and the splenocolic ligament is dissected. Omentectomy is performed just below the gastroepiploic vessels and, unless infiltrated by the tumour, left gastroepiploic vessels are preserved. The embryologic adhesion is cleared between the stomach and the transverse mesocolon and the lesser sac is identified. Continued dissection to the dorsal and lateral aspects joins the previously dissected surgical planes.

Choice of technique

There are two aspects to the choice of surgical technique which can be used for colonic cancer resection.

Firstly, is the choice of method of access. An extensive discussion of the pros and cons of open versus laparoscopic versus robotic access for colectomy is outside the scope of this chapter and readers are referred to the chapter by Siddila and Siddiqui in a previous edition of this book [29].

With respect to CME, open surgery is traditionally performed since MIS CME is a technically demanding procedure and requires a steep learning curve. Robot-assisted CME is potentially easier to master than laparoscopic CME and intra-corporeal anastomosis but is more expensive. The stability of the operating platform, the 3D operating view and the dexterity achieved with endowrist instruments makes the robotic approach very attractive.

Studies which compare open with laparoscopic CME surgery have shown that laparoscopic CME has a longer operative time, comparable complication rates and earlier recovery compared to the open CME group with similar overall survival and disease-free survival rates [6,22].

There are few studies available comparing the robotic CME with other techniques. The studies that do compare robotic CME with another technique show comparable results, with longer operating times and higher costs involved [7,30,31].

Secondly, the surgeon must choose between operative CME techniques for right-sided tumours. The SMV first and sub-ileal approaches are described earlier and individual surgeons will prefer one technique having considered the salient points of each procedure.

Complications of complete mesocolic excision

Because the procedure is more complex than traditional hemicolectomy, there is an increased risk of severe complications. This may be one of the reasons why the uptake of CME has been relatively slow.

Bleeding

The most common reason for intraoperative bleeding in CME for right sided colon cancer is injury to the gastrocolic trunk, SMV or central vessels. Some possible mechanisms of SMV injury include anatomic variations and avulsion of the MCV due to excessive traction. For left sided CME, bleeding may occur due to avulsion/traction injury to the IMV. High ligation of the IMA at the aorta may cause bleeding if the vessel is not controlled adequately.

Nerve damage

The coeliac nerve plexus surrounds the SMA and may be damaged by CVL, with the potential risk of refractory postoperative diarrhoea. The SMA is also surrounded by the superior mesenteric nerve plexus, which is a continuation of the coeliac nerve plexus and ganglions. It has been suggested that central lymph node dissection in CME could injure the plexus, which might increase the risk of neurogenic diarrhoea with subsequent worsening of quality of life (QOL) [22].

Chyle leak

More extensive lymphadenectomy increases the risk of chyle leakage. Bae et al reported that chyle leakage occurred less frequently in patients undergoing laparoscopic, rather than open, CME. They attributed this difference to the use of an ultrasound scalpel or vessel-sealing device for perivascular lymph node dissection and a magnified view provided by laparoscopy [31].

Geographical differences in techniques of complete mesocolic excision surgery

Although, the purpose of CME surgery is the same worldwide, some technical aspects and terminology vary, particularly between Western and Japanese practice. The CME with CVL, as we know it in the Western world, is comparable with the D3 lymphadenectomy as practiced in Japan. D3 or high tie or central lymph node dissection in Japan is recommended for clinical stage T3-4 or pN1-2 tumours, but the root of the IMA may be preserved in some left-sided tumours. A D2 resection or standard low tie is recommended for early stage tumours. The key principle, according to Japanese guidelines, is to resect 5 cm beyond the feeding arterial vessel in the direction of lymph flow and 10 cm away from the tumour in the opposite direction. This 10 cm-rule is based on Japanese studies [2,16,32,25] which have shown that longitudinal spread greater than 10 cm beyond the tumour is extremely rare, at 1–4% for right sided tumours and 0% for left-sided tumours.

FUTURE STUDIES AND TRIALS

Although, the trails listed in **Table 15.1** showed promising results, it has not yet been possible to prove that CME surgery has better long-term oncological outcomes than conventional colonic resection. Therefore, there are numerous trials (both observational and randomised) in progress at the time of writing. These are shown in **Table 15.2**.

CONCLUSION

The removal of the complete mesocolic envelope around a colonic cancer is an important part of colorectal cancer surgery. CME has become more popular as a surgical technique since the importance of an adequate clearance of the vascular supply and lymphatic drainage of a tumour has been recognised both as a marker of surgical quality and as an aid to improved prognosis. It is essential to understand the anatomy and embryology of the colon and its blood supply before embarking on CME operations. Open, laparoscopic and robotic approaches to CME have all been reported and there are on going trials as to the exact indications and considerations for each method. There are variations in surgical technique for operations on the right colon and individual surgeons will usually settle on one method in the light of their own training, experience, and preference. Because of the more extensive nature of CME surgery, there are risks of collateral damage to surrounding structures, particularly blood vessels and nerves. It is important for surgeons to monitor and record the technical and longer term oncological outcomes of CME surgery, either within local databases or within clinical trials where appropriate.

Key points for clinical practice

- A detailed knowledge of the anatomy of the colon along with its blood supply and lymphatic drainage is required before embarking on CME
- Meticulous preoperative planning and surgical technique are essential for good outcomes from CME surgery
- Complete mesocolic excision surgery generates a large colonic resection specimen with increased lymph node harvest compared to conventional surgery
- Clinical studies have reported improved oncological outcomes (reduced local recurrence and improved survival) after CME surgery but robust clinical trials are required in order to demonstrate improved long-term survival

Table 15.2 Current trials on complete mesocolic excision (CME)

Name trial	Country	Study type	Recruitment target	Aim study	Inclusion	Primary end point	Reference number
D3/CME	Norway	RCT, 2 centres	218	Open D3 right colectomy vs Lap CME	Right-sided colon cancer	2 and 5 years survival	NCT03776591
5 years oncological outcome after CME for sigmoid colon cancer	Denmark	Observational, population	920	CME	Sigmoid cancer	5 years survival	NCT03774134
5 years oncological outcome after CME for right-sided colon cancer	Denmark	Observational, population	1069	CME	Right-sided colon cancer	5 years survival	NCT03754075
SLRC	China	RCT	582	CME (with D2) vs Right hemi (with D3)	Right-sided colon cancer	3 years survival	NCT02942238
DILEMMA	Russia	RCT	1381	D2 vs D3	Left-sided colon cancer	5 years survival	NCT04364373
RELARC	China	RCT	1072	CME vs D2	Right-sided colon cancer	3 years survival	NCT02619942
A novel technique of HALS with CME and CVL for RCC	China	RCT	60	HALS* CME vs conventional Lap CME	Right-sided colon cancer	3 years survival	NCT02625272
T-Rex	Japan	Observational	4000	Distribution metastasis lymph nodes	Colon cancer	Distribution metastases lymph nodes	NCT02938481
RICON	Russia	RCT	239	D2 vs D3	Right-sided colon cancer	5 years survival	NCT03200834
OLCMECC	China	RCT	1080	Open versus Lap CME	Locally advanced colon cancer	5 years survival	NCT02682589
LCME	China	RCT	99	Lap CME versus D3 lap colectomy	Colon cancer	Lymph nodes yield	NCT01628250

(HALS: hand-assisted laparoscopic surgery; RCT: randomised controlled trial; CME: complete mesocolic excision; CVL: central vascular ligation; LCME: laparoscopic complete mesocolic excision; SLRC: superior laparoscopic right hemicolectomy; OLCMECC: open versus laparoscopic complete mesocolic excision for locally advanced colon cancer; RICON: right colon cancer; RELARC: radical extent of lympadenectomy; D2 dissection versus complete mesocolic excision of laparoscopic right colectomy for right-sided colon cancer)

REFERENCES

1. World Cancer Research Fund. Colorectal cancer statistics: Colorectal cancer is the third most common cancer worldwide. [online] Available from https://www.wcrf.org/dietandcancer/cancer-trends/colorectal-cancer-statistics. [Last Accessed December, 2020].
2. West NP, Kobayashi H, Takahashi K, et al. Understanding optimal colonic cancer surgery: comparison of Japanese D3 resection and European complete mesocolic excision with central vascular ligation. J Clin Oncol 2012; 30:1763–1769.
3. SEER. Stat Statistical Software (Cancer). [online] Available from www.seer.cancer/gov/seerstat. [Last Accessed December, 2020].
4. Van der Pas MH, Haglind E, Cuesta MA, et al. Laparoscopic versus open surgery for rectal cancer (COLR II): short-term outcomes of a randomised, phase 3 trial. Lancet Oncol 2013; 14:210–218.
5. Guillou PJ, Quirke P, Thorpe H, et al. MRC CLASICC trial group. Short-term endpoints of conventional versus laparoscopic-assisted surgery in patients with colorectal cancer (MRC CLASICC trial): multicentre, randomised controlled trial. Lancet 2005; 365:1718–1726.
6. Spinoglio G, Bianchi PP, Marano A, et al. Robotic Versus Laparoscopic Right Colectomy with Complete Mesocolic Excision for the Treatment of Colon Cancer: Perioperative Outcomes and 5-Year Survival in a Consecutive Series of 202 Patients. Ann Surg Oncol 2018; 25:3580–3586.
7. Ozben V, Aytac E, Atasoy D, et al. Totally robotic complete mesocolic excision for right-sided colon cancer. J Robot Surg 2019; 13:107–114.
8. Heald RJ, Ryall RD. Recurrence and survival after total mesorectal excision for rectal cancer. Lancet 1986; 1:1479–1482.
9. Miles WE. A method of performing abdomino-perineal excision for carcinoma of the rectum and of the terminal portion of the pelvic colon (1908). CA Cancer J Clin 1971; 21:361–364.
10. Wibe A, Møller B, Norstein J, et al. A national strategic change in treatment policy for rectal cancer—implementation of total mesorectal excision as routine treatment in Norway. A national audit. Dis Colon Rectum 2002; 45:857–866.
11. Glimelius B, Beets-Tan R, Blomqvist L, et al. Mesorectal fascia instead of circumferential resection margin in preoperative staging of rectal cancer. J Clin Oncol 2011; 29:2142–2143.
12. Vather R, Sammour T, Kahokehr A, et al. Lymph node evaluation and long-term survival in Stage II and Stage III colon cancer: a national study. Ann Surg Oncol 2009; 16:585–593.
13. Kapiteijn E, Putter H, van de Velde CJ. Impact of the introduction and training of total mesorectal excision on recurrence and survival in rectal cancer in the Netherlands. Br J Surg 2002; 89:1142–1149.
14. Emmanuel A, Haji A. Complete mesocolic excision and extended (D3) lymphadenectomy for colonic cancer: is it worth that extra effort? A review of the literature. Int J Colorectal Dis 2016; 31:797–804.
15. Ueno H, Sugihara K. Japanese D3 Dissection. In: Kim N, Sugihara K, Liang JT, (Eds) Surgical Treatment of Colorectal Cancer. Singapore: Springer 2018. pp. 259–266.
16. Hohenberger W, Weber K, Matzel KT, et al. Standardized surgery for colonic cancer: complete mesocolic excision and central ligation--technical notes and outcome. Colorectal Dis 2009; 11:354–364.
17. Strey CW, Wullstein C, Adamina M, et al. Laparoscopic right hemicolectomy with CME: standardization using the "critical view" concept. Surg Endosc 2018; 32:5021–5030.
18. Benz S, Tannapfel A, Tam Y, et al. Proposal of a new classification system for complete mesocolic excison in right-sided colon cancer. Tech Coloproctol 2019; 23:251–257.
19. Søndenaa K, Quirke P, Hohenberger W, et al. The rationale behind complete mesocolic excision (CME) and a central vascular ligation for colon cancer in open and laparoscopic surgery: proceedings of a consensus conference. Int J Colorectal Dis 2014; 29:419–428.
20. West NP, Morris EJ, Rotimi O, et al. Pathology grading of colon cancer surgical resection and its association with survival: a retrospective observational study. Lancet Oncol 2008; 9:857–865.
21. Bokey EL, Chapuis PH, Dent OF, et al. Surgical technique and survival in patients having a curative resection for colon cancer. Dis Colon Rectum 2003; 46:860–866.
22. Storli KE, Søndenaa K, Furnes B, et al. Outcome after introduction of complete mesocolic excision for colon cancer is similar for open and laparoscopic surgical treatments. Dig Surg 2013; 30:317–327.
23. Olofsson F, Buchwald P, Elmståhl S, et al. No benefit of extended mesenteric resection with central vascular ligation in right-sided colon cancer. Colorectal Dis 2016; 18:773–778.
24. Kotake K, Mizuguchi T, Moritani K, et al. Impact of D3 lymph node dissection on survival for patients with T3 and T4 colon cancer. Int J Colorectal Dis 2014; 29:847–852.

25. Bertelsen CA, Neuenschwander AU, Jansen JE, et al. Short-term outcomes after complete mesocolic excision compared with 'conventional' colonic cancer surgery. Br J Surg 2016; 103:581–589.
26. Siani LM, Pulica C. Laparoscopic complete mesocolic excision with central vascular ligation in right colon cancer: Long-term oncologic outcome between mesocolic and non-mesocolic planes of surgery. Scand J Surg 2015; 104:219–226.
27. Kitano S, Inomata M, Mizusawa J, et al. "Survival outcomes following laparoscopic versus open D3 dissection for stage II or III colon cancer (JCOG0404): a phase 3, randomised controlled trial. Lancet Gastroenterol Hepatol 2017; 2:261–268.
28. Karachun A, Panaiotti L, Chernikovskiy I, et al. Short-term outcomes of a multicentre randomized clinical trial comparing D2 versus D3 lymph node dissection for colonic cancer (COLD trial). Br J Surg 2020; 107:499–508.
29. Siddila A, Siddiqui S. The use of Robotics in Colorectal Surgery. In: Taylor I (Ed). Recent Advances in Surgery 37. New Delhi: Jaypee Brothers Medical Publishers (P) Ltd.; 2015. pp. 120–125.
30. Yozgatli TK, Aytac E, Ozben V, et al. Robotic Complete Mesocolic Excision Versus Conventional Laparoscopic Hemicolectomy for Right-Sided Colon Cancer. J Laparoendosc Adv Surg Tech A 2019; 29:671–676.
31. Bae SU, Saklani AP, Lim DR, et al. Laparoscopic-assisted versus open complete mesocolic excision and central vascular ligation for right-sided colon cancer. Ann Surg Oncol 2014; 21:2288–2294.
32. Kim NK, Kim YW, Han YD, et al. Complete mesocolic excision and central vascular ligation for colon cancer: Principle, anatomy, surgical technique, and outcomes. Surg Oncol 2016; 25:252–262.

Section 8

Clinical trials

Chapter 16

Major randomized controlled trials in surgery in the last five years

Akriti Nanda

INTRODUCTION

The performance of high-quality randomised controlled trials (RCTs) within the field of surgery has historically posed its own unique difficulties compared to medicine [1] resulting in the field of surgical research filled with studies at high risk of bias (e.g. retrospective reviews and case series). RCTs remain the gold standard of evidence-based medicine; therefore, in recent years, investigators have adapted RCT methodology to the field of surgery. With new precedents and guidance in the last 5 years, there has been a rapid increase in the number of large multicenter RCTs in surgery. In this chapter, RCTs influencing general surgical practice over the last 5 years are reviewed.

GENERAL SURGERY

Appendicitis

The long-term outcomes of antibiotics for appendicitis were evaluated in this 5-year follow-up paper of the APPAC (Appendicitis Acuta) trial [2] in Finland. Around 530 adults with computed tomography (CT)-confirmed uncomplicated acute appendicitis were randomised to either receive antibiotic therapy (n = 257) or appendectomy (n = 273). About 70/256 patients who initially received antibiotics underwent appendectomy within the 1st year [27.3% (95% CI 22.0–33.2)] and another 30/186 additional antibiotic-treated patients [16.1% (95% CI 11.2–22.2)] underwent appendectomy between 1 and 5 years. Of the 85 patients in the antibiotic group that underwent appendectomy, only two had complicated appendicitis. At 5 years, the complication rate [surgical site infections (SSIs), incisional hernias, abdominal pain, and obstructive symptoms] was 24.4% [(95% CI 19.2–30.3) (n = 60/246)] in the appendectomy group and 6.5% [(95% CI 3.8–10.4) (n = 16/246)] in antibiotic group (p < 0.001). There was no difference between groups for length of hospital stay, but there was a significant increase of 11 days in sick leave for the surgery group. Most appendectomies were open, the complication rate and hospital stay may have been lower with the standard laparoscopic approach. The authors write favourably about the success of antibiotics as initial treatment, but the chosen ones used were ertapenem, levofloxacin, and metronidazole and may be considered excessive and risk unintended antibiotic resistance. This long-term follow-up shows that the likelihood of recurrence decreases over time but over one-third of those treated with antibiotics will have recurrent appendicitis within 5 years.

Hernia

The hernia operation is one of the oldest in a general surgeon's repertoire. In recent years, RCTs have focussed on robotic-assisted minimally invasive techniques and the use of various mesh types. The impact of robotic compared to laparoscopic repair for ventral hernias on days in hospital was assessed in a multicenter, blinded RCT in hernia clinics in Houston, USA [3]. Adults with a ventral hernia defect < 12 cm deemed appropriate for elective minimally invasive hernia repair were randomised to either robotic ventral hernia repair (n = 65) versus laparoscopic ventral hernia repair (n = 59). There was no difference in days in hospital within 90 days postsurgery between the two groups (median 0 in both; RR 0.90; 95% CI 0.37–2.19; p = 0.82) nor in emergency department visits, wound complications, hernia recurrence, or reoperation. The only significant outcome found was that robotic repair had a longer operative duration [141 vs. 77 min; mean difference 62.89 (45.75–80.01); p ≤ 0.001] and increased healthcare costs [$15,865 vs. $12,955; cost ratio 1.21 (1.07–1.38); p = 0.004]. Two patients with robotic ventral hernia repair had an enterotomy compared with zero in laparoscopic repair–the study is not adequately powered to find significance in this. This first of its kind RCT, shows robotic ventral hernia repair confers no benefit but incurs operating room time and cost. Applicability to repairs of larger sized hernias, with placement of mesh in spaces other than intra-peritoneally (e.g. preperitoneal or retro-rectus) or by nonexpert surgeons is limited and further research into this is needed before adoption of the robotic technique.

The impact of mesh compared to suture repair for umbilical hernias was explored in a double-blind RCT in 12 hospitals across Europe [4]. Around 300 adults with primary umbilical hernias of 1–4 cm were randomised equally to either suture or mesh repair by surgeons trained in standardised techniques for both approaches. The primary outcome of hernia recurrence (assessed by physical examination and/or ultrasound at 2 months) was significantly less in the mesh than in the suture group [6/146 (4%) vs. 17/138 (12%); hazard ratio (HR) 0·31; 95% CI 0·12–0·80; p = 0·01]–giving a number needed to treat of 12.8. Differences in other common postoperative complications like seroma [1 (< 1%) in the suture group vs. 5 (3%) in the mesh group], haematoma [2 (1%) vs. 3 (2%)], and wound infection [1 (< 1%) vs. 3 (2%)] were similar. This RCT supports the use of mesh repair for small umbilical hernias.

The effectiveness and placement of mesh reinforcement to prevent incisional hernias in high-risk patients was evaluated in PRIMA [5]–a double-blind RCT in 11 hospitals across Austria, Germany, and the Netherlands. About 480 adults undergoing an elective midline laparotomy for an abdominal aortic aneurysm (AAA) repair or had a body mass index (BMI) > 27 kg/m^2 were randomised to closure with primary suture (n = 107); onlay mesh (n = 188), or sublay mesh (n = 185) reinforcement. The primary outcome of incisional hernia after 2 years was significantly less in both mesh groups. There were 33 (30%) with primary suture, 25 (13%) with onlay mesh reinforcement, and 34 (18%) with sublay mesh reinforcement (onlay vs. suture; OR 0.37; 95% CI 0.20–0.69; p = 0.0016 and sublay vs. suture; OR, 0.55; 95% CI 0.30–1.00; p = 0.05). Seromas were more frequent in patients with the onlay mesh versus primary suture and sublay mesh (18% vs. 7% vs. 7%; p = 0.002) though the study is not powered to determine this. The incidence of wound infection did not differ between groups (13% primary suture; 13% onlay mesh reinforcement; 10% sublay mesh reinforcement) though follow-up of 2 years is short to assess complications like chronic infection and fistula formation. The authors conclude that due to a significant reduction in incidence of incisional hernia with onlay mesh reinforcement should be the standard treatment to prevent incisional hernias for high-risk patients undergoing midline laparotomy but critics of the conclusion argue initial mesh use will make subsequent hernia repairs more complex. Further support for mesh use was found in the study of stoma site closures in the ROCSS (Reinforcement of Closure of Stoma Site) trial [6] across seven hospitals in three European countries (35 UK, 1 Denmark, 1 Netherlands). Total 790 patients were randomised to biological mesh or standard suture closure. After 2 years, incisional hernia was detected in 12% of patients in the mesh group and 20% of controls (RR 0.62; 95% CI 0.43–0.9; p = 0.012). Rates of wound infection, adverse events, and quality of life (QOL) were similar in both groups. Further follow-up at 5 years is awaited.

The impact of varying bite size for fascial closure in abdominal midline incisions on hernia incidence was evaluated in STITCH [7]–a prospective, multicenter, double-blind, well-powered RCT in 10 hospitals in the Netherlands. Total 560 adults underwent elective abdominal surgery with midline laparotomy and were randomised to either small tissue bites of 5 mm every 5 mm with UPS 2-0 PDS (n = 276) or large bites of 1 cm every 1 cm with thicker PDS 1-loop (n = 284). Randomisation was stratified by center and between surgeons and residents with a minimisation procedure to ensure balanced allocation. The primary outcome of incisional hernia at 1 year was significantly less in the small bites group 35/268 (13%) versus 57/277 (21%) in the large bite group [adjusted odds ratio (aOR) 0.52; 95% CI 0.31–0.87; p = 0.0131]. Expectedly, there was a higher ratio of suture length to wound length in the small bite group [5.0 (1.5) vs. 4.3 (1.4); p < 0.0001] and increased closure time [14 (6) vs. 10 (4) min; p < 0.0001]. There was no significant difference in rates of adverse events such as ileus, pneumonia, SSI, and burst abdomen. This RCT shows smaller bites are better for the prevention of incisional hernia in midline incisions and not associated with higher rates of adverse events–though the use of different sized needle and suture materials between the two groups may contribute to the results.

The safety of low-cost mesh made from sterilised mosquito meshes was compared against standard commercial mesh for groin hernia repair in a double-blind RCT in eastern Uganda [8]. Total 302 men with groin hernias operated electively by four surgeons were randomised equally to either mosquito mesh. There was no significant difference in neither the primary outcome of hernia recurrence with 1 (0.7%) in the mosquito mesh and 0 in the commercial group (RD 0.7%; 95% CI –1.2 to 2.6; p = 1.0) nor postoperative complications (including haematoma, swelling, and infection)–44 patients in both groups (30.8% vs. 29.7%; RD 1%; 95% CI –9.5 to 11.6; p = 1.0). This RCT shows this low-cost mesh made of mosquito net is noninferior to commercial mesh for groin repair in men electively. This finding is particularly impactful for cost saving in low- and middle-income countries.

BREAST SURGERY

Intra-operative radiotherapy

the impact of intraoperative radiotherapy during lumpectomy on 5-year outcomes was evaluated in the TARGIT-A trial [9]–a prospective, open-label, RCT across 32 centres in 10 countries. About 2,298 women with invasive ductal carcinoma up to 3.5 cm in size, cN0-N1, were randomised to either targeted intraoperative radiotherapy [TARGIT-IORT (n = 1,140)] or external beam radiotherapy [EBRT (n = 1,158)], which consisted of a standard daily fractionated course (3–6 weeks) of whole breast radiotherapy. TARGIT-IORT was supplemented by EBRT when postoperative histopathology found unsuspected higher risk factors (20% of patients). In longer term follow-up (median, 8.6 years; maximum, 18.90 years; IQR 7.0–10.6), no statistically significant difference was found in local recurrence-free survival (HR 1.13; 95% CI 0.91–1.41; p = 0.28), mastectomy-free survival (HR 0.96; 95% CI 0.78–1.19; p = 0.74), distant disease-free survival (HR 0.88; 95% CI 0.69–1.12; p = 0.30), overall survival (HR 0.82; 95% CI 0.63–1.05; p = 0.13) or breast cancer mortality (HR 1.12; 95% CI 0.78–1.60; p = 0.54). TARGIT-IORT resulted in 14 fewer deaths compared with EBRT (42/1,140 vs. 56/1,158). Mortality from other causes was significantly lower with TARGIT-IORT (HR, 0.59; 95% CI 0.40–0.86; p = 0.005). This landmark trial shows TARGIT-IORT during lumpectomy is an effective alternative to EBRT, with comparable long-term efficacy for cancer control and lower nonbreast cancer mortality. Although conventional EBRT has changed since the TARGIT-A trial randomised its first patient (March, 2000), with shorter treatment schedules and smaller breast treatment volumes, it still requires multiple treatment fractions with rate of late normal tissue effects continuing to increase over time. Compared to EBRT, TARGIT-IORT is delivered to the tumour bed as a single fraction during surgery and should therefore be discussed with all eligible patients when breast-conserving surgery is planned.

Anaesthetic

The feasibility and impact of recurrence of breast cancer by regional versus general anaesthesia during surgery was assessed in a large international RCT in at 13 hospitals in eight countries [10]. Around 2,132 women undergoing curative breast cancer surgery were randomised to either regional anaesthesia (paravertebral blocks ± propofol) or general anaesthesia (sevoflurane). There was no difference in local recurrence among women regional anaesthesia-analgesia, 102 (10%) compared with 111 (10%) in the general anaesthesia group (HR 0·97; 95% CI 0.74–1.28; p = 0.84). The frequency, severity, and persistence of breast pain were unaffected by anaesthetic technique. Although the results are significant, the trial was underpowered, slow to recruit, and did not standardise the regional technique used, and therefore is not a conclusive trial applicable and generalisable to change practice but warrants further study.

Pre-operative imaging

Two studies looked at preoperative imaging to help plan the extent of surgical resection. The IRCIS [11] trial evaluated the addition of magnetic resonance imaging (MRI) and the SenSzi [12] trial for lymphoscintigraphy (LSG). About 358 women with ductal carcinoma in situ (DCIS) undergoing breast-conserving surgery were randomised to MRI group (n = 178) or the control arm (n = 174). The addition of MRI did not reduce the rate of early reintervention: OR 0.68; 95% CI 0.41–1.1; p = 0.13. Mastectomy rates were also similar. MRI conferred no significant surgical improvement with the use of preoperative MRI for DCIS staging. In the SenSzi prospective multicenter, phase III RCT [12], surgeons operating on 1,198 patients with cN0 early breast cancer or extensive/high-grade DCIS planned for standard radioactive-labelled colloid LSG with subsequent sentinel lymph node biopsy (SLNB) were randomly assigned to know the results of the LSG or not. Knowledge of the LSG did not increase the mean number of histologically detected sentinel lymph nodes (SLNs) of 2.21 with LSG and 2.26 without LSG (difference 0.05; stratified 95% CI −0.18 to infinity). LSG does not improve SLNB surgery, negatively impacts the patient pathway and increases cost. These trials show no benefit of either of these extra imaging methods to the surgical management of breast cancer. Future novel imaging modalities should also be considered in this way, in terms of their clinical impact.

Axilla

Two studies presented 10-year follow-up data for management of the axilla. The ACOSOG Z0011 trial [13] is a phase III, multicenter, RCT that randomised women with clinical T1 or T2 invasive breast cancer, no palpable axillary adenopathy, and 1 or 2 SLNs containing metastases to either lumpectomy with SLN dissection (SLND) and axillary lymph node dissection [ALND (n = 445)] or just SLNB [SLND (n = 446)]. At a median follow-up of 9.3 years, neither the 10-year overall survival [86.3% in the SLND alone group and 83.6% in the ALND group (HR 0.85; 95% CI 0–1.16; p = 0.02)] nor 10-year disease-free survival [80.2% in the SLND alone group and 78.2% in the ALND group (HR 0.85; 95% CI 0.62–1.17; p = 0.32)] was significantly different. There is unclear applicability for patients with hormone receptor negative tumours and young women due to under enrolment in these groups. This landmark study supports the use of conservative axillary management as an alternative to axillary node dissection, for women with low burden axillary involvement, tumours under 5 cm, who undergo whole-breast radiation with systemic adjuvant treatment. Though questions remain as to the role of ALND given other factors such as hormone status, immunochemical and gene profile risk stratification, and neoadjuvant treatment (excluded in this trial).

The international IBCSG [14] was a similar trial for women with sentinel node micrometastases. After 10 years, disease-free survival was no better after axillary dissection (74.9%) than after no dissection (76.8%). About 76.8% (95% CI 72.5–81.0) in the no axillary dissection group compared with 74.9% (95% CI 70.5–79.3) in the axillary dissection group (HR 0.85; 95% CI 0.65–1.11; log-rank p = 0.24; p = 0.0024 for noninferiority). These two RCTs support the practice of avoiding an axillary dissection in patients with early breast cancer and low burden axillary disease, who receive systemic adjuvant treatment.

Cavity shave margins

The impact of cavity shave margins during partial mastectomy for breast cancer was evaluated in this RCT [15]. About 235 patients with stage 0–III breast cancer undergoing partial mastectomy, with or without resection margins, were randomised equally to have further cavity shave margins (shave) or no further shave (no-shave). The rate of positive margins after partial mastectomy (before randomisation) was not significantly different between the shave group and no-shave group (36% and 34%, respectively; p = 0.69). After randomisation, patients in the shave group had a significantly lower rate of positive margins than those in the no-shave group (19% vs. 34%, p = 0.01), as well as a lower rate of second surgery for margin clearance (10% vs. 21%, p = 0.02). There was no significant difference in complications between the two groups. Cavity shaving halved the rate of positive margins and consequently reduced the re-excision rate.

Resection of the primary tumour in patients with metastatic breast cancer

The impact of locoregional management of the primary tumour in metastatic breast cancer was evaluated in this single center RCT in Mumbai [16]. About 350 women with previously untreated metastatic breast cancer were randomised to receive chemotherapy and locoregional treatment directed at their primary breast tumour and axillary lymph nodes (n = 173), or chemotherapy and no locoregional treatment (n = 177). Locoregional treatment consisted of either modified radical mastectomy or simple or breast-conserving treatment plus radiotherapy. At time of cutoff (median time 23 months), there were 235 deaths; 118 in the locoregional treatment and 117 in the no locoregional group. There was no significant different in the 2-year overall survival, which was 41.9% (95% CI 33.9–49.7) in the locoregional treatment group and 43.0% (395% CI 5.2–50.8) in the no locoregional treatment group. This study found no evidence for primary tumour treatment in metastatic breast cancer.

Breast reconstruction

The safety [17] and impact on patient-reported outcome measures (PROMs) [18] of one-stage implant-based breast reconstruction (IBBR) with an acellular dermal matrix (ADM) versus two-stage breast reconstruction was assessed in the BRIOS trial in eight hospitals in this multicenter, open-label RCT in the Netherlands. Around 142 women about to undergo skin-sparing mastectomy with IBBR were randomised to either one-stage IBBR with ADM (n = 69) or two-staged approach (n = 73). The one-stage group was associated with significantly higher risk of surgical complications (OR 3.81; 95% CI 2.67–5.43; p < 0.001), reoperation (OR 3.38; 95% CI 2.10–5.45; p < 0.001), and removal of implant (OR 8.80; 95% CI 8.24–9.40; p < 0·001). There was no significant difference in Breast-Q QOL domains, including physical well-being [one-stage mean 78.0 (SD 14.1) vs. two-stage 79.3 (12.2), p = 0.60], psychosocial well-being [72.6 (17.3) vs. 72.8 (19.6), p = 0.95], and sexual well-being [58.0 (17.0) vs. 57.1 (19.5), p = 0·82], or in the patient-reported satisfaction with breasts [63.4 (15.8) vs. 60.3 (15.4), p = 0.35]. This study showed one-stage IBBR with ADM compared to two-stage IBBR does not improve PROMs but significantly increases risks for adverse outcomes. Patient selection, risk factors, and surgical and postsurgical procedures for reconstruction require further research.

UPPER GASTROINTESTINAL SURGERY

Achalasia

The role of per-oral endoscopic myotomy (POEM) for idiopathic achalasia was compared to the standard laparoscopic Heller's myotomy (LHM), was evaluated in this multicenter RCT [19]. Total 221 patients were randomised to either POEM (n = 112) or LHM plus Dor's fundoplication (n = 109). At 2-year clinical success, defined as Eckdart symptom score of 3 or less/12 without further treatment required, was achieved in 83.0% of patients in the POEM group and 81.7% of patients in the LHM group (difference, 1.4 percentage points; 95% CI –8.7 to 11.4; p = 0.007 for noninferiority). Though clinical success was equivalent; serious adverse events were significantly reduced in the POEM group 2.7% compared to 7.3% in the LHM group. However, POEM resulted in more reflux oesophagitis at 3 months 57% vs. 20%, which reduced to 44% and 29%, respectively. There was no difference in oesophageal sphincter function nor in gastrointestinal (GI) QOL index. POEM was noninferior compared to LHM in controlling symptoms of achalasia at 2 years with fewer severe complications but more common gastro-oesophageal reflux disease.

Oesophageal cancer

The role of hybrid minimally invasive oesophagectomy for oesophageal cancer was assessed in this French trial [20]. About 103 patients with resectable middle or lower thirds oesophageal cancer were randomised to either the hybrid-procedure group (n = 103), or to the standard open-procedure group (n = 104). The hybrid surgery comprised of a two-field abdominal-thoracic operation (also known as Ivor Lewis procedure) with laparoscopic gastric mobilisation and open right thoracotomy. Surgical quality assurance was implemented by checking surgeon credentials, standardisation of technique, and monitoring of performance. Hybrid surgery reduced the rate of major postoperative complications (mostly pulmonary) from 64% in the open group to 36% (OR 0.31; 95% CI 0.18–0.55; p < 0.001), and improved overall and disease-free 3-year survival from 55 to 67%, 48 to 57%, respectively.

Gastric cancer

Similarly, a minimally invasive laparoscopic approach was compared to open gastrectomy for advance gastric cancer in three trials: KLASS-01 [21], CLASS-01 [22], and another Chinese multicenter RCT [23]. The KLASS-01 was a phase III, open-label noninferiority RCT that included 15 surgeons from 13 institutes in South Korea. Total 1,416 patients were randomised to wither laparoscopic distal gastrectomy (n = 705) or open distal gastrectomy (n = 711). The 5-year overall survival rates were 94.2% in the laparoscopic group and 93.3% in the open surgery group (p = 0.64). Disease-free survival was also similar (97.1% in the laparoscopic group and 97.2% in the open surgery group, p = 0.91; difference, –0.03 percentage points; 97.5% CI –1.8 to infinity). These results were supported by the findings of the two other RCTs conducted in China that confirmed 3-year survival [22] and postoperative morbidity and mortality [23] were similar for both techniques.

To assess whether removal of the primary tumour would be of any benefit in metastatic gastric cancer, the open label, randomised, phase III REGATTA [24] trial was conducted at 44 centers or hospitals in Japan, South Korea, and Singapore. Total 175 patients with advanced gastric cancer with a single noncurable factor confined to either the liver (H1), peritoneum (P1), or para-aortic lymph nodes (16a1/b2) were randomly assigned to chemotherapy alone (n = 86) or gastrectomy followed by chemotherapy (n = 89). Chemotherapy consisted of oral S-1 80 mg/m^2/day on days 1–21 and cisplatin 60 mg/m^2 on day 8 of every 5-week cycle and gastrectomy was restricted to D1 lymphadenectomy without any resection of metastatic lesions. At 2 years, overall survival was 31.7% (95% CI 21.7–42.2) for patients assigned to chemotherapy alone compared with 25.1% (16.2–34.9) for those assigned to gastrectomy plus chemotherapy and median survival time was 16.6 months (95% CI 13.7–19.8) and 14.3 months (11.8–16.3), respectively (HR 1.09; 95% CI 0.78–1.52; one-sided p = 0.70). The study was halted due to futility as the predictive probability of overall survival being significantly higher in the gastrectomy plus chemotherapy group became 13.2%. Chemotherapy-associated adverse events such as leucopoenia, anorexia, nausea, and hyponatraemia were higher in the gastrectomy plus chemotherapy group. The role of chemotherapy administered orally also may have adversely affected the gastrectomy group. This study shows for metastatic gastric cancer; the addition of gastrectomy to chemotherapy confers no survival or morbidity benefit.

Bariatric surgery

Bariatric surgery is increasing dramatically in recent years in both caseload and research.

Techniques in bariatric surgery were studied in two studies. The efficacy and safety of one anastomosis gastric bypass (OAGB) versus Roux-en-Y gastric bypass (RYGB) was assessed in the YOMEGA [25] prospective, noninferiority RCT across nine obesity centers in France. Around 261 patients with BMI > 40 kg/m^2 or > 35kg/m^2 and at least one comorbidity (type 2 diabetes mellitus (T2DM), high blood pressure, obstructive sleep apnoea, dyslipidaemia, or arthritis) and with no oesophageal reflux disease were randomly assigned to OAGB (n = 129) or RYGB (n = 124). RYGB consisted of a 150-cm alimentary limb and a 50-cm biliary limb and OAGB of a single gastro-jejunal anastomosis with a 200-cm biliopancreatic limb. After 2 years, the mean percentage excess BMI loss was −87.9% in the OAGB group and −85.8% in the RYGB group (mean difference −3.3%; 95% CI −9.1 to 2.6), confirming noninferiority. There were 24 serious adverse events in the RYGB group versus 42 in the OAGB group (p = 0.042), of which 9 (21.4%) were nutritional complications versus 0 in the RYGB group (p = 0.0034). Although OAGB was found to be noninferior to RYGB regarding weight loss and metabolic improvement at 2 years it resulted in higher incidences of diarrhoea, steatorrhoea, and nutritional adverse events.

The routine closure of mesenteric defects in laparoscopic gastric bypass surgery was evaluated in a two-arm, parallel design done at 12 centres for bariatric surgery in Sweden [26]. Total 2,507 patients planned for laparoscopic gastric bypass surgery were randomised to closure of the mesenteric defects beneath the jejunojejunostomy and at Petersen's space (n = 1,259) or non-closure (n = 1,248). At 3 years, reoperation within 3 years for small bowel obstruction was more common in patients who did not have mesenteric closure (HR 0.56; 95% CI 0.41–0.76; p = 0.0002). However, the closure of mesenteric defects increased the risk of severe post-operative complications (4.3% vs. 2.8% OR 1.55; 95% CI 1.01–2.39; p = 0.044) which may be due to kinking of jejunostomy.

The medical impact of bariatric surgery was studied in two RCTs. The GATEWAY [27] trial looked at the effect of RYGB on hypertension and the STAMPEDE trial long-term follow-up data looked at diabetes. GATEWAY is a single-centre, non-blinded trial that randomised 100 patients with hypertension (using ≥ 2 medications at maximum doses or > 2 at moderate doses) and a BMI between 30.0 and 39.9 kg/m^2 to either medical management (n = 47) or medical management plus RYGB (n = 49). There was an increased reduction of ≥ 30% of the total number of antihypertensive medications while maintaining controlled blood pressure in the RYGB group 41/49 (83.7%) compared with the control 6/47 patients (12.8%) [rate ratio of 6.6 (95% CI 3.1–14.0); p < 0.001]. Waist circumference, BMI, fasting plasma glucose, glycohaemoglobin, low-density lipoprotein cholesterol, triglycerides, high-sensitivity C-reactive protein, and 10-year Framingham risk score were all lower in the gastric bypass than in the control group. This trial adds to the mounting body of high-level evidence that shows benefits of bariatric surgery beyond weight loss. The long-term results of the STAMPEDE trial [28], which randomly assigned 150 patients with T2DM and a BMI of 27–43 to receive intensive medical therapy alone or intensive medical therapy plus RYGB or sleeve gastrectomy. At 5 years, bariatric surgery increased the rate of those achieving excellent glycaemic control (HbA1c ≤ 42 mmol/mol; ≤ 6.0%) from 5% in the control to 29% in the RYGB and 23% in the gastrectomy group (adjusted p = 0.03). Changes from baseline seen in the gastric bypass and sleeve gastrectomy groups were also superior to those seen in the medical therapy group with respect to body weight, triglyceride and HDL-C levels, use of insulin, and QOL measures. No major late surgical complications were reported except for one reoperation. Long-term survival data is a key outcome that is still awaited from this study. As the RCT is a single-center, single-surgeon study generalisability is therefore limited and further multicenter RCTs would be recommended.

The RYGB was compared to sleeve gastrectomy in three RCTs. The effect on BMI loss was assessed in the SM-BOSS [29] and SLEEVEPASS [30] trials. T2DM was evaluated in the SLEEVEPASS [30] and the Osberg [31] trials. The SM-BOSS trial [29] randomised 217 morbidly obese patients to laparoscopic sleeve gastrectomy (n = 107) or laparoscopic RYGB (n = 110). At 5-year follow-up, there was no significant difference in excess BMI loss in patients who had sleeve gastrectomy (61.1%) versus those who had gastric bypass (68.3%) (absolute difference, –7.18%; 95% CI –14.30 to 0.06%; p = 0.22). There was more reflux remission associated with the gastric bypass (60.4%) than after sleeve gastrectomy (25.0%) and less gastric reflux worsening 6.3% versus 31.8%. Sleeve gastrectomy patients also more frequently required reoperations 16/101 (15 8%) versus 23/104 (22.1%). The authors concluded that there was no difference in BMI loss and other associated outcomes that make RYGB superior. These findings were conflicting to the SLEEVEPASS [30] trial with 240 patients and 5-year follow-up. They found excess weight loss at 5 years was 49% (95% CI 45–52%) after sleeve gastrectomy and 57% (95% CI 53–61%) after gastric bypass [difference, 8.2 percentage units (95% CI 3.2–13.2%), higher in the gastric bypass group], which did not meet criteria for equivalence but this result was not statistically significant. There was no significant difference in complete or partial remission of T2DM seen in 37% (n = 15/41) after sleeve gastrectomy and in 45% (n = 18/40) after gastric bypass (p > 0.099). Medication for dyslipidaemia was discontinued in 47% (n = 14/30) after sleeve gastrectomy and 60% (n = 24/40) after gastric bypass (p = 0.15). QOL between groups was no different (p = 0.85) and no treatment-related mortality was observed. At 5 years, the overall morbidity rate was 19% (n = 23) for sleeve gastrectomy and 26% (n = 31) for gastric bypass (p = 0.19). However, a greater reduction in hypertension was seen with the RYGB group in 29% (n = 20/68) and 51% (n = 37/73) (p = 0.02). The Osberg [31] triple-blind RCT in Norway looked at T2DM specifically comparing RYGB and sleeve gastrectomy. One hundered nine patients with T2DM were randomised to gastric bypass (n = 54) or sleeve gastrectomy (n = 55). After 1-year follow-up, diabetes remission rates were higher in the gastric bypass group than in the sleeve gastrectomy group [RD 27%; 95% CI 10–44; relative risk (RR) 1·57 (1.14–2.16), p = 0.0054]. At 1-year after surgery, RYGB appears superior for remission of T2DM. The SLEEVEPASS study had no longer term data and so this difference may become nonsignificant in later follow-up. Combining the RCT data shows bypass is likely superior to sleeve gastrectomy for other medical impacts compared to sleeve gastrectomy, but both perform similarly at 5 years in terms of BMI loss.

LOWER GASTROINTESTINAL SURGERY

Bowel preparation

The role of mechanical and oral antibiotic bowel preparation (MOABP) to prevent SSIs in elective colectomy was evaluated in the MOBILE multicenter, single-blinded RCT [32]. About 396 participants were randomised to MOABP (2 L of polyethylene glycol, 1 L of clear fluid before 6 PM on the day before surgery, 2 g of neomycin at 7 PM, and 2 g of metronidazole at 11 PM the day before surgery) (n = 196), or no bowel preparation (NBP) (n = 200). The primary outcome of SSI within 30 days was detected in 13 (7%) patients randomised to MOABP, and 21 (11%) to NBP (OR 1·65; 95% CI 0·80–3·40; p = 0·17). The study was powered to detect an 8% difference in SSI rates but only detected 4% and was, therefore, underpowered. This could be due to the low overall rates of SSIs in clean laparoscopic surgery as in this study. The authors conclude "MOABP does not reduce SSIs or the overall morbidity of colon surgery compared with NBP". Given these findings, the current recommendations of using MOABP for colectomies to reduce SSIs or morbidity should be reconsidered.

Rectal cancer

Two RCTs have investigated laparoscopic surgery compared to open surgery for rectal cancer. The ACOSOG [33] multicentre, noninferiority RCT in USA and Canada randomised 486 patients with stage 2 or 3 rectal cancer within 12 cm of the anal verge after completion of neoadjuvant therapy to laparoscopic (n = 240) or open resection (n = 222). The primary outcome was a composite of circumferential radial margin > 1 mm, distal margin without tumour, and completeness of total mesorectal excision. Successful resection occurred in 81.7% of laparoscopic resection cases (95% CI 76.8–86.6%) and 86.9% of open resection cases (95% CI 82.5–91.4%). Laparoscopic resection failed to meet the noninferiority margin of 6%. Conversion to open resection occurred in 11.3% of patients and the operative time was significantly longer for laparoscopic resection (266.2 vs. 220.6 min; p < 0.001). There was no significant difference in length of stay, readmission or severe complications between the groups. These findings were similar to the ALaCaRT trial [34], which randomised 475 patients with T1–T3 rectal cancers across multiple sites in Australia and New Zealand to open laparotomy and rectal resection (n = 237) or laparoscopic rectal resection (n = 238). Successful resection was achieved in 194 patients (82%) in the laparoscopic surgery group and 208 patients (89%) (RD –7%) in the open surgery group which failed to meet their margin of 8% for noninferiority. In laparoscopic surgery, the circumferential resection margin was clear in 4% fewer patient (93% vs. 97%), 5% less for total mesorectal excision (87% vs. 92%) but equivocal at 99% for distal margin clearance. The conversion rate from laparoscopic to open surgery was 9%. Both trials show there is not enough evidence for the routine use of laparoscopic surgery for rectal cancer.

To study whether the risk of conversion to open in rectal cancer surgery was reduced using robot assistance the ROLARR [35] international multicentre trial compared the two. About 471 patients with rectal adenocarcinoma suitable for curative resection were randomised to robotic-assisted (n = 237) or conventional (n = 234) laparoscopic rectal cancer resection. There was also no significant difference between the two in positive cancer resection margins (CRM+)–14/244 (6.3%) in the conventional group and 12/235 (5.1%) in the robotic-assisted group (aOR 0.78; 95% CI 0.35–1.76; p = 0.56). These CRM+ rates are significantly lower than in the other trials, suggesting patient selection and surgeon experience for minimally invasive techniques is key.

In rectal cancer management further support for traditional total mesorectal excision comes from the GRECCAR 2 trial [36]. The prospective, randomised, open-label, multicentre phase III trial randomised 145 patients to either local excision (n = 74) or total mesorectal (n = 71) excision. In the local excision, a completion mesorectal excision was undertaken if tumour stage was ypT2-3. The trial failed to show superiority of local excision because 26/74 patients in that group went on to have completion total mesorectal excision. The composite outcome that included death, recurrence, and morbidity at 2 years was similar in both groups (OR 1·33; 95% CI 0.62–2.86; p = 0.43). More research is needed to identify which patients will benefit from local excision and can avoid unnecessary completion total mesorectal excision. Currently, no benefit has been shown for postchemotherapy rectal cancer organ preservation.

Haemorrhoids

Whether haemorrhoidal artery ligation (HAL) or rubber band ligation(RBL) is the optimal surgical intervention for low-grade haemorrhoids, was evaluated within the HubBLe [37] open-label RCT across 17 UK trusts. About 337 participants were randomised to either HAL (n = 161) or RBL (n = 176). For the primary outcome at 1-year postprocedure, 87/176 (49%) in the RBL group and 48/161 (30%) in the HAL group had haemorrhoid recurrence (aOR 2.23; 95% CI 1·42–3·51; p = 0.0005) and more patients who had banding required a further procedure (14% vs. 32%). However, HAL was more painful postoperatively (p = 0.0002) and resulted in more frequent serious adverse events (7% vs. 1%).

Diverticulitis

The role of laparoscopic lavage for acute perforated diverticulitis was evaluated in the SCANDIV RCT in 21 centres across Sweden and Norway [38]. About 199 participants with perforated colonic diverticulitis were randomised to laparoscopic lavage (n = 101) or primary resection (n = 98). All patients with faecal peritonitis (15 patients in lavage vs. 13 in colon resection group) underwent colon resection. Mortality at 90 days [13.9% lavage group vs. 11.5% resection group (difference, 4.7%; 95% CI –7.9 to 17.0%; p = 0.53)] and major complications (30.7% vs. 26%, respectively) were similar in both groups. Length of operation was significantly shorter in the lavage group but this did not translate to a difference in length of stay in hospital potentially due to the increased rate of reoperations in the lavage group (15/74; 20.3%) than in the colon resection group [4/70; 5.7% (difference, 14.6%; 95% CI 3.5–25.6%; p = 0.01]. Notably, four sigmoid carcinomas were missed with laparoscopic lavage. Given no reduction in mortality and the increased rate of reoperation and missed diagnoses; the findings do not support laparoscopic lavage as standard of care for perforated diverticulitis.

HEPATO-PANCREATO-BILIARY SURGERY

Pancreatitis

The impact of early surgical treatment on chronic pancreatitis was assessed in the ESCAPE [39] trial in 30 Dutch hospitals. About 88 patients with painful chronic pancreatitis were randomised equally to pancreatic drainage surgery or the endoscopy-first approach group, who underwent medical treatment, endoscopy including lithotripsy if needed, and surgery if needed. In the 18-month follow-up period, patients in the early surgery group had a lower pain score than patients in endoscopy-first group [37 vs. 49; between-group difference, – 12 points (95% CI –22 to –2); p = 0.02]. The early surgery group also required fewer overall number of interventions (median, 1 vs. 3; p < 0.001). Treatment complications, mortality, hospital admissions, pancreatic function, and QOL were not significantly different between the interventions. Given the small number of recruited patients, further studies are needed to confirm these findings and evaluate persistence of symptoms long-term.

The role of partial pancreatoduodenectomy compared to duodenum-preserving pancreatic head resection (DPPHR) was evaluated in the ChroPac trial [40]. In this double-blind, parallel-group superiority trial done across Europe; 226 patients were analysed in the DPPHR (n = 115) or partial pancreatoduodenectomy (n = 111) groups. There were no differences in major adverse events (64% in the DPPHR and 52% after partial pancreatectomy), or QOL after 2 years. This differs from other recent single-centre trials showing superiority of DPPHR.

For acute necrotising pancreatitis, the standard surgical step-up approach of percutaneous catheter drainage followed, if necessary, by retroperitoneal debridement was compared to endoscopic ultrasound-guided transluminal drainage followed, if necessary, by endoscopic necrosectomy in this multicentre RCT in the Netherlands [41]. About 98 patients were equally assigned to each group. Rates of death or major complication within 6 months: 43% in the endoscopy group versus 45% in the surgery group [risk ratio (RR), 0.97; 95% CI 0.62–1.51; p = 0.88] and mortality rates (18% vs. 6%; RR 1.38; 95% CI 0.53–3.59; p = 0.50) were similar between the groups. In patients with infected necrotising pancreatitis, the endoscopic step-up approach was not inferior to the surgical step-up approach in reducing major complications or death. The endoscopic approach was associated with a lower rate of pancreatic fistulas and shorter hospital stay but further better powered trials are needed to confirm these findings.

The role of same admission versus interval cholecystectomy for mild gallstone pancreatitis was evaluated in the PONCHO trial [42]. At 23 hospitals in the Netherlands, 266 inpatients were randomly assigned to interval cholecystectomy (n = 137) or same-admission cholecystectomy (n = 129). The primary endpoint was a composite of readmission for recurrent gallstone-related complications (pancreatitis, cholangitis, cholecystitis, choledocholithiasis needing endoscopic intervention, or gallstone colic) or mortality within 6 months after randomisation. This occurred in 23 (17%) patients in the interval group and in 6 (5%) in the same-admission group (RR 0.28; 95% CI 0.12–0.66; p = 0.002). This trial showed in patients with mild biliary pancreatitis, same admission cholecystectomy safely reduces the risk of recurrent pancreatitis and other gallstone-related sequelae. It must be noted these results cannot be applied to patients who either have local complications of pancreatitis (which can increase the difficulty of cholecystectomy) or have significant comorbidities as such patients were excluded from this trial.

Cholecystitis

The CHOCOLATE [43] trial assessed treatment for high-risk patients with acute calculous cholecystitis in a RCT in 11 hospitals. About 142 patients at high risk, as per an APACHE II score > 7, were randomised to laparoscopic cholecystectomy (n = 66) or to percutaneous catheter drainage (n = 68). The trial was concluded early after a planned interim analysis because although the rate of death did not differ between the laparoscopic cholecystectomy and percutaneous catheter drainage groups (3% vs. 9%, p = 0.27), there were significantly more major complications in the percutaneous drainage group [44/86 (65%) vs. 8/66 (12%)] (RR 0.19; 95% CI 0.10–0.37; p < 0.001). Almost 66% of the drainage group required reintervention compared with 12% in the cholecystectomy group (p < 0.001). Recurrent biliary disease occurred more often in the percutaneous drainage group (53% vs. 5%, p < 0.001), and the median length of hospital stay was longer (9 days vs. 5 days, p < 0.001). Laparoscopic cholecystectomy is superior to percutaneous drainage in high-risk patients with cholecystitis.

TRANSPLANT SURGERY

Many sub-optimal potential donor organs do not tolerate conventional cold storage and there is no reliable way to assess organ viability preoperatively. A novel normothermic machine perfusion maintains the liver in a physiological state, avoids cooling, and allows recovery and functional testing. The role of this machine on harvested livers was evaluated in the UK [44]. About 270 harvested livers were randomised to normothermic perfusion (n = 137) or standard cold storage (n = 133). This normothermic machine perfusion resulted in a 50% lower level of graft injury compared to standard cooling [measured by AST enzyme release, 484.5 (406.4–577.6) vs. 937.7 (795.2–1192.3), p < 0.001], a 50% lower rate of organ discard (11.7% vs. 24.1%, p = 0.008) and 54% longer mean preservation time (11 h 54 min vs. 7 h 45 min, p < 0.001). There was no significant difference in bile duct complications, graft survival or survival of the recipient. This landmark study demonstrates the potential of this novel technology in clinical practice and could dramatically increase the numbers of viable liver transplants.

CONCLUSION

Clinical trials in surgery continue to provide evidence of the effectiveness of new techniques for diagnosis and treatment. Although surgical oncology and vascular surgery lead the way with a long history of surgical clinical trials, this chapter has also included trials form areas of surgery where randomisation and other aspects of trial conduct are more difficult, such as emergency or bariatric procedures. Many of the surgical trials reported here are multicentre and multinational and the surgical community is to be commended for this collaborative effort. It is essential that the results of well conducted clinical trials are translated into clinical surgical practice.

Key points for clinical practice

General surgery

- Appendicitis treated with antibiotics has a 39% recurrence rate within 5 years.
- The use of a low-cost mesh for groin hernias was found to be noninferior to standard commercial mesh.
- The use of mesh is beneficial in the treatment of umbilical hernias.
- Small suture bites and prophylactic mesh reinforcement both reduce the incidence of incisional and parastomal hernias in abdominal surgery.

Breast surgery

- Intraoperative compared to external radiotherapy for early breast cancer has comparable long-term safety and lower nonbreast cancer mortality.
- Regional anaesthesia-analgesia does not reduce breast cancer recurrence nor breast pain after potentially curative surgery.

- There is no significant surgical improvement with the use of preoperative MRI for DCIS or SLNBs.
- In patients with low or intermediate axillary tumour burden, SLNB alone is noninferior and can avoid axillary nodal clearance (ANC).
- Cavity shaving halves the rates of positive margins and re-excision with partial mastectomy.
- Locoregional treatment of the primary tumour confers no overall survival benefit in metastatic breast cancer.
- One-stage with ADM when compared to two-stage IBBR does not improve patient-reported QOL but increases risks of adverse outcomes.

Upper gastrointestinal surgery

- Endoscopic management of achalasia is superior to the traditional LHM with Dor's fundoplication.
- Hybrid minimally invasive esophagectomy has a lower incidence of intraoperative and post-operative major complications without compromising overall and disease-free survival.
- Laparoscopic distal gastrectomy has comparable morbidity and mortality and long-term survival compared to the open approach for advanced gastric cancer.
- There is no benefit to primary tumour removal for metastatic gastric cancer.
- OAGB is non-inferior to RYGB for weight loss but results in more adverse events.
- The routine closure of mesenteric defects in laparoscopic gastric bypass surgery reduces long-term small bowel obstruction but may increase early complications.
- Bariatric surgery in addition to medical therapy is beneficial in hypertension and T2DM.
- Gastric bypass is superior to sleeve gastrectomy for remission T2DM at 1 year, but the evidence is conflicting for effect on BMI and other medical conditions long-term.

Lower gastrointestinal surgery

- MOABP compared with NBP for elective colectomies does not reduce surgical site infections (SSIs).
- In rectal cancer management, more research is needed to identify patients who will benefit from local excision and can avoid total mesorectal excision.
- The laparoscopic approach is inferior to open resection for achieving oncological resection in rectal cancer—the robotic-assisted laparoscopic technique confers no additional benefit in terms of excision and conversion to open.
- HAL was associated with lower recurrence but was more painful and less preferable than repeat RBL.
- For perforated diverticulitis, laparoscopic lavage did not reduce severe post-operative complications and resulted in more reoperations compared to primary resection.

Hepato-pancreato-biliary surgery

- Same-admission cholecystectomy compared with interval cholecystectomy for mild gallstone pancreatitis is not associated with higher operative complications but reduces gallstone-related complications.
- Endoscopic step-up approach is non-inferior to standard surgical approach in mortality and major complications for infected necrotising pancreatitis.
- In chronic pancreatitis, early surgical drainage is beneficial in managing pain.
- Partial pancreatoduodenectomy and DPPHR for chronic pancreatitis result in similar improvement in QOL and complications.

- Laparoscopic cholecystectomy is superior to percutaneous catheter drainage in high-risk patients with acute cholecystitis.

Transplant surgery
- The use of the novel technique of normothermic perfusion is safe and may increase the number of viable liver transplants.

REFERENCES

1. McCulloch P, Taylor I, Sasako M, et al. Randomised trials in surgery: problems and possible solutions. BMJ 2002; 324:1448–1451.
2. Salminen P, Tuominen R, Paajanen H, et al. Five-year follow-up of antibiotic therapy for uncomplicated acute appendicitis in the APPAC randomized clinical trial. JAMA 2018; 320:1259–1265.
3. Olavarria OA, Bernardi K, Shah SK, et al. Robotic versus laparoscopic ventral hernia repair: multicenter, blinded randomized controlled trial. BMJ 2020; 370:m2457.
4. Kaufmann R, Halm JA, Eker HH, et al. Mesh versus suture repair of umbilical hernia in adults: a randomised, double-blind, controlled, multicentre trial. Lancet 2018; 391:860–869.
5. Jairam AP, Timmermans L, Eker HH, et al. Prevention of incisional hernia with prophylactic onlay and sublay mesh reinforcement versus primary suture only in midline laparotomies (PRIMA): 2-year follow-up of a multicentre, double-blind, randomised controlled trial. Lancet 2017; 390:567–576.
6. Reinforcement of Closure of Stoma Site (ROCSS) Collaborative and West Midlands Research Collaborative. Prophylactic biological mesh reinforcement versus standard closure of stoma site (ROCSS): a multicentre, randomised controlled trial. Lancet 2020; 395:417–426.
7. Deerenberg EB, Harlaar JJ, Steyerberg EW, et al. Small bites versus large bites for closure of abdominal midline incisions (STITCH): a double-blind, multicentre, randomised controlled trial. Lancet 2015; 386:1254–1260.
8. Löfgren J, Nordin P, Ibingira C, et al. A randomized trial of low-cost mesh in groin hernia repair. N Engl J Med 2016; 374:146–153.
9. Vaidya JS, Bulsara M, Baum M, et al. Long-term survival and local control outcomes from single dose targeted intraoperative radiotherapy during lumpectomy (TARGIT-IORT) for early breast cancer: TARGIT-A randomised clinical trial. BMJ 2020; 370:m2836.
10. Sessler DI, Pei L, Huang Y, et al. Recurrence of breast cancer after regional or general anaesthesia: a randomised controlled trial. Lancet 2019; 394:1807–1815.
11. Balleyguier C, Dunant A, Ceugnart L, et al. Preoperative breast magnetic resonance imaging in women with local ductal carcinoma in situ to optimize surgical outcomes: results from the randomized phase III trial IRCIS. J Clin Oncol 2019; 37:885–892.
12. Kuemmel S, Holtschmidt J, Gerber B, et al. Prospective, multicenter, randomized phase III trial evaluating the impact of lymphoscintigraphy as part of sentinel node biopsy in early breast cancer: SenSzi (GBG80) trial. J Clin Oncol 2019; 37:1490–1498.
13. Giuliano AE, Ballman KV, McCall L, et al. Effect of axillary dissection vs. no axillary dissection on 10-year overall survival among women with invasive breast cancer and sentinel node metastasis: the ACOSOG Z0011 (Alliance) randomized clinical trial. JAMA 2017; 318:918–926.
14. Galimberti V, Cole BF, Viale G, et al. Axillary dissection versus no axillary dissection in patients with breast cancer and sentinel-node micrometastases (IBCSG 23-01): 10-year follow-up of a randomised, controlled phase 3 trial. Lancet Oncol 2018; 19:1385–1393.
15. Chagpar AB, Killelea BK, Tsangaris TN, et al. A randomized, controlled trial of cavity shave margins in breast cancer. N Engl J Med 2015; 373:503–510.
16. Badwe R, Hawaldar R, Nair N, et al. Locoregional treatment versus no treatment of the primary tumour in metastatic breast cancer: an open-label randomised controlled trial. Lancet Oncol 2015; 16:1380–1388.
17. Dikmans RE, Negenborn VL, Bouman MB, et al. Two-stage implant-based breast reconstruction compared with immediate one-stage implant-based breast reconstruction augmented with an acellular dermal matrix: an open-label, phase 4, multicentre, randomised, controlled trial. Lancet Oncol 2017; 18:251–258.

18. Negenborn VL, Young-Afat DA, Dikmans RE, et al. Quality of life and patient satisfaction after one-stage implant-based breast reconstruction with an acellular dermal matrix versus two-stage breast reconstruction (BRIOS): primary outcome of a randomised, controlled trial. Lancet Oncol 2018; 19:1205–1214.
19. Werner YB, Hakanson B, Martinek J, et al. Endoscopic or surgical myotomy in patients with idiopathic achalasia. N Engl J Med 2019; 381:2219–2229.
20. Mariette C, Markar SR, Dabakuyo-Yonli TS, et al. Hybrid minimally invasive esophagectomy for esophageal cancer. N Engl J Med 2019; 380:152–162.
21. Kim HH, Han SU, Kim MC, et al. Effect of laparoscopic distal gastrectomy vs. open distal gastrectomy on long-term survival among patients with stage I gastric cancer: the KLASS-01 randomized clinical trial. JAMA Oncol 2019; 5:506–513.
22. Yu J, Huang C, Sun Y, et al. Effect of laparoscopic vs. open distal gastrectomy on 3-year disease-free survival in patients with locally advanced gastric cancer: the CLASS-01 randomized clinical trial. JAMA 2019; 321:1983–1992.
23. Hu Y, Huang C, Sun Y, et al. Morbidity and mortality of laparoscopic versus open D2 distal gastrectomy for advanced gastric cancer: a randomized controlled trial. J Clin Oncol 2016; 34:1350–1357.
24. Fujitani K, Yang HK, Mizusawa J, et al. Gastrectomy plus chemotherapy versus chemotherapy alone for advanced gastric cancer with a single non-curable factor (REGATTA): a phase 3, randomised controlled trial. Lancet Oncol 2016; 17:309–318.
25. Robert M, Espalieu P, Pelascini E, et al. Efficacy and safety of one anastomosis gastric bypass versus Roux-en-Y gastric bypass for obesity (YOMEGA): a multicentre, randomised, open-label, non-inferiority trial. Lancet 2019; 393:1299–1309.
26. Stenberg E, Szabo E, Ågren G, et al. Closure of mesenteric defects in laparoscopic gastric bypass: a multicentre, randomised, parallel, open-label trial. Lancet 2016; 387:1397–1404.
27. Schiavon CA, Bersch-Ferreira AC, Santucci EV, et al. Effects of bariatric surgery in obese patients with hypertension: the GATEWAY randomized trial (Gastric Bypass to Treat Obese Patients with Steady Hypertension). Circulation 2018; 137:1132–1142.
28. Schauer PR, Bhatt DL, Kirwan JP, et al. Bariatric surgery versus intensive medical therapy for diabetes—5-year outcomes. N Engl J Med 2017; 376:641–651.
29. Peterli R, Wölnerhanssen BK, Peters T, et al. Effect of laparoscopic sleeve gastrectomy vs. laparoscopic Roux-en-Y gastric bypass on weight loss in patients with morbid obesity: the SM-BOSS randomized clinical trial. JAMA 2018; 319:255–265.
30. Salminen P, Helmiö M, Ovaska J, et al. Effect of laparoscopic sleeve gastrectomy vs. laparoscopic Roux-en-Y gastric bypass on weight loss at 5 years among patients with morbid obesity: the SLEEVEPASS randomized clinical trial. JAMA 2018; 319:241–254.
31. Hofsø D, Fatima F, Borgeraas H, et al. Gastric bypass versus sleeve gastrectomy in patients with type 2 diabetes (Oseberg): a single-centre, triple-blind, randomised controlled trial. Lancet Diabetes Endocrinol 2019; 7:912–924.
32. Koskenvuo L, Lehtonen T, Koskensalo S, et al. Mechanical and oral antibiotic bowel preparation versus no bowel preparation for elective colectomy (MOBILE): a multicentre, randomised, parallel, single-blinded trial. Lancet 2019; 394:840–848.
33. Fleshman, J. et al. Effect of laparoscopic-assisted resection vs. open resection of stage II or III rectal cancer on pathologic outcomes: the ACOSOG Z6051 randomized clinical trial. JAMA 2015; 314:1346–1355.
34. Stevenson AR, Solomon MJ, Lumley JW, et al. Effect of laparoscopic-assisted resection vs. open resection on pathological outcomes in rectal cancer: the ALaCaRT randomized clinical trial. JAMA 2015; 314:1356–1363.
35. Jayne D, Pigazzi A, Marshall H, et al. Effect of robotic-assisted vs. conventional laparoscopic surgery on risk of conversion to open laparotomy among patients undergoing resection for rectal cancer: the ROLARR randomized clinical trial. JAMA 2017; 318:1569–1580.
36. Rullier E, Rouanet P, Tuech JJ, et al. Organ preservation for rectal cancer (GRECCAR 2): a prospective, randomised, open-label, multicentre, phase 3 trial. Lancet 2017; 390:469–479.
37. Brown SR, Tiernan JP, Watson AJ, et al. Haemorrhoidal artery ligation versus rubber band ligation for the management of symptomatic second-degree and third-degree haemorrhoids (HubBLe): a multicentre, open-label, randomised controlled trial. Lancet 2016; 388:356–364.
38. Schultz JK, Yaqub S, Wallon C, et al. Laparoscopic lavage vs. primary resection for acute perforated diverticulitis: the SCANDIV randomized clinical trial. JAMA 2015; 314:1364–1375.
39. Issa Y, Kempeneers MA, Bruno MJ, et al. Effect of early surgery vs. endoscopy-first approach on pain in patients with chronic pancreatitis: the ESCAPE randomized clinical trial. JAMA 2020; 323:237–247.

40. Diener MK, Hüttner FJ, Kieser M, et al. Partial pancreatoduodenectomy versus duodenum-preserving pancreatic head resection in chronic pancreatitis: the multicentre, randomised, controlled, double-blind ChroPac trial. Lancet 2017; 390:1027–1037.

41. van Brunschot S, van Grinsven J, van Santvoort HC, et al. Endoscopic or surgical step-up approach for infected necrotising pancreatitis: a multicentre randomised trial. Lancet 2018; 391:51–58.

42. da Costa DW, Bouwense SA, Schepers NJ, et al. Same-admission versus interval cholecystectomy for mild gallstone pancreatitis (PONCHO): a multicentre randomised controlled trial. Lancet 2015; 336:1261–1268.

43. Loozen CS, van Santvoort HC, van Duijvendijk P, et al. Laparoscopic cholecystectomy versus percutaneous catheter drainage for acute cholecystitis in high-risk patients (CHOCOLATE): multicentre randomised clinical trial. BMJ 2018; 363:k3965.

44. Nasralla D, Coussios CC, Mergental H, et al. A randomized trial of normothermic preservation in liver transplantation. Nature 2018; 557:50–56.